WALTER J. BO, Ph.D.

Professor of Anatomy

ISADORE MESCHAN, M.D.

Professor of Radiology

WAYNE A. KRUEGER, Ph.D.

Associate Professor of Anatomy

Illustrations Coordinated by

GEORGE C. LYNCH

Professor of Medical Illustration

BOWMAN GRAY SCHOOL OF MEDICINE
WAKE FOREST UNIVERSITY
WINSTON-SALEM, NORTH CAROLINA

BASIC ATLAS of CROSS-SECTIONAL ANATOMY

W.B. Saunders Company

Philadelphia London Toronto Mexico City Rio de Janeiro Sydney Tokyo

W. B. Saunders Company: West Washington Square
Philadelphia, PA   19105

1 St. Anne's Road
Eastbourne, East Sussex BN21 3UN, England

1 Goldthorne Avenue
Toronto, Ontario M8Z 5T9, Canada

Apartado 26370 — Cedro 512
Mexico 4, D.F., Mexico

Rua Coronel Cabrita, 8
Sao Cristovao Caixa Postal 21176
Rio de Janeiro, Brazil

9 Waltham Street
Artarmon, N.S.W. 2064, Australia

Ichibancho, Central Bldg., 22-1 Ichibancho
Chiyoda-Ku, Tokyo 102, Japan

Library of Congress Cataloging in Publication Data

Bo, Walter J

Basic atlas of cross-sectional anatomy.

1. Anatomy, Human — Atlases.   I. Meschan, Isadore, joint
author.   II. Krueger, Wayne A., joint author.   III. Title.
[DNLM: 1. Anatomy — Atlases. QS17 B662b]
QM25.B65   611'.0022'2   79–66032
ISBN 0–7216–1767–0

Basic Atlas of Cross-Sectional Anatomy   ISBN   0-7216-1767-0

Last digit is the print number: 9   8   7   6   5

Dedicated to our wives
Jeanice Bo, Rachel Meschan, M.D., and Doris Krueger
for their support in this endeavor

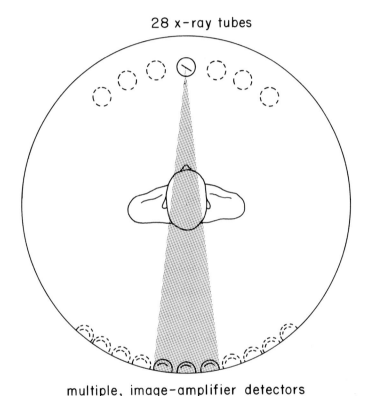

28 x-ray tubes

multiple, image-amplifier detectors

Figure 2E.   Multiple stationary x-ray tubes and image-amplifier dectectors.

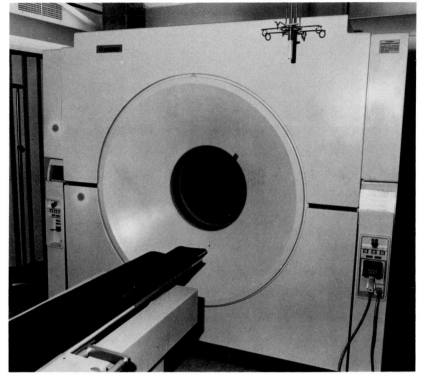

Figure 3.   Gantry and cot on which patient lies while being inserted into the gantry opening.

on an arbitrary basis—now called Hounsfield units. In general, if we accept water as being 0, air and fat are at the lower end of the scale; bone is at the higher end of the scale. Because of the delimitation of scattered radiation, even the central gray matter of the brain may be differentiated from the white matter by a range of 15 to 20 units. Increased calcium in the gray matter results in greater density.

Contrast enhancement used in conjunction with computed tomography allows for better and more accurate images to be obtained. Special contrast agents may be employed in such structures as the blood vessels, the gastrointestinal tract, and the collecting system of the urinary tract.

With some of the commercial CT units now available, special algorithmic capabilities allow the reproduction of sagittal sections on the cathode ray oscilloscope or television screen after several cross sections have been obtained. Sagittal sections, therefore, have already achieved clinical usefulness. For this reason, this atlas includes an appendix of cadaveric sagittal sections.

Ambrose J, and Hounsfield G: Computerized transverse axial tomography. Br J Radiol 46:148–149, 1973

Meschan I, Bo WJ, and Krueger WA: The utilization of xeroradiography for radiography of cross-section of thin cadaveric slices. Invest Radiol 14:97–102, 1979.

New PFJ, and Scott WR: Computed tomography of the brain and orbit (EMI Scanning). Williams and Wilkins Co., Baltimore, 1975.

Preface

Cross-sectional anatomy is utilized occasionally in the study of gross anatomy, but only recently, with the advent of computed tomography and ultrasound, has knowledge of cross-sectional anatomy assumed great clinical importance. The purpose of this atlas is to present cross-sectional anatomy in a meaningful manner to students of gross anatomy and to clinicians and technologists who are interested in correlations between cross-sectional anatomy and computed tomography and ultrasonography. Sagittal sections have been included because they often make it easier for the student, physician, and technologist to grasp contiguous cross-sectional relationships.

Anatomy has always been important as a basis for clinical radiology, but this dimension now requires an additional emphasis. For students of gross anatomy, the atlas presents a three-dimensional concept of the body that is usually not obtained from dissection or audiovisual material. For clinicians and technologists, it offers information that is valuable in daily practice.

Cross sections of the head, neck, and torso are presented serially to portray accurately the progression of structures. Selected cross-sections of the extremities and selected sagittal sections of the head, neck, and torso show the essential features of these regions. Cross sections are viewed from below, since this has been the convention for computed tomographs and ultrasonographs. Sagittal sections are viewed from the right. A position drawing is included with each illustration, indicating the location of the section.

Xeroradiographs of cadaveric cross sections have been included to portray the ultimate in the detection of differences in absorption coefficients of both normal and abnormal tissues and the ultimate in "edge enhancement" of the junction of tissues with different absorption coefficients. Xeroradiography is not presented for what it offers as a clinical tool in this instance; rather, we offer it as a learning tool and as a vision of desirable capabilities in future generations of computed tomographic (CT) equipment.

Accompanying each cross section are textual comments that stress important details and call attention to relationships of structures. Clinical comments are presented in the introduction to each chapter and with each cross section of the head, neck, and torso.

Selected CT scans are presented to show the clinical applicability of cross-sectional anatomy.

The nomenclature adopted represents that of the "Nomina Anatomica" of 1967 combined with the English nomenclature commonly employed in most medical schools and clinical applications today. It has been our experience in teaching anatomy that students at times prefer to use the English nomenclature rather than the Latin and *vice versa,* when it better suits the purposes of communication to do so.

Acknowledgments

We are extremely grateful to Dr. Richard Janeway, Dean of the Bowman Gray School of Medicine of Wake Forest University, for his interest in cross-sectional anatomy and for awarding us a venture grant for the initial study in this area.

Many other individuals had a significant role in the development of this atlas.

To Mr. Robert Bowden, Anatomy Technologist, we express our greatest appreciation for the preparation of the sections and for his dedication in his work.

Our sincere thanks to Mr. George Lynch, Director of Audiovisual Resources, for coordinating the illustrations and overseeing many phases of this work and for his interest throughout the project.

For preparing the label overlays for the illustrations, we extend special thanks to Ms. Linda Bentley, Graphic Artist.

We are indebted to Mrs. Jeanice Bo for the final typing of the text material.

We express our gratitude to Dr. Rachel Meschan for her great help in checking the accuracy of the clinical material.

To Mr. Bruce Coats, Mr. Jack Dent, and Ms. Ellen Hinsen, we are grateful for the preparation of the illustrations.

We express our thanks to Mrs. Betty Royal, Radiologic Technologist, for preparing the xeroradiographs; Mrs. Nadeene Temple and Mrs. Carolyn Shaver for the initial typing of the clinical material; and Mr. Orville Ilgner, Photographer for the Radiology Department, for the photographs of the computed tomographic scanner.

We appreciate the contributions of the following people, who furnished us with the computed tomographic scans: Drs. Neil Wolfman, James Ball, and Marshall Ball and Mrs. Bonnie Landreth, all of the Department of Radiology, Bowman Gray School of Medicine, Wake Forest University; Dr. Sadek Hilal, Department of Radiology, Columbia University; Dr. George Flouty, Pfizer Corporation, New York, New York; and Mr. Timothy J. Keane, General Electric, Milwaukee, Wisconsin.

We are extremely grateful to Mr. John Hanley, Vice-President and Publisher, and Mrs. Roberta Kangilaski, Associate Medical Editor, W. B. Saunders Company, Publishers, for their assistance in the preparation of this atlas. The assistance offered by W. B. Saunders has indeed made this atlas possible.

Contents

Introduction

A total of six specimens, five males and one female, provided the cross-sectional material for this atlas. Three male specimens were included in Chapter 1; one of these three was also used for Chapter 2. The fourth male specimen was used in Chapters 3 and 4 and the fifth for Chapters 6 and 7. The female specimen was used in Chapter 5.

We used three specimens, two males and one female, for the sagittal sections (see Appendix) as follows: a male specimen for the head and neck and the pelvis; the other male specimen for the thorax and abdomen; and the female specimen for the pelvis.

The specimens were embalmed with a solution of formalin, glycerin, and phenol (1.5 : 1.5 : 1) and then frozen at minus-20°C for at least 1 week prior to sectioning. The frozen specimens were sectioned using a commercial band saw. Sections through the orbit were cut 0.5 cm thick; all others were cut at 1.0 cm thickness. The sections were lightly sanded, using a fine grain sandpaper, and allowed to thaw. They were then fixed in Kaiserling's solution* for 3 days, washed in running water for 6 to 8 hours, and immersed in 80 per cent alcohol for 1 hour prior to photographing.

A black rectangular shadowless copy box, approximately 2 feet deep, was used in the photographic procedure. A sheet of plate glass covered the top of the box and served as the surface on which the section was placed.

The box was lighted with two 3200°K tungsten klieg lights positioned approximately 2 feet to each side of the box and 2 feet above the section, so that the light did not fall on the background, resulting in a black background around the body section. The film used was 4 × 5 plus-X sheet film exposed for 1½ seconds at a lens opening of f/4.5; the camera used was a 4 × 5 Linhof view camera with Schneider optics. After the film was processed and printed, a graphic artist prepared label overlays for the illustrations.

To avoid overcrowding the illustrations with labels and lines, an attempt was made to label structures that were clearly visible, and bilateral structures were generally labeled only once. Some of the structures, such as vessels and nerves, could not be identified because they either were collapsed or blended in with the surrounding connective tissue. We chose not to have an artist draw in these structures because we wanted to depict the anatomy as it truly exists in the section. At times, individual muscles were difficult to distinguish; therefore, they were grouped in labeling (for example, transversospinal muscles of the back).

Xeroradiographs of the cadaveric slices are included because the marked edge enhancement characteristic of xeroradiographic images serves as a useful tool in delineating anatomic parts (Meschan et al., 1979). The equipment employed was a CGR Cinegraph with a 0.6-mm molybdenum tube target. A xeroradiograph is the photographic image of a thin layer of selenium on a rigid aluminum support on which a uniform electrostatic charge has been "disturbed" by remnant radiation passing through an anatomic part. A latent image is first produced and this is then made visible by spraying the rearranged selenium particles with an electrically charged blue image powder. This powdered image is transferred to a charged paper, whereupon it is fused to the paper by heat.

The xeroradiographic cassettes were often too small to contain an entire cross section. It became necessary to obtain overlapping xeroradiographs and then to piece them together to produce the initial gross specimen for comparative purposes. Right and left sides were reversed to conform to the present convention of the right side appearing on the reader's left, although typically the reverse is true of a xeroradiographic image. In some instances, the lumina of hollow viscera, spinal canal, and blood vessels were enhanced by a black background to make them readily discernible. Occasionally even a 1-cm thickness would not show the small glandular structures seen on gross specimens and these required "retouching" by an artist. One example of this may be found in the pampiniform plexus of veins.

CLINICAL APPLICATIONS. Cross-sectional anatomy first became a clinical tool in daily application with the advent of diagnostic ultrasound, and later with the discovery of computed tomography. The clinical emphasis of this atlas, however, is on computed tomography. In computed tomography, as in conventional radiography, technical factors can be standardized; but in ultrasonography, image quality and consequently diagnostic accuracy depend to a great extent upon the skill of the physician or technologist performing the procedure. Appropriate references to ultrasonography are included in this atlas when applicable (Chapters 3 and 5), but very little emphasis is placed on

---

*Kaiserling's solution: formalin 400 cc, water 2000 cc, potassium nitrate 30 gm, potassium acetate 60 gm

ultrasonic applications. The examples of abnormalities are largely portrayed through computed tomography. Nevertheless, it is our feeling that the student must be aware that ultrasonography is developing rapidly and may have much greater clinical usefulness in the future.

COMPUTED TOMOGRAPHIC SCANNING. The pioneering publication in computed tomography was by Ambrose and Hounsfield in 1973. Numerous textbooks on this subject have since been written. Basically, the technique involves passing a pencil-like beam of x-rays through the body, which contains tissues of different densities. The beam of x-rays is attenuated in accordance with the absorption coefficient of these tissues.

A cross section of tissues is theoretically divided into volume elements, which usually measure 1.3 cm by 1.3 cm by 0.4 cm or 0.5 cm, as required. Each of these small volumes of the cross section is spoken of as a "voxel" (abbreviation for volume element). As the slitlike beam of x-rays is rotated around the patient at 1-degree increments in the first scanners used in a clinical setting, each voxel becomes a storehouse of photons, depending upon the different angles from which the voxel is "viewed." The total number of photons collected by each voxel from each of these 1-degree rotational increments is transferred to a computer, which in essence stores a profile of the attenuation of x-rays in the tissues traversed in the cross section, at 180-degree angles. The computer "reconstructs" the tomographic section by appropriate algorithms (Fig. 1).

Initially, the highly collimated x-ray beam scanned the patient in one direction. It was indexed to move 1 degree at a time through this 180-degree arc (Fig. 2A). A later design incorporated two collimated beams, each striking a separate scintillation detector device. This was called the "translate-rotate scanner." Gas tube detectors (usually xenon) were also employed.

A second type of apparatus involved the rotation of both the x-ray beam and the detector devices around the patient in a 360-degree arc with multiple detector devices and a single fan-shaped x-ray beam (Fig. 2B). Earlier models of this unit utilized gas detectors of xenon, which have been retained in some of the computed tomograph units of today. This design is called the "rotating fan beam with rotating detectors."

A third type of machine was designed with a rotating tube, several hundred detectors (in order of 600), and a fan beam (Fig. 2C). The x-ray tube in these instruments can rotate at various arc increments, usually 10 degrees or more, thus diminishing the time for obtaining the cross-sectional "picture" to 1 or 2 seconds. Other types of machines employ multiple x-ray tubes (Fig. 2D) as well as multiple detector devices (Fig. 2E).

In each instance, the supportive device for the x-ray tube and detector devices is spoken of as the "scanner gantry." There is an opening in this gantry for the patient's body or body part (Fig. 3).

The data stored by the computer is transferred to a cathode ray tube or television screen as desired for photography and reconversion into an anatomic depiction. Several photographs of CT scans have been included in this atlas particularly to demonstrate abnormalities that can be detected clinically by this modality. In the display, the most radiodense materials appear white at peak; those least dense appear black.

CT apparatus includes a control for "window width," which permits selection of the range of absorption coefficients or units between the black and the white peaks displayed on the cathode ray tube. There is also a "window level" control to determine the center of the range selected by the window width control. In most units this range may be from plus-1000 to minus-1000

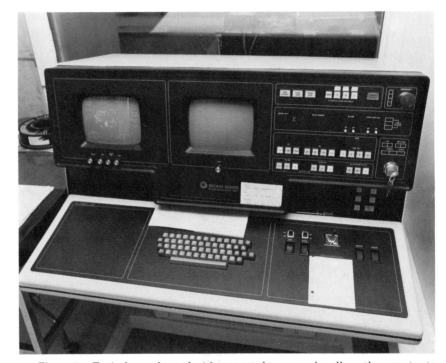

Figure 1. Typical console used with computed tomography allows the operator to control window width, window level, and the various other input devices that appear on the ultimate cathode ray oscilloscope reconstruction of the scan.

x-ray tube

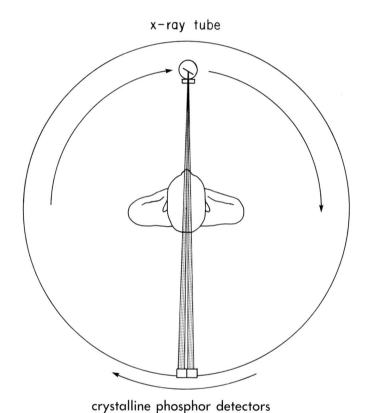

crystalline phosphor detectors

Figure 2A. Movement of tube and detectors: 180° at 1° increments.

x-ray tube

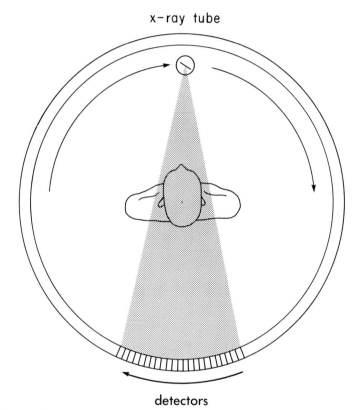

detectors

Figure 2B. Movement of tube and detectors: 180° in 10° arc increments. Detectors are crystalline phosphors or xenon gas tubes.

x-ray tube

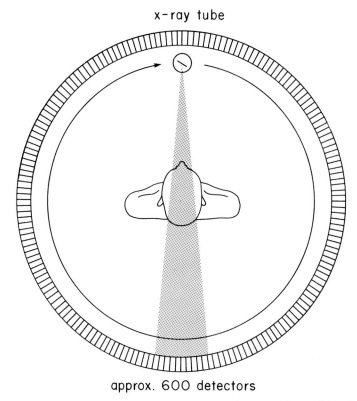

approx. 600 detectors

Figure 2C. X-ray tube moves (360°); stationary detectors of crystalline phosphors or xenon gas tubes.

28 x-ray tubes

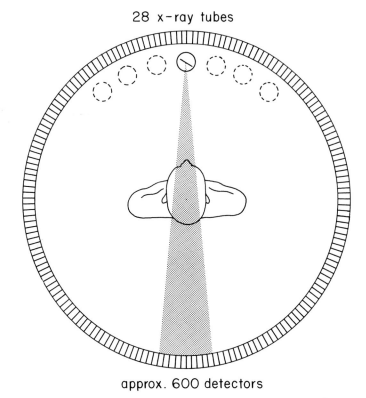

approx. 600 detectors

Figure 2D. Stationary tubes and detectors. Detectors are crystalline phosphors or xenon gas tubes.

1

Head and Neck

INTRODUCTION

Three specimens were used in preparing the illustrations for this chapter. Sections 1–1 to 1–11 were cut at a thickness of 1 cm at a plane 30 degrees to Reid's base line. Reid's base line passes from the inferior margin of the orbit through the center of the external auditory meatus. These sections were cut at a 30-degree angle, since the anatomy of this area is viewed in this manner in conventional computed tomography. Sections 1–12 to 1–25 were cut parallel to Reid's base line; they extend from the superior margin of the orbit to the intervertebral disc between C5 and C6. The sections through the orbit (1–12 to 1–18) were cut 0.5 cm thick in order to identify as many structures as possible in this compact area. The remaining sections (1–19 to 1–25) were cut at a 1-cm thickness. The third specimen (Sections 1–26 to 1–28) is the same one that was used for the thorax (Chapter 2). The sections here extend from the intervertebral disc between C5 and C6 to the vertebral body of C7.

The computed tomography of the orbit is carried out with thinner sections so that the intricate detail of the anatomy of the orbit may be best portrayed. These cuts are parallel to Reid's base line. For study of the supratentorial contents of the cranium, it is usually best to cut the sections 25 to 30 degrees to Reid's base line, as indicated in the diagram. The anatomy of the supratentorial structures is most advantageously shown in this manner. On the other hand, "cuts" that are used for the orbit and its contents may also be used for the posterior fossa to provide another perspective of that structure. Similar orientation of "cuts" is best used with regard to the facial bones.

Possible Sources of Error and Artifacts in Interpretation of Computed Tomographs

The most important possible sources of error and artifacts in CT scanning are movement by the patient and high differential attenuation values of adjacent tissues, giving rise to a black interface between these tissues. With rapid scanning, motion is less likely to occur, but with a very cooperative patient, even a 4.5-minute scan can be an excellent one. In the uncooperative patient sedation must always be considered.

High attenuation differential artifacts occur at interfaces such as air and bone, air and brain, bone and brain, and metal and brain. These result from computer "overloads" due to the high differential values, and they produce a streaking of the image. Surgical clips, metallic clips, Holter valves used in shunting procedures, and metal reservoirs can produce such streaking. Pneumoencephalography air can itself produce streaking at the air-fluid interface. On the other hand, air or contrast enhancement of the ventricles can be very useful.

Other artifacts result from improper selection by the operator of window level and width, improper photography of the televised image, improper patient positioning, and, due to the averaging effect within the small volume elements themselves, misinterpretation of the image. Magnification factors for measurement must be accurately calculated; fortunately, in most of the newer instruments, actual measurements are given with the magnification factor corrected by the computer.

Other sources of error include misinterpretation of anatomy. For example, the jugular tubercle, when it is prominent and invaginated, may simulate a tumor.

Applications of Computed Tomography

Computed tomography is capable of the following procedures:
1. Depiction of the cerebrospinal fluid–filled structures and spaces, such as the ventricles and sulci of the brain, as differentiated from the brain parenchyma.
2. Visualization of areas of blood-brain barrier breakdown or high vascularity, facilitated by injection of an appropriate contrast agent.
3. Visualization of orbital structures.
4. Detection of clotted and unclotted blood, as well as cerebral calcifications, which may not be visible on conventional skull radiographs.
5. More accurate definition of the component parts of the sella turcica than is obtainable by any other method of study.
6. Separation in most recent equipment of gray matter from white matter and even of such structures as the basal ganglia.
7. Algorithmic translation of a series of axial views into a sagittal projection.
8. Detection of cranial vault abnormalities.

Brain abnormalities that can be diagnosed by conventional computed tomography without the aid of contrast enhancement include cerebral atrophy, wherein the ventricles are large and the sulci of the brain appear very prominent; subdural or epidural hematomas, which may appear rarefied in their early phase but in their later phases quite dense; tuberous sclerosis; and some brain tumors, particularly those that contain calcification.

Some disorders are primarily of vascular origin and require contrast enhancement by the infusion of a contrast agent. Very often angiography is helpful as a supplementary study in these instances, particularly with aneurysms, vascular malformations, and highly vascular tumors.

Computed tomography displays orbital anatomy and pathology with considerable clarity (Momose et al., 1975; Vermess et al., 1978; Wende et al., 1977), but one must not overlook the possible applicability of ultrasonography in detection of orbital abnormalities such as a detached retina (Momose and Dallow, 1975). Radiation to the eye must, of course, be considered, but in the usual ranges of exposure with computed tomography there is no danger. Repeated examinations of the eye, however, must certainly be entertained with caution.

In the normal orbit, the globe and optic nerve as well as the retrobulbar fat are clearly defined. In addition, the medial and lateral rectus muscles, as well as the other muscles surrounding the eye and the ethmoid sinuses, may be clearly seen. The lens of the eye can usually be detected without difficulty.

Radiographic evaluation of diseases of the face and neck has profited considerably from an understanding of cross-sectional anatomy by computed tomography (Gould et al., 1977; Pullen, 1977; Wolf et al., 1977; Zimmerman and Bilaniuk, 1977).

With regard to the paranasal sinuses, computed tomography is particularly valuable in revealing extension of a lesion into the orbit, even disclosing involvement of the orbit and the facial area *per se*. Extension into the cranial cavity and infratemporal fossa can similarly be predicted. Of course, any bone or soft tissue extension can be clearly defined.

In trauma victims, conventional radiographic techniques are valuable in cataloging the type of fracture, particularly of facial bones. These same patients, however, may also have epidural or subdural hematomas, which are best analyzed by means of computed tomography.

Computed tomography and transverse study of the skeletal system are potentially valuable in the study of skeletal trauma and in the evaluation of trauma to the skull, the face, or the cervical spine, in which visualization by more conventional methods may be difficult. The associated soft tissue abnormalities are much better depicted. Thus, the entire clinical picture can be reconstructed to better advantage.

Disease entities involving the nasal cavities, nasopharynx, and oropharynx are especially difficult to assess by clinical examination and conventional radiographic techniques. At times even biopsy may lead to profound bleeding, as in the case of hemangioma or hemangiofibroma of the nasopharynx. Since these and other lesions may be associated with intraorbital or intracranial extension, computed tomography of all types becomes of considerable value; with contrast enhancement, it may even replace angiography as a means of study.

Tumors involving the salivary glands and soft tissues of the neck may also be investigated by computed tomography, even though the salivary glands may be studied by sialography, which involves the injection of the salivary duct with a contrast agent followed by radiography. Sialography alone, however, may not suffice. The tumor may extend to the infratemporal fossa, for example, or to the base of the skull; in either case assessment is difficult without this special modality.

With thyroid and parathyroid glands, conventional modalities will usually yield a satisfactory answer. At times, however, computed tomography may be very helpful, as in cases of carcinomas wherein the full extent of the lesion is difficult to ascertain. With parathyroid lesions particularly, mediastinal extension may be diagnosed by computed tomography (Doppman et al., 1977).

Computed tomography can also play a significant role with regard to the larynx and hypopharynx, as illustrated with Section 1–26. Unfortunately, it is difficult to suspend swallowing for long periods of time; hence, the instruments particularly valuable for such procedures are those capable of 1- or 2-second scans. A significant contribution may be made by computed tomography when there is an anticipated or actual spread of the tumor into the paraepiglottic space.

Computed tomography may actually be superior to conventional radiography in the evaluation of soft tissues as well as bone lesions of the neck, provided appropriate window settings are used. The high density of the bone requires a higher window level and wider window width for adequate visualization (McLeod et al., 1978).

Doppman JL, Brennan MF, Koehler JO, and Marx SJ: Computed tomography for parathyroid localization. J Computer Assisted Tomography 1:30–36, 1977.

Gould LV, Cummings CW, Rabuzzi DD, Reed GF, and Chung CT: Use of computerized axial tomography of head and neck region. Laryngoscope 87:1270–1276, 1977.

McLeod RA, Stephens DH, Beabout JW, Sheedy PF, and Hattery RR: Computed tomography of the skeletal system. Sem Roentgenol 13:235–247, 1978.

Momose KJ and Dallow RL: Comparison in the use of computerized axial tomography with ultrasonography in the investigation of orbital lesions. Thirteenth Annual Meeting —American Society of Neuroradiology, Vancouver, B.C., June 3–7, 1975.

Momose KJ, New PFJ, Grove AS Jr, and Scott WR: The use of computed tomography in ophthalmology. Radiology 115:361–368, 1975.

Pullen FW: The use of computerized tomography in otolaryngology. Trans Am Acad Ophthalmol Otolaryngol 84:622–627, 1977.

Vermess M, Haynes BF, Fauci AS, and Wolff SM: Computer-assisted tomography of orbital lesions in Wegener's granulomatosis. J Computer Assisted Tomography 2:45–48, 1978.

Wende S, Aulich A, Nover A, Lanksch W, Kazner E, Steinhoff H, Meese W, Lange S, and Grumme T: Computed tomography of orbital lesions: Cooperative study of 210 cases. Neuroradiology 13:123–134, 1977.

Wolf BS, Nakagawa H, and Yeh HC: Visualization of the thyroid gland with computed tomography. Radiology 123:368, 1977.

Zimmerman RA, and Bilaniuk LT: Computed tomography of sphenoid sinus tumors. Computed Axial Tomography 1:25–32, 1977.

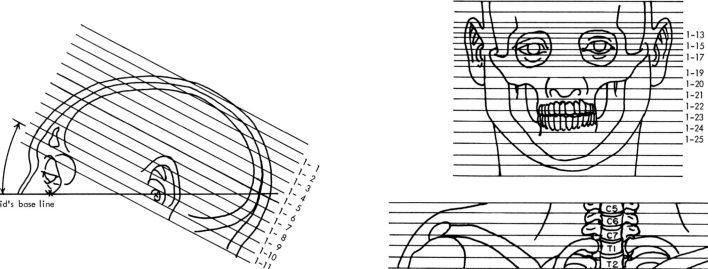

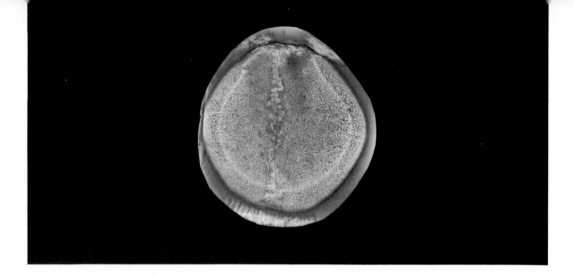

enlargement (New and Scott, 1975). Cala and Mastaglia (1976) showed additional optic nerve lesions in multiple sclerosis. These lesions may show contrast enhancement and subside after treatment with adrenocorticotropic hormone.

In young children, shrinkage of the hemispheres, widening of the sulci, ventricular enlargement, and softening of large areas of white matter (Greenfield and Norman, 1963) is called "Schilder's disease." The occipital lobes particularly become involved and symmetry is rare; contrast enhancement assists in the demonstration.

Loss of brain tissue with the formation of cysts is referred to as "porencephalic cysts"; they usually communicate with a ventricle, frequently dilated. This occurs particularly with external trauma or surgery.

A diffuse decrease in white matter density constitutes "progressive multifocal leukoencephalopathy" and may be observed in lymphoma, leukemia, sarcoidosis, and tuberculosis, as well as in advanced age.

The falx cerebri is a very rigid structure and even in the presence of a space-occupying lesion may remain in the midline. It cannot be relied upon clinically to demonstrate a shift from one side to the other.

Cala LA and Mastaglia FL: Computerized axial tomography in multiple sclerosis. Letter to the Editor, Lancet 1:689, 1976.

Fox JH, Ramsey RG, Huckman MS, and Proske AE: Cerebral ventricular enlargement in chronic alcoholics examined by computed tomography. JAMA 236:365–368, 1976.

Gath I, Jorgenson A, Sjaastad O, and Berstad J: Pneumoencephalographic findings in Parkinsonism. Arch Neurol 32:769–773, 1975.

Greenfield JG and Norman RM: Demyelinating diseases. In Greenfield's Neuropathology. Blackwood W. et al. (Editors): Williams and Wilkins Co., Baltimore, 1963, 475–519.

Hachinski VC, Lassen NA, and Marshall J: Multi-infarct dementia: A cause of mental deterioration in the elderly. Lancet 2:207–210, 1974.

Huckman MS, Fox JH, and Topel J: The validity of criteria for the evaluation of cerebral atrophy by computed tomography. Radiology 116:85–92, 1975.

New PFJ, and Scott WR: Computed Tomography of the Brain and Orbit — EMI Scanning. The Williams and Wilkins Co., Baltimore, 1975.

SECTION

1–1

Through the top of the calvaria, 9 cm above the plane that is at a 30-degree angle to Reid's base line

Anatomic Considerations

The scalp, which can be seen in this section and in several of the following ones, covers the cranium and extends from the eyebrows to the superior nuchal line. The scalp is composed of five layers; from superficial to deep these are skin, connective tissue, aponeurosis, loose areolar tissue, and periosteum. The three superficial layers are bound tightly together. The skin is quite thick, and the connective tissue layer is dense and contains numerous blood vessels. The third layer is a musculoaponeurotic sheet; the occipital and frontal bellies of the occipitofrontalis muscle are located at the posterior and anterior aspects of this layer, and the strong aponeurosis between the muscles in the galea aponeurotica. The loose areolar tissue, the fourth layer, allows the superficial layers of the scalp to move easily; this layer contains the emissary veins. The periosteum (pericranium) is the deepest layer of the scalp. It covers the bones of the cranium and is continuous with the outer layer of dura mater through the sutures and foramina.

Clinical Considerations

From the clinical standpoint, the main applications of this section pertain to (1) the integrity of the scalp; (2) the visualization of an intact parietal bone; and (3) the diagnosis of the various types of brain atrophy. Pneumoencephalography has been virtually replaced by CT for the demonstration of large cortical sulci, fissures, cisterns, and ventricles. The accuracy of computed tomography in the diagnosis of brain atrophy is comparable to that of the gross pathologic examination of the brain (Huckman et al., 1975). It should not be presumed that all patients with dementia have these radiographic signs of cerebral atrophy.

Arteriosclerosis may at times produce a dementia-like syndrome in the elderly, and grossly this is associated with softening of the cortex and basal ganglia and multiple small infarcts (Hachinski et al., 1974).

Diffuse cortical atrophy is also a frequent finding in Parkinson's disease (Gath et al., 1975) and chronic alcoholism (Fox et al., 1976).

With regard to multiple sclerosis, computed tomographic findings reveal irregularly distributed loss of cerebral substance with regions of ventricular

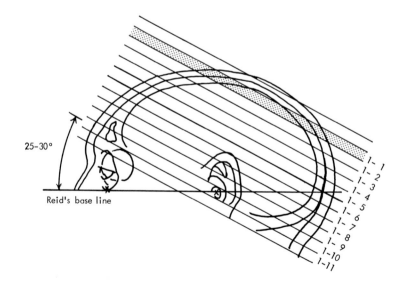

25-30°

Reid's base line

1-1
1-2
1-3
1-4
1-5
1-6
1-7
1-8
1-9
1-10
1-11

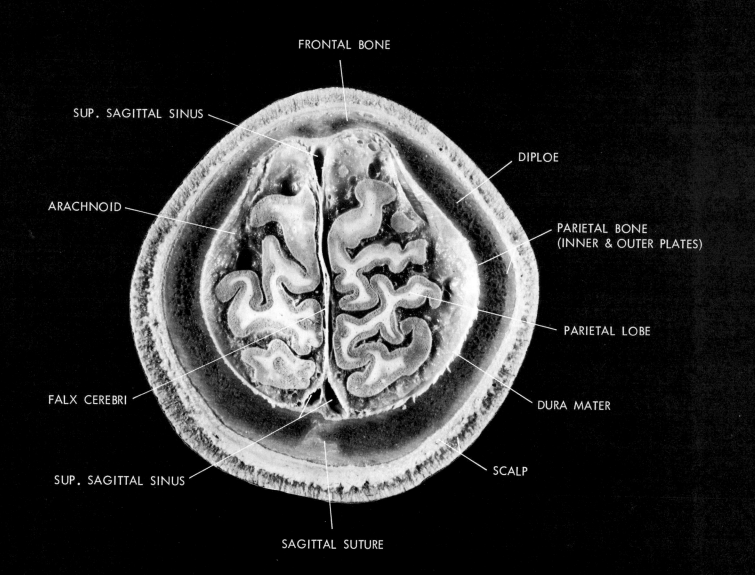

FRONTAL BONE

SUP. SAGITTAL SINUS

DIPLOE

ARACHNOID

PARIETAL BONE
(INNER & OUTER PLATES)

PARIETAL LOBE

FALX CEREBRI

DURA MATER

SUP. SAGITTAL SINUS

SCALP

SAGITTAL SUTURE

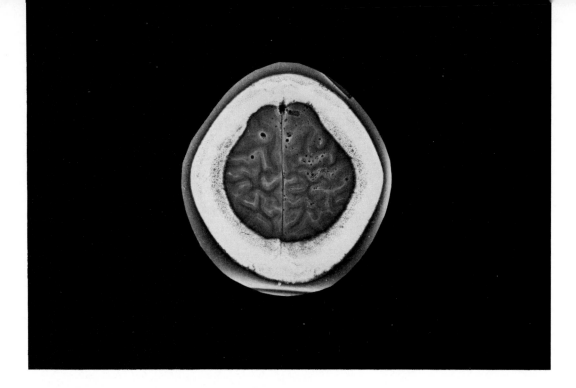

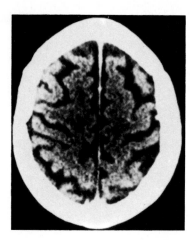

In general, the clinical considerations that have been described for Section 1–1 also apply to Section 1–2, since in this cadaveric section the major findings relate to the scalp, the integrity of the bone, and the sulci, as well as the relative proportion of gray and white matter.

SECTION

1–2

Through the skull, 1 cm below the preceding section

Anatomic Considerations

The bones that make up the calvaria are the frontal, two parietal, and the occipital. The coronal suture is located between the frontal and parietal bones; the sagittal suture is between the two parietal bones; and the lambdoidal suture is between the parietal bones and the occipital. The bregma is located at the junction of the sagittal and coronal sutures; the lambda is located at the junction of the sagittal and lambdoidal sutures.

The calvaria consists of an outer and an inner layer of compact bone and a layer of spongy bone (diploë) between the compact layers. The four diploic veins on each side — frontal, anterior temporal, posterior temporal, and occipital — communicate with the meningeal veins and sinuses of the dura mater and veins of the pericranium.

On the inner surface of the calvaria are markings due to the meningeal arteries, the superior sagittal sinus, and the arachnoid granulations.

Clinical Considerations

This CT scan demonstrates the vertex of the head with moderately enlarged sulci and an interhemispheric fissure due to moderate cerebral atrophy. (Courtesy of Dr. George Flouty and Dr. Sadek Hilal.)

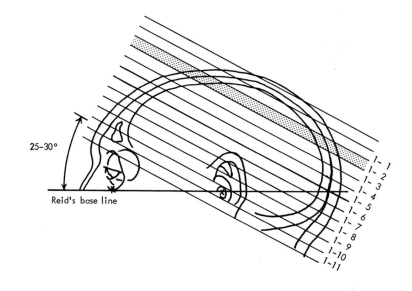

25-30°

Reid's base line

1– 1
1– 2
1– 3
1– 4
1– 5
1– 6
1– 7
1– 8
1– 9
1–10
1–11

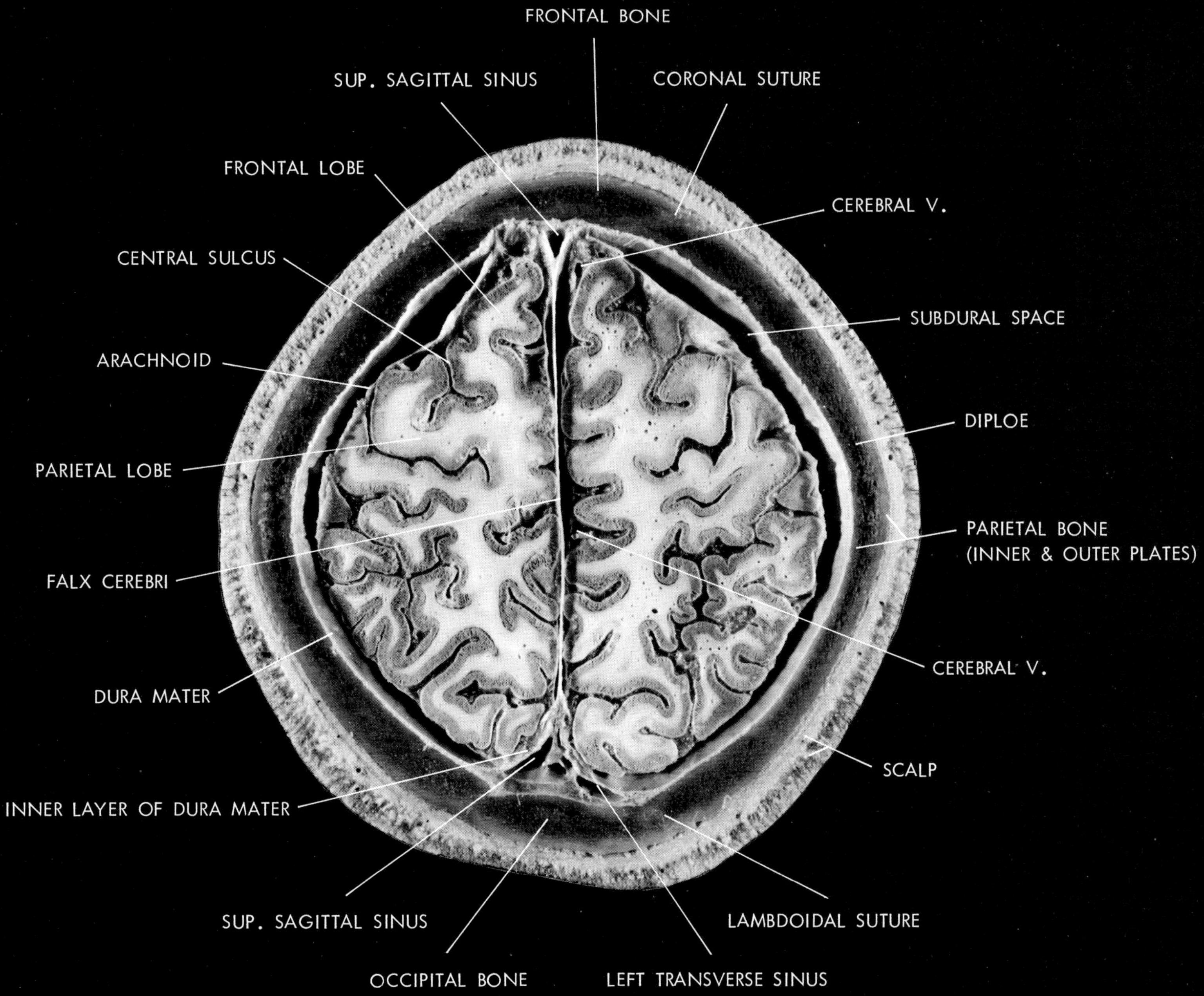

FRONTAL BONE

SUP. SAGITTAL SINUS

CORONAL SUTURE

FRONTAL LOBE

CEREBRAL V.

CENTRAL SULCUS

SUBDURAL SPACE

ARACHNOID

DIPLOE

PARIETAL LOBE

PARIETAL BONE
(INNER & OUTER PLATES)

FALX CEREBRI

CEREBRAL V.

DURA MATER

SCALP

INNER LAYER OF DURA MATER

SUP. SAGITTAL SINUS

LAMBDOIDAL SUTURE

OCCIPITAL BONE

LEFT TRANSVERSE SINUS

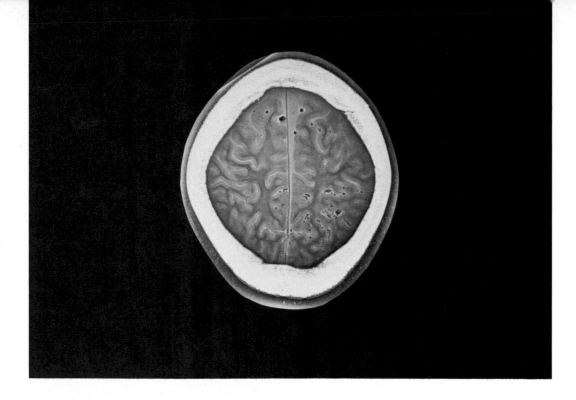

variable and may mimic neoplasm, inflammation, the demyelinating diseases, contusions, or arteriovenous malformation. When the infarct is acute, the areas show a diminished absorption coefficient associated with the tissue edema and a midline shift of the brain away from the new lesion; over one half the cases show fairly well-defined margins. This mass effect usually subsides by 3 weeks and the brain shifts toward the lesion. A cavity may result by 4 to 8 weeks.

Contrast enhancement is of considerable value in serial CT studies of infarction. This finding is most demonstrable between 7 and 21 days. It is during this phase that neoplasm or arteriovenous malformation may be simulated. Hemorrhage may also occur into an infarct, and computed tomography demonstrates this by contrast enhancement and by the different absorption coefficient of the clot. In addition, angiography may be necessary.

Arteriovenous malformations (AVM) may occur in highly variable situations and may have different etiologies and sizes. Very often, the AVM is in close association with one of the venous sinuses and may contain calcium or clotted blood. Prior to contrast enhancement, the appearance may not be readily perceptible. If it is a large AVM, it may "steal" blood from adjoining brain tissue and result in a very confusing picture.

Neoplasms can occur in many areas of the brain and are usually readily detected radiographically. Parasagittal meningiomas and gliomas may be indistinguishable by computed tomography. Other diagnoses may be entertained, particularly if angiography is not performed. These are the parasellar, cerebellopontine angle, and intraventricular tumors and the cerebral metastases, particularly if they are dural and involve the cranial vault.

Since almost any area of the brain may be involved by gliomas, it would be more appropriate to describe the clinical considerations in respect to gliomas in other areas of the brain.

SECTION

1–3

Through the skull, 1 cm below the preceding section

Anatomic Considerations

The brain is enclosed by three membranes; from within outward these are the pia mater, arachnoid, and dura mater. The pia mater is the vascular membrane that invests and is intimately attached to the entire surface of the brain since it follows the convolutions of the cerebral cortex. The arachnoid is a delicate weblike membrane that lies outside the pia membrane. Cerebrospinal fluid is found just deep to the arachnoid layer. The dura mater of the cranial cavity consists of two layers: the outer layer of dura forms the internal periosteum (endosteum) of the cranial cavity, while the inner layer corresponds to the dura of the spinal cord. The inner layer forms four inward-projecting reduplicated folds, the falx cerebri, the falx cerebelli, the tentorium cerebelli, and the diaphragma sellae. The falx cerebri, which can be observed in this illustration and in several adjacent sections, is the midline sickle-shaped projection between the cerebral hemispheres. The falx cerebelli is a small fold that projects between the cerebellar hemispheres. The tentorium cerebelli can be seen in Sections 1–6 and 1–7. This partition is located between the cerebellum and the occipital and posterior portions of the temporal lobes of the cerebrum. The diaphragma sellae (Section 1–8) bridges over the sella turcica and covers the pituitary gland.

Clinical Considerations

Section 1–3 shows evidence of a cerebral infarct. This could have been clearly identified by computed tomography; unfortunately, this demonstration is

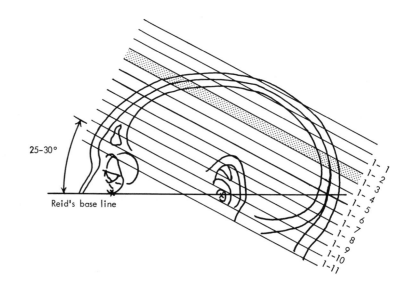

25-30°

Reid's base line

1–1
1–2
1–3
1–4
1–5
1–6
1–7
1–8
1–9
1–10
1–11

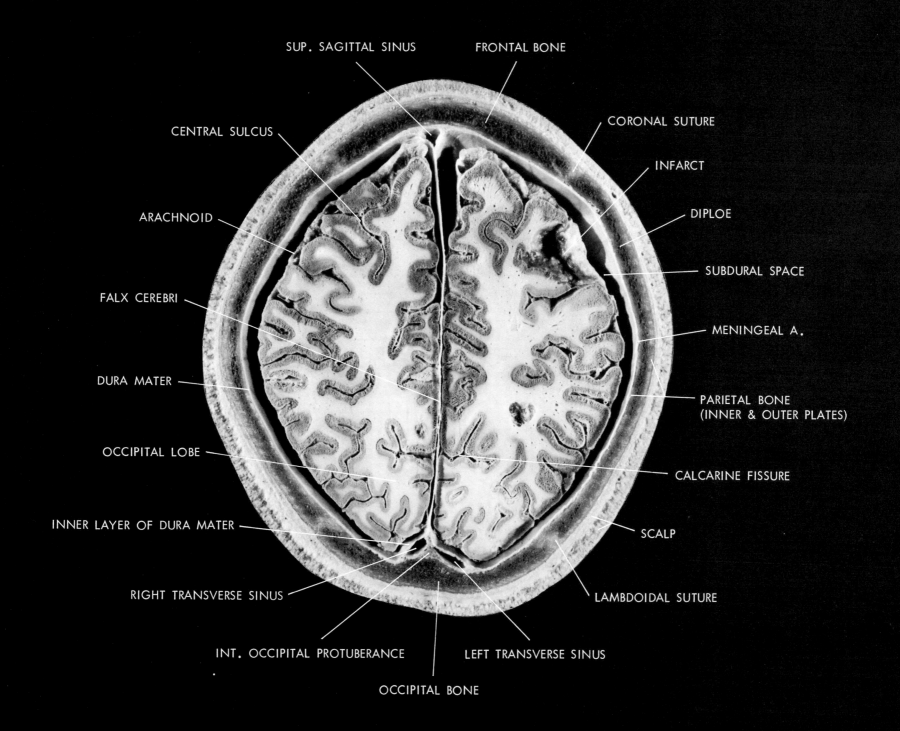

SUP. SAGITTAL SINUS

FRONTAL BONE

CENTRAL SULCUS

CORONAL SUTURE

INFARCT

ARACHNOID

DIPLOE

SUBDURAL SPACE

FALX CEREBRI

MENINGEAL A.

DURA MATER

PARIETAL BONE
(INNER & OUTER PLATES)

OCCIPITAL LOBE

CALCARINE FISSURE

INNER LAYER OF DURA MATER

SCALP

RIGHT TRANSVERSE SINUS

LAMBDOIDAL SUTURE

INT. OCCIPITAL PROTUBERANCE

LEFT TRANSVERSE SINUS

OCCIPITAL BONE

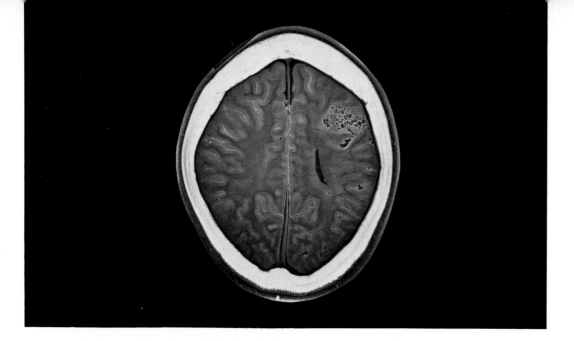

contrast material to perfuse through to the center of the solid tumor (Davis, 1977). An infarct usually has more regular edges and is wedge-shaped, but even this appearance occasionally occurs with gliomas. Moreover, like a glioma, infarction is confined to a specific vascular territory and usually has little mass effect. Gliomas may even be difficult to differentiate from meningiomas, particularly when they are peripheral, especially without contrast enhancement or angiography.

In this section we are beginning to see the lateral ventricle lined by ependyma. Ependymomas, as visualized by computed tomography, are often similar in their appearance to malignant gliomas, except that their intraventricular location allows differentiation.

Oligodendrogliomas allow a more specific CT appearance. They are usually intracerebral, and often frontal, but may be extensive; cystic degeneration occurs in about 20 per cent (Mansuy et al., 1975). Dense calcification occurs in about 70 per cent of these tumors, but the calcification is demonstrable by ordinary radiologic means in only about 50 per cent of cases. This lesion should thus be suspected when the CT scan with contrast enhancement discloses high-density areas due to calcification interspersed with low-density areas, with faint enhancement surrounding the lesion. Hemorrhage may complicate the appearance.

It can be noted that the central sulcus begins to make its appearance on this section, as does the lateral ventricle. But the ventricular system is better shown in subsequent sections, and lesions that pertain thereto will be described later. These concern particularly suspected metastatic disease, head trauma, intracranial inflammatory disease, and visual disturbances, even though visual disturbances may be produced by disorders involving the calcarine fissure.

Davis DO: CT in the diagnosis of supratentorial tumors. Semin Roentgenol 12:97–108, 1977.

Mansuy L, Thierry A, and Tommasi M: Oligodendrogliomas. In Handbook of Clinical Neurology, Vol. 18. P. J. Vinken and G. W. Bruyn (Editors): North Holland Publishing Co., Amsterdam, 1975, pp. 81–103.

Weisberg LA, Nice C, and Katz M: Cerebral Computed Tomography: A Text-Atlas. W. B. Saunders Co., Philadelphia, 1978, p. 131.

SECTION 1–4

Through the skull, 1 cm below the preceding section

Anatomic Considerations

The venous sinuses of the cranial cavity are found between the layers of dura mater. They receive the veins from the brain and communicate with the meningeal and diploic veins and with the veins external to the cranium. The sinuses terminate directly or indirectly into the internal jugular vein and are either paired or unpaired. The paired ones are the transverse, sigmoid, occipital, cavernous, sphenoparietal, and superior and inferior petrosal. The unpaired sinuses are the superior sagittal, inferior sagittal, straight, intercavernous, and basilar (plexus of veins).

The paired sinuses that can be observed in these sections are the transverse (Sections 1–2 to 1–5, 1–14, and 1–15), sigmoid (Sections 1–6 to 1–8 and 1–14 to 1–17), cavernous (Section 1–9), and occipital (Sections 1–5 and 1–6).

The unpaired sinuses that can be seen in these sections are the superior sagittal (Sections 1–1 to 1–7), the inferior sagittal (Section 1–4), and the straight (Section 1–5).

Clinical Considerations

The venous sinuses, partially in view here, are subject to two main clinical abnormalities: (1) obstruction by thrombosis or invasion by tumor, and (2) arteriovenous malformation.

With respect to involvement of the brain in this and other sections by gliomas, it is generally agreed now that the incidence of low-grade gliomas is shown by CT studies to be 20 to 30 per cent of all gliomas, compared with 5 to 7 per cent demonstrated with conventional studies (Weisberg et al., 1978). The more malignant gliomas are much more variable in appearance and generally show a greater degree of ventricular displacement as the ventricles come into view in CT scans.

Approximately 15 per cent of glioblastomas show computed tomographic evidence of calcification (Weisberg et al., 1978). Unfortunately, a ring of enhancement is not at all specific for a malignant glioma, since it may occur with infarction, hematoma, abscess, or metastases. Usually, however, a malignant glioma has a ring of variable thickness and even a central low absorption coefficient core as in a cyst. The latter may be due to a failure of

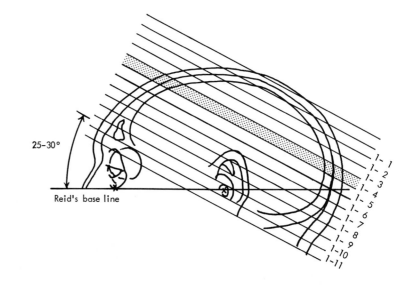

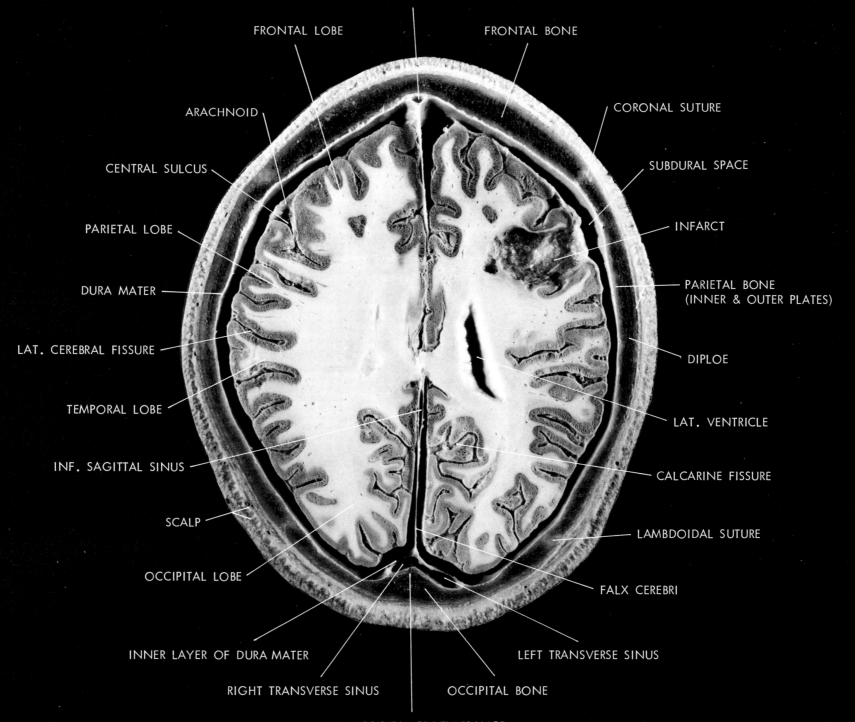

SUP. SAGITTAL SINUS

FRONTAL LOBE

FRONTAL BONE

ARACHNOID

CORONAL SUTURE

CENTRAL SULCUS

SUBDURAL SPACE

PARIETAL LOBE

INFARCT

DURA MATER

PARIETAL BONE
(INNER & OUTER PLATES)

LAT. CEREBRAL FISSURE

DIPLOE

TEMPORAL LOBE

LAT. VENTRICLE

INF. SAGITTAL SINUS

CALCARINE FISSURE

SCALP

LAMBDOIDAL SUTURE

OCCIPITAL LOBE

FALX CEREBRI

INNER LAYER OF DURA MATER

LEFT TRANSVERSE SINUS

RIGHT TRANSVERSE SINUS

OCCIPITAL BONE

INT. OCCIPITAL PROTUBERANCE

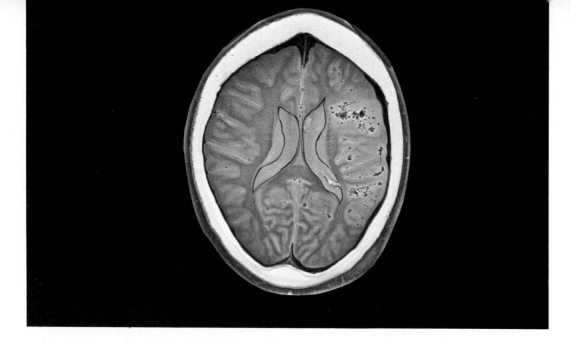

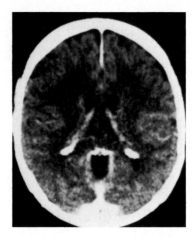

Anatomic Considerations

In Sections 1–4 to 1–8 the different portions of the ventricular system of the brain can be observed. The ventricular system is a series of cavities in the brain containing cerebrospinal fluid that is secreted by the choroid plexus. The lateral ventricles are located in each of the cerebral hemispheres. Each is connected to the third ventricle of the diencephalon by the interventricular foramen. The cerebral aqueduct of the midbrain connects the third ventricle with the fourth, which is located in the pons and medulla. The fourth ventricle communicates with the central canal of the spinal cord and with the subarachnoid space by way of the foramina of Luschka and the foramen of Magendie. The cerebrospinal fluid enters the venous circulation by diffusing through the arachnoid granulations into the superior sagittal sinus.

Clinical Considerations

In the CT scan of the head, note the large supracerebellar cistern. There is excellent delineation also of the choroid plexus of the lateral ventricle. (Courtesy of Dr. George Flouty and Dr. Sadek Hilal.)

The anterior horn of the lateral ventricle is bounded by the caudate nucleus. This area of the brain is involved particularly in early degeneration and atrophy in Huntington's disease, a disorder that causes patients to develop abnormal movements (chorea) and associated mental deterioration.

Ordinarily, the ratio of maximum distance between the frontal horns to intercaudate distance becomes smaller (less than 2 cm) owing to a localized form of atrophy (Sax and Menzer, 1977).

In this section the thalamus makes its appearance. In general, tumors involving this area may simulate many other lesions. With computed tomography, preoperative diagnosis may be possible, as well as definition of the full extent of the lesion (Messina et al., 1976).

One can identify the great cerebral vein, which is the centrum into which the internal cerebral veins drain.

The posterior horns of the lateral ventricles may be readily identified and are clinically useful in measuring dilatation of the ventricular system.

It will be noted that the middle cerebral artery is "buried" in the lateral cerebral fissure and sweeps out of the fissure over the parietal lobe. The position of the insula plays a very important part, particularly in angiography.

The posterior horn of the lateral ventricle forms a portion of the so-called trigone of the lateral ventricle, which represents a junction of the body, the posterior horn, and the temporal horn of the lateral ventricle. Just lateral to the thalamus is the posterior limb of the internal capsule, which can barely be identified by its change in shading on the present section. The hippocampus is just identifiable as it produces an indentation on the medial posterior floor of the posterior horn of the lateral ventricle.

Messina AV, Potts G, Sigel RM, and Liebeskin AL: Computed tomography: Evaluation of the posterior or third ventricle. Radiology 119:581–592, 1976.
Sax DS and Menzer L: CT in Huntington's disease. Neurology 27:388, 1977.

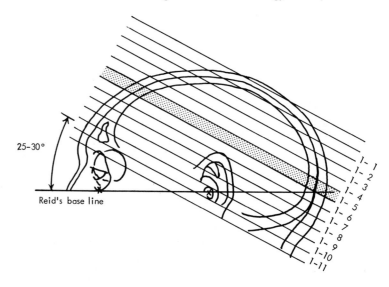

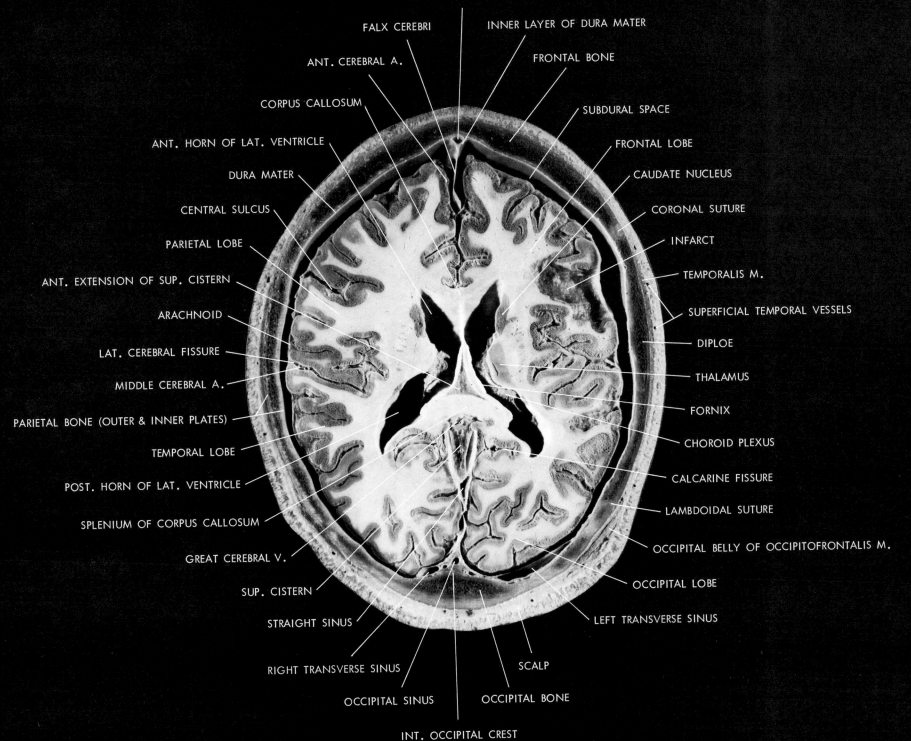

SUP. SAGITTAL SINUS

FALX CEREBRI

INNER LAYER OF DURA MATER

ANT. CEREBRAL A.

FRONTAL BONE

CORPUS CALLOSUM

SUBDURAL SPACE

ANT. HORN OF LAT. VENTRICLE

FRONTAL LOBE

DURA MATER

CAUDATE NUCLEUS

CENTRAL SULCUS

CORONAL SUTURE

PARIETAL LOBE

INFARCT

ANT. EXTENSION OF SUP. CISTERN

TEMPORALIS M.

ARACHNOID

SUPERFICIAL TEMPORAL VESSELS

LAT. CEREBRAL FISSURE

DIPLOE

MIDDLE CEREBRAL A.

THALAMUS

PARIETAL BONE (OUTER & INNER PLATES)

FORNIX

TEMPORAL LOBE

CHOROID PLEXUS

POST. HORN OF LAT. VENTRICLE

CALCARINE FISSURE

SPLENIUM OF CORPUS CALLOSUM

LAMBDOIDAL SUTURE

GREAT CEREBRAL V.

OCCIPITAL BELLY OF OCCIPITOFRONTALIS M.

SUP. CISTERN

OCCIPITAL LOBE

STRAIGHT SINUS

LEFT TRANSVERSE SINUS

RIGHT TRANSVERSE SINUS

SCALP

OCCIPITAL SINUS

OCCIPITAL BONE

INT. OCCIPITAL CREST

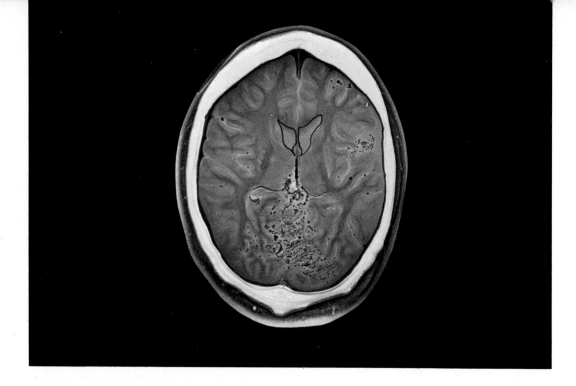

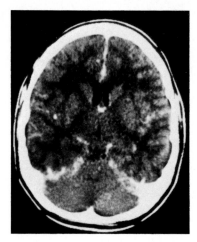

and optic radiation, which pass to the temporal and occipital cortices. In this cadaveric section, one sees the cut edge of the tentorium cerebelli as well as the cerebellar hemispheres. The caudal parts of the lateral lobes of the cerebellum are called the cerebellar tonsils and lie on each side of the midline just dorsal to the medulla and above the posterior part of the foramen magnum. Downward displacement from hydrocephalus and dilatation of the supratentorial ventricles is an indication of increased intracranial pressure. Measurements of the third ventricle, when dilated, suggest hydrocephalus.

The cistern, just above the cerebellum, is often spoken of as the cistern of the quadrigeminal plate with a cavity anteriorly and contains important venous structures. The rounding of the cornua of the lateral ventricles becomes an important roentgen sign of dilatation of the ventricular system.

SECTION
1–6

Through the skull, 1 cm below the preceding section

Anatomic Considerations

The brain can be divided into the (1) cerebral hemispheres, or telencephalon, (2) diencephalon, (3) midbrain, (4) pons and cerebellum, and (5) medulla oblongata. Numerous structures of the brain can be observed in these illustrations, which were sectioned at a 30-degree angle to Reid's base line, and, in some of the sections parallel to Reid's base line.

The cerebral hemispheres compose the majority of the brain; portions of the cerebrum can be seen in Sections 1–1 to 1–10 and in Sections 1–12 to 1–16. The cerebral cortex is divided into well-defined areas: the frontal, parietal, occipital, and temporal lobes. The lobes lie approximately deep to the bones with corresponding names. The frontal and temporal lobes can be observed in this section; these lobes are separated by the lateral cerebral fissure.

Clinical Considerations

The CT scan shows the head with excellent separation of the central white and gray matter. The caudate nucleus and the basal ganglia are clearly seen. (Courtesy of Dr. George Flouty and Dr. Sadek Hilal.)

The caudate nucleus, lentiform nucleus, and intervening internal capsule are called the corpus striatum. The lentiform and caudate nuclei are part of the extrapyramidal motor system, which, if impaired, gives rise to a palsy or paralysis of the contralateral side.

The posterior limb of the internal capsule contains fibers controlling movements of the tongue, arms, and legs, as well as fibers of the auditory

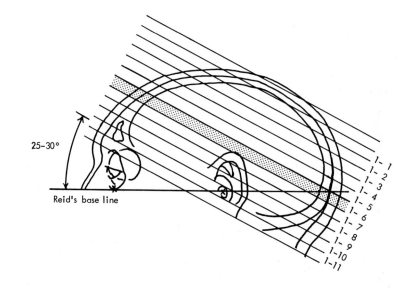

25–30°

Reid's base line

1–1
1–2
1–3
1–4
1–5
1–6
1–7
1–8
1–9
1–10
1–11

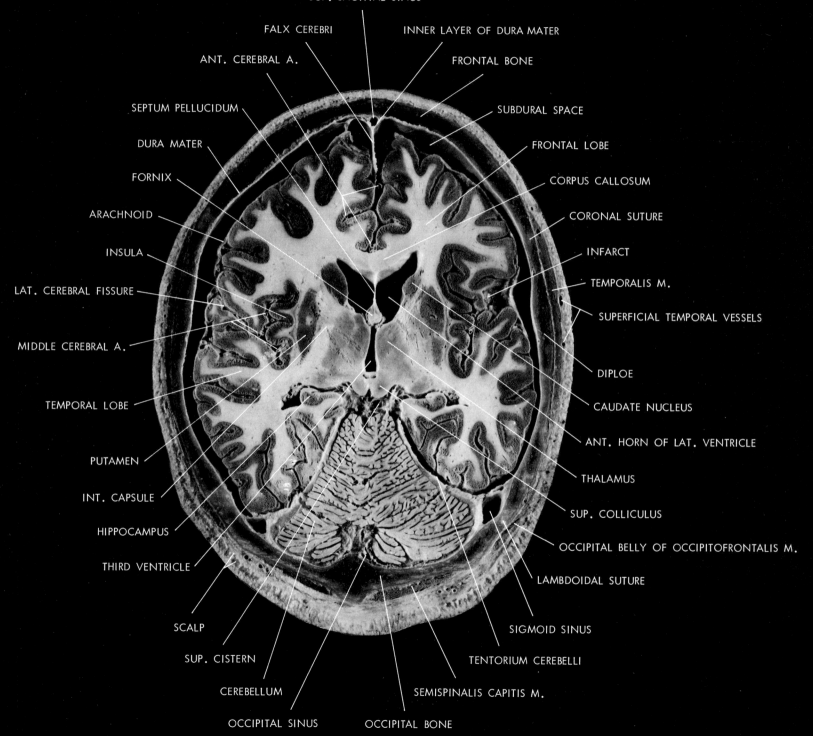

SUP. SAGITTAL SINUS

FALX CEREBRI

INNER LAYER OF DURA MATER

ANT. CEREBRAL A.

FRONTAL BONE

SEPTUM PELLUCIDUM

SUBDURAL SPACE

DURA MATER

FRONTAL LOBE

FORNIX

CORPUS CALLOSUM

ARACHNOID

CORONAL SUTURE

INSULA

INFARCT

LAT. CEREBRAL FISSURE

TEMPORALIS M.

SUPERFICIAL TEMPORAL VESSELS

MIDDLE CEREBRAL A.

DIPLOE

TEMPORAL LOBE

CAUDATE NUCLEUS

ANT. HORN OF LAT. VENTRICLE

PUTAMEN

THALAMUS

INT. CAPSULE

SUP. COLLICULUS

HIPPOCAMPUS

OCCIPITAL BELLY OF OCCIPITOFRONTALIS M.

THIRD VENTRICLE

LAMBDOIDAL SUTURE

SCALP

SIGMOID SINUS

SUP. CISTERN

TENTORIUM CEREBELLI

CEREBELLUM

SEMISPINALIS CAPITIS M.

OCCIPITAL SINUS

OCCIPITAL BONE

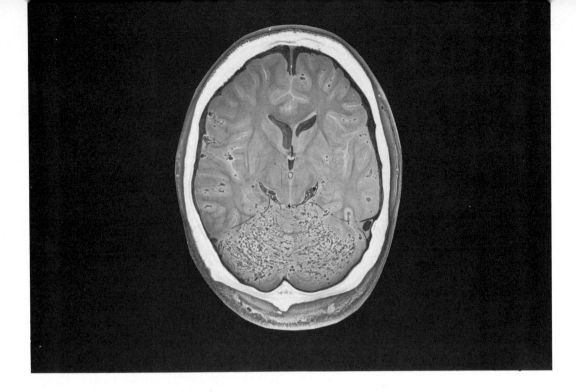

SECTION 1-7

Through the skull, 1 cm below the preceding section

Anatomic Considerations

The cerebellum is the largest part of the hindbrain and is found in the posterior cranial fossa. As can be seen in the illustration, it is composed of two lateral cerebellar hemispheres and a median vermis. The cerebellum is connected to the brain stem by three pairs of cerebellar peduncles: the superior pair connects it to the midbrain; the middle pair to the pons (shown in the following section); and the inferior pair to the medulla oblongata. The cerebellum is the portion of the brain involved in regulation of posture, muscle tone, and coordination.

Clinical Considerations

The CT scan of the head demonstrates the central white and gray matter. The caudate nuclei are very distinct. The posterior medial choroidal artery is visualized in the quadrigeminal cistern (arrow). (Courtesy of Dr. George Flouty and Dr. Sadek Hilal.)

The contour of the lateral ventricle should be carefully noted, since measurements of the lateral ventricles in this view become of increasing importance in determining enlargement. Various measurements have been proposed (Meschan, 1975).

As the result of trauma, hemorrhage into the basal ganglia may also occur, with unconsciousness and numerous neurologic deficits resulting. Since the internal capsule is the great axial projection system connecting the cerebral cortex with lower brain centers and since it is intimately related to the thalamus, caudate nucleus, and lentiform nucleus, this section of the brain is particularly important.

Mass lesions in this area may also involve the third ventricle at this level and, by causing an obstruction of the third ventricle, result in hydrocephalus.

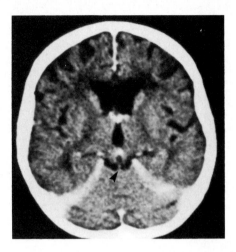

Any mass that produces an obstruction of the outlet of the third ventricle may be responsible for a progressive mental deterioration, dementia, and erosion of the dorsum sellae.

The midbrain, tentorium cerebelli, and cerebellum and its vermis are particularly important in all age groups, but especially the younger individuals, who are subject to such posterior fossa tumors as ependymomas responsible for headaches, ataxia, nystagmus, and bilateral papilledema. The medulloblastoma and the astroblastoma are particularly common among the brain tumors involving patients in younger age groups. One should, however, also think of lesions of this type in individuals who are older, even in the third and fourth decades. The cerebellum may also contain cystic astrocytomas, which produce a symptomatology similar to that already mentioned for the posterior fossa tumors.

Meschan I: An Atlas of Anatomy Basic to Radiology. W. B. Saunders Co., Philadelphia, 1975, p. 383.

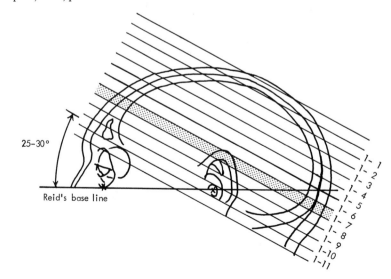

25–30°

Reid's base line

1–1
1–2
1–3
1–4
1–5
1–6
1–7
1–8
1–9
1–10
1–11

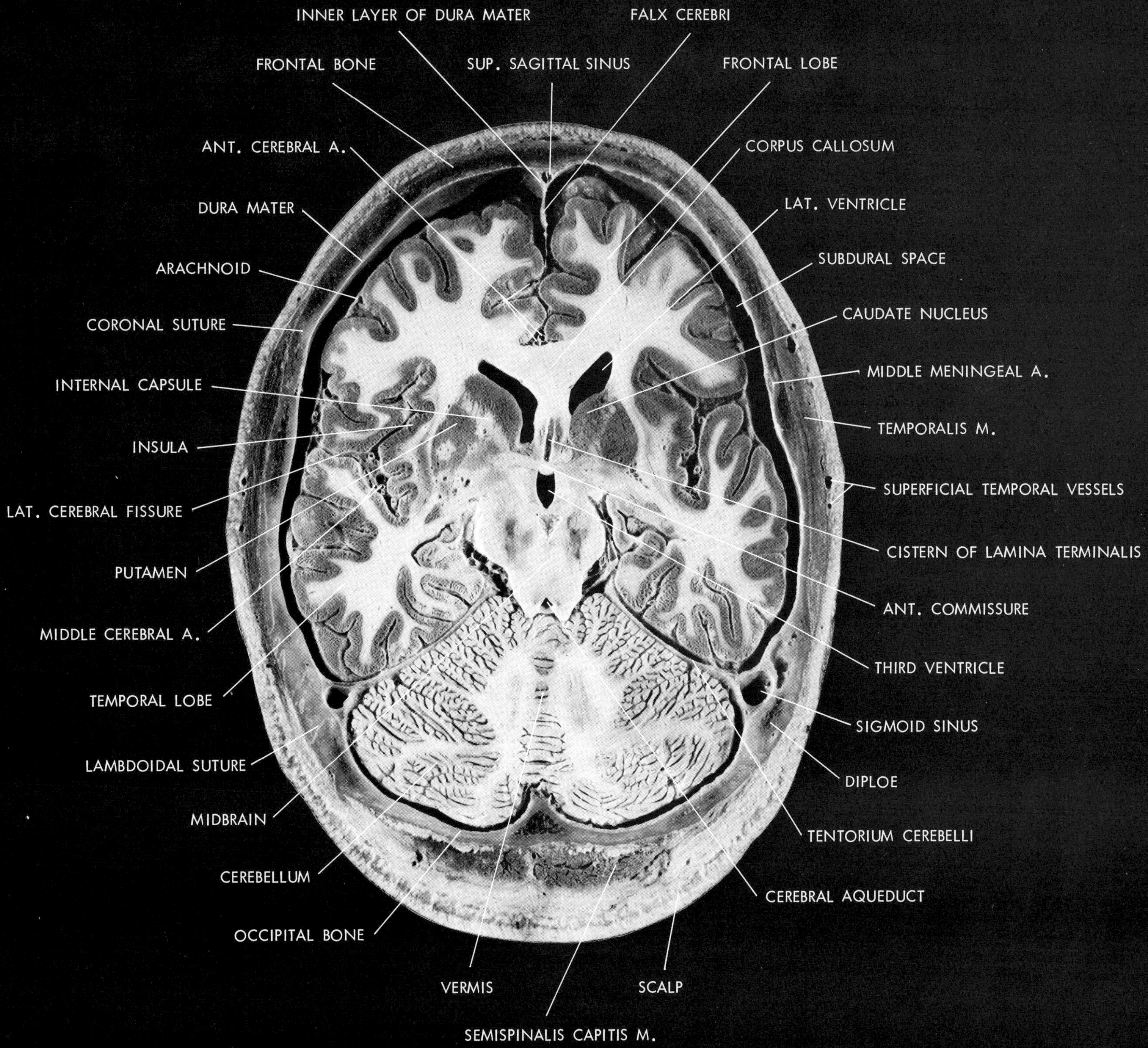

INNER LAYER OF DURA MATER   FALX CEREBRI

FRONTAL BONE   SUP. SAGITTAL SINUS   FRONTAL LOBE

ANT. CEREBRAL A.   CORPUS CALLOSUM

DURA MATER   LAT. VENTRICLE

ARACHNOID   SUBDURAL SPACE

CORONAL SUTURE   CAUDATE NUCLEUS

INTERNAL CAPSULE   MIDDLE MENINGEAL A.

INSULA   TEMPORALIS M.

LAT. CEREBRAL FISSURE   SUPERFICIAL TEMPORAL VESSELS

PUTAMEN   CISTERN OF LAMINA TERMINALIS

MIDDLE CEREBRAL A.   ANT. COMMISSURE

TEMPORAL LOBE   THIRD VENTRICLE

LAMBDOIDAL SUTURE   SIGMOID SINUS

MIDBRAIN   DIPLOE

CEREBELLUM   TENTORIUM CEREBELLI

OCCIPITAL BONE   CEREBRAL AQUEDUCT

VERMIS   SCALP

SEMISPINALIS CAPITIS M.

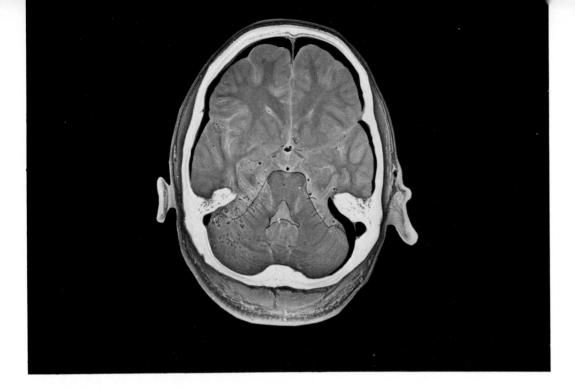

optic nerves, the optic chiasm, the cavernous sinus, and numerous vascular structures contained in the circle of Willis.

Lesions contained within the sella turcica might be those affecting the pituitary gland or hypothalamus proper; small adenomas, for example, may have very important relevance to clinical symptomatology.

In this section also is the petrous portion of the temporal bone. This area is therefore very intimately involved with the auditory mechanism and the trigeminal nerve. Individuals with mass lesions in this locus may suffer from hearing loss, ataxia, and even neuralgia, particularly in relation to the trigeminal nerve.

Because the bony structures are so clearly identified, even lesions arising elsewhere, such as in the parotid gland, and producing a destruction of the skull base may extend posteriorly to involve the cerebellum in one or the other of its hemispheres; such lesions may produce headache, nausea, vomiting, and vertigo, as well as palsies of the seventh and eighth nerves. One must certainly be alert to pontine gliomas, which may grow forward to obstruct the cistern just anterior to the pons.

Apart from mass lesions of neoplastic origin, the petrous portion of the temporal bone is also a site for extension of inflammatory processes arising in the ear mechanism; abscesses at the region of the cerebellopontine angle are not at all uncommon, and give rise to somewhat similar symptomatology.

SECTION
1-8

Through the skull, 1 cm below the preceding section

Anatomic Considerations

In Sections 1–8 and 1–13 portions of the circle of Willis can be observed.

The blood supply to the brain is derived from the vertebral and internal carotid arteries. The vertebral arteries pass into the cranial cavity through the foramen magnum and form the basilar artery. The internal carotid artery passes through the carotid canal, along the upper part of the foramen lacerum, and into the cavernous sinus. It pierces the roof of the sinus and terminates close to the optic foramen by dividing into the anterior cerebral and middle cerebral arteries.

The circle of Willis is formed by the anterior cerebral arteries; the anterior communicating artery, which connects the two anterior cerebral arteries; the middle cerebral arteries; the posterior cerebral arteries, which arise from the basilar artery; and the posterior communicating arteries, which join the middle cerebral and posterior cerebral arteries.

Clinical Considerations

Of primary importance in this section is the visualization of the structures adjoining the sella turcica. These include such important elements as the

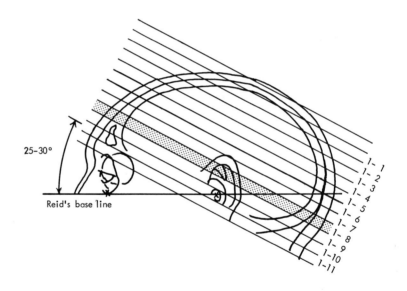

25-30°

Reid's base line

1-1
1-2
1-3
1-4
1-5
1-6
1-7
1-8
1-9
1-10
1-11

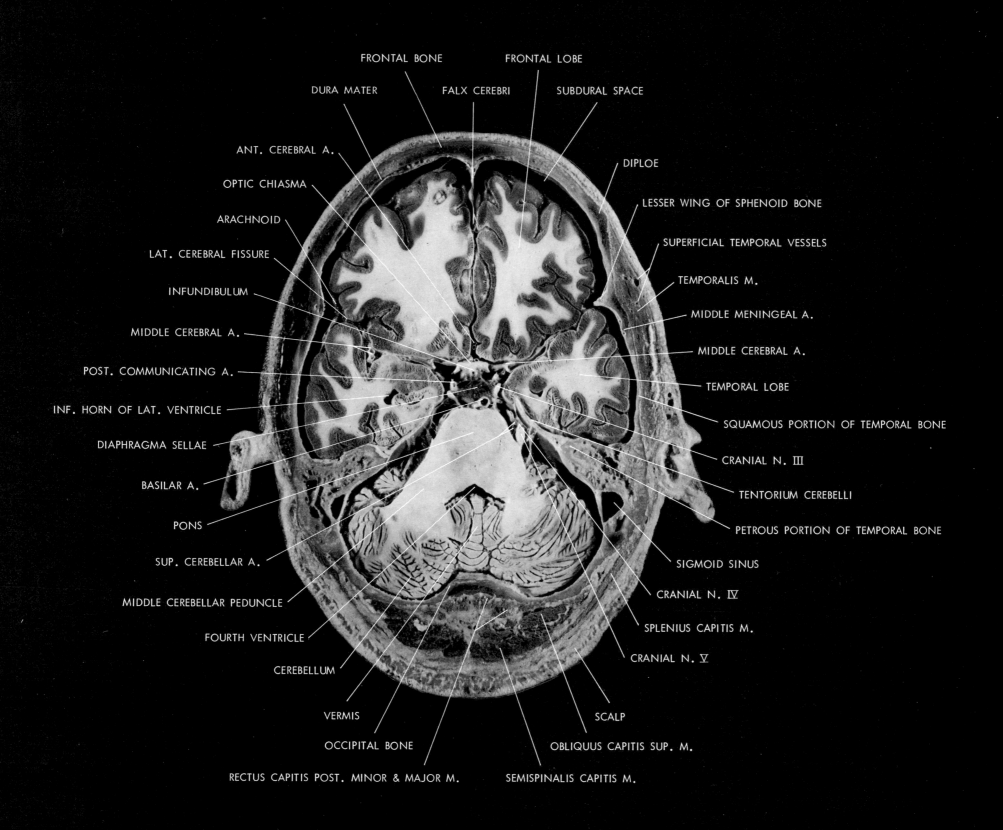

FRONTAL BONE   FRONTAL LOBE

DURA MATER   FALX CEREBRI   SUBDURAL SPACE

ANT. CEREBRAL A.   DIPLOE

OPTIC CHIASMA   LESSER WING OF SPHENOID BONE

ARACHNOID   SUPERFICIAL TEMPORAL VESSELS

LAT. CEREBRAL FISSURE   TEMPORALIS M.

INFUNDIBULUM   MIDDLE MENINGEAL A.

MIDDLE CEREBRAL A.   MIDDLE CEREBRAL A.

POST. COMMUNICATING A.   TEMPORAL LOBE

INF. HORN OF LAT. VENTRICLE   SQUAMOUS PORTION OF TEMPORAL BONE

DIAPHRAGMA SELLAE   CRANIAL N. III

BASILAR A.   TENTORIUM CEREBELLI

PONS   PETROUS PORTION OF TEMPORAL BONE

SUP. CEREBELLAR A.   SIGMOID SINUS

MIDDLE CEREBELLAR PEDUNCLE   CRANIAL N. IV

FOURTH VENTRICLE   SPLENIUS CAPITIS M.

CEREBELLUM   CRANIAL N. V

VERMIS   SCALP

OCCIPITAL BONE   OBLIQUUS CAPITIS SUP. M.

RECTUS CAPITIS POST. MINOR & MAJOR M.   SEMISPINALIS CAPITIS M.

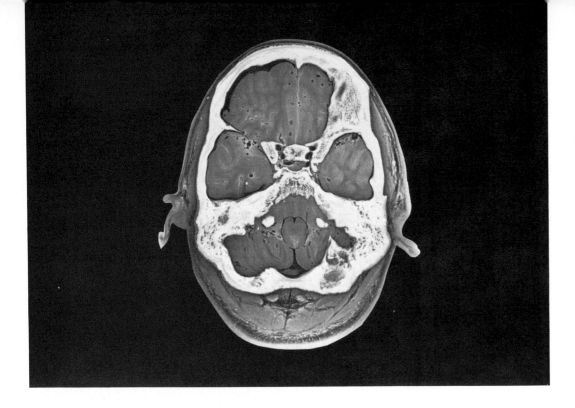

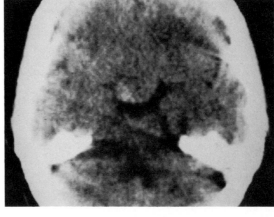
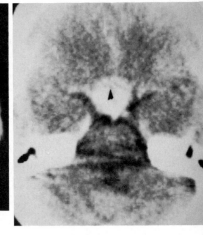

Anatomic Considerations

The hypophysis cerebri (pituitary gland) is observed in this section and in Section 1–14. It is located in the hypophyseal fossa or sella turcica of the sphenoid bone and is roofed by the diaphragma sellae. Through a small opening in the diaphragma sellae, the infundibulum connects the hypophysis cerebri with the tuber cinereum of the floor of the third ventricle.

The hypophysis has important relations and some of them can be observed in these illustrations. The sphenoid sinus is located in front of and inferior to it, whereas the cavernous sinuses are found laterally. The internal carotid artery traverses the cavernous sinus. In the lateral wall of the sinus, cranial nerves III, IV, and V can be seen. In addition to these structures, cranial nerve VI also traverses the sinus, but it is not evident in these sections. In this illustration, the divisions of cranial nerve V are not distinguishable. The optic chiasma (Section 1–8) is separated from the hypophysis by the diaphragma sellae.

Clinical Considerations

The CT scan shows a chromophobe adenoma of the pituitary (arrow) before (A) and after (B) contrast enhancement.

In this cadaveric section, the major additional features that come into view are the sphenoid sinus, the medulla oblongata, the various structures already mentioned in respect to the petrous portion of the temporal bone,

and the mastoids. Many of the cranial nerves are in view, as indicated here, and each may be subject to one or another major pathologic process. The brain stem is particularly important, of course, since it contains many vital centers involved in breathing, temperature control, and control of the cerebrovascular system. Brain stem herniation downward through the foramen magnum as a result of pressure above will give rise very often to posterior fossa symptomatology such as ataxia.

Mass lesions involving the sphenoid sinus, extend upward to the brain, to involve the sella turcica and its adjoining structures, or downward into the nasopharynx, causing some destruction at the base of the skull and involvement of the respiratory air passages immediately adjoining.

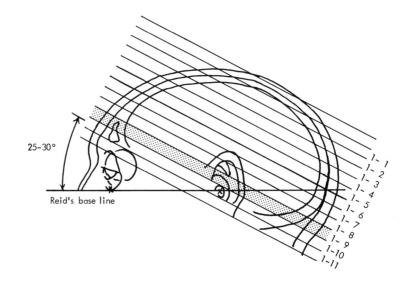

25–30°

Reid's base line

1–1
1–2
1–3
1–4
1–5
1–6
1–7
1–8
1–9
1–10
1–11

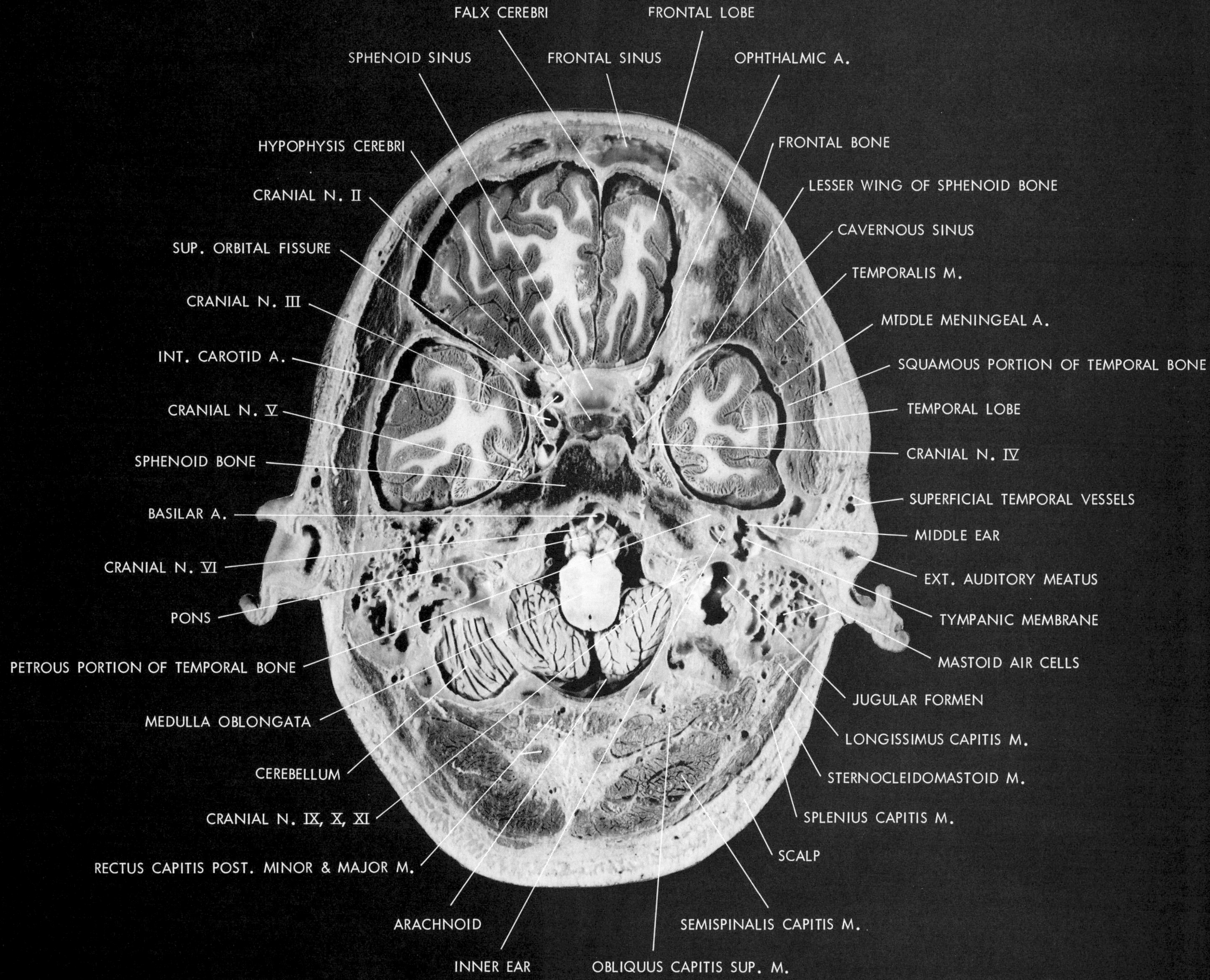

FALX CEREBRI

FRONTAL LOBE

SPHENOID SINUS

FRONTAL SINUS

OPHTHALMIC A.

HYPOPHYSIS CEREBRI

FRONTAL BONE

CRANIAL N. II

LESSER WING OF SPHENOID BONE

SUP. ORBITAL FISSURE

CAVERNOUS SINUS

TEMPORALIS M.

CRANIAL N. III

MIDDLE MENINGEAL A.

INT. CAROTID A.

SQUAMOUS PORTION OF TEMPORAL BONE

CRANIAL N. V

TEMPORAL LOBE

SPHENOID BONE

CRANIAL N. IV

BASILAR A.

SUPERFICIAL TEMPORAL VESSELS

MIDDLE EAR

CRANIAL N. VI

EXT. AUDITORY MEATUS

PONS

TYMPANIC MEMBRANE

PETROUS PORTION OF TEMPORAL BONE

MASTOID AIR CELLS

MEDULLA OBLONGATA

JUGULAR FORMEN

LONGISSIMUS CAPITIS M.

CEREBELLUM

STERNOCLEIDOMASTOID M.

CRANIAL N. IX, X, XI

SPLENIUS CAPITIS M.

RECTUS CAPITIS POST. MINOR & MAJOR M.

SCALP

ARACHNOID

SEMISPINALIS CAPITIS M.

INNER EAR

OBLIQUUS CAPITIS SUP. M.

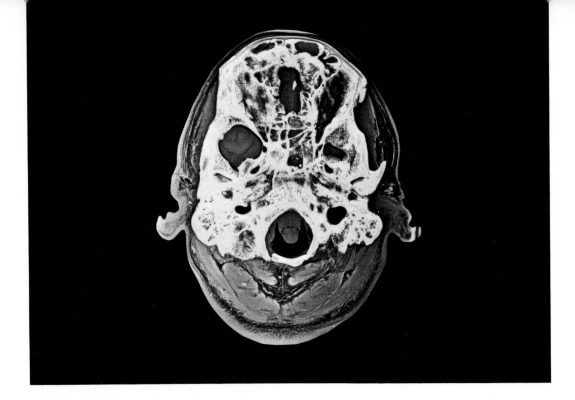

hypophysis, inferiorly to the nose and nasopharynx, and laterally to the cavernous sinuses. Each opens into the sphenoethmoidal recess.

The maxillary sinus is the largest of the paranasal sinuses and is located in the body of the maxilla. It is inferior to the orbit, anterior to the pterygopalatine and infratemporal fossae, lateral to the nasal cavity, and superior to the molar and premolar teeth. The infraorbital nerve and vessels pass in the roof of the sinus. The sinus opens into the hiatus semilunaris of the middle meatus.

Clinical Considerations

The orbits and their contents will be described more fully in respect to clinical considerations in the sections parallel to Reid's base line rather than in these, which are angulated.

In this section, the nasal air passages, the crista galli, the ethmoid air cells, some sphenoid air cells, and more of the medulla oblongata, as well as the base of the skull, come into view. The close relationship of the occipital bone to the lateral aspect of the atlas is likewise clearly demonstrated and is pertinent to injuries in the vicinity that involve the first and second cervical segments in particular. Mass or infectious lesions involving the various paranasal sinuses will produce changes herein; mass lesions involving the base of the skull and traumatic lesions involving the atlas and the brain stem are of particular importance in this section.

SECTION
1–10

Through the external auditory meatus at a 30-degree angle to Reid's base line, 1 cm below the preceding section

Anatomic Considerations

The four pair of paranasal sinuses are the frontal, ethmoidal, sphenoidal, and maxillary. They are air-filled cavities that are produced by evaginations of the mucous membrane of the nose into the adjacent bones. The mucoperiosteum has a ciliated epithelium that is continuous with that of the nasal cavity. All the sinuses open into this cavity.

The frontal sinuses (Section 1–9 to 1–13) are located in the frontal bone near the midline, and their sizes are variable. Each opens in the middle meatus through the infundibulum.

The ethmoidal sinuses (Sections 1–10 and 1–11 and 1–14 to 1–16) consist of numerous air cells forming the ethmoidal labyrinth and are located between the orbit and upper part of the nasal cavity. Each sinus is divided into anterior, middle, and posterior groups. The anterior and middle groups open into the middle meatus by way of the infundibulum and bulla ethmoidalis, respectively. The posterior group opens into the superior meatus.

The sphenoid sinuses are seen in the preceding illustration, in this section, in Section 1–11, and in Sections 1–14 to 1–17. They are located side by side in the body of the sphenoid bone, separated by a septum that is not usually in the midline. Each is related anteriorly to the nasal cavity and ethmoid sinuses, posteriorly to the posterior cranial fossa, superiorly to the

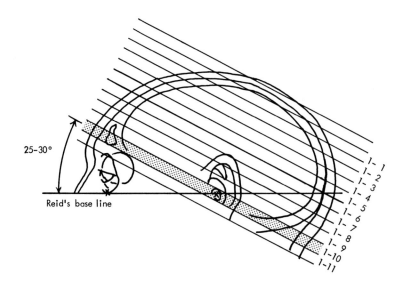

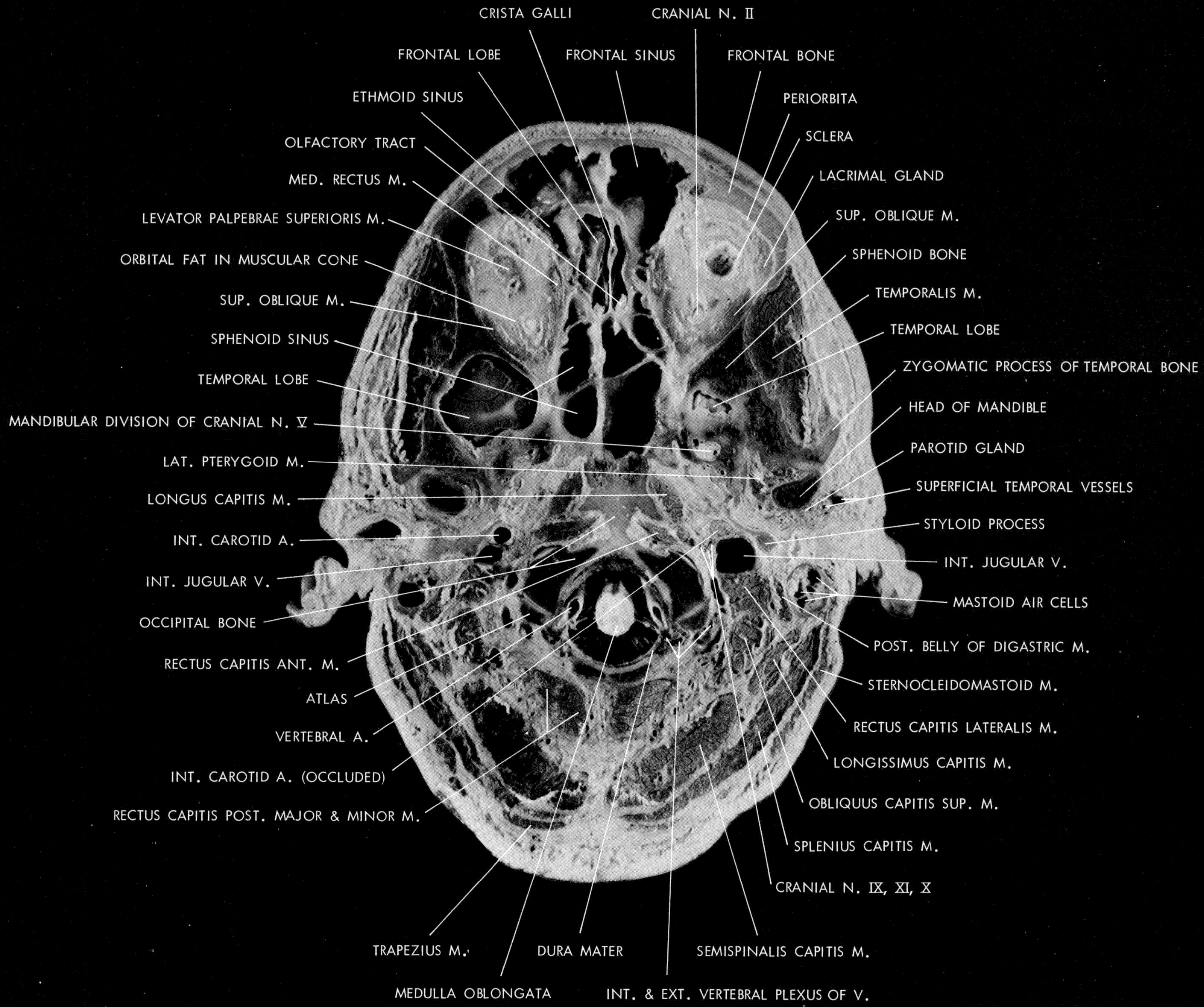

CRISTA GALLI
CRANIAL N. II
FRONTAL LOBE
FRONTAL SINUS
FRONTAL BONE
ETHMOID SINUS
PERIORBITA
OLFACTORY TRACT
SCLERA
MED. RECTUS M.
LACRIMAL GLAND
LEVATOR PALPEBRAE SUPERIORIS M.
SUP. OBLIQUE M.
ORBITAL FAT IN MUSCULAR CONE
SPHENOID BONE
SUP. OBLIQUE M.
TEMPORALIS M.
SPHENOID SINUS
TEMPORAL LOBE
TEMPORAL LOBE
ZYGOMATIC PROCESS OF TEMPORAL BONE
MANDIBULAR DIVISION OF CRANIAL N. V
HEAD OF MANDIBLE
LAT. PTERYGOID M.
PAROTID GLAND
LONGUS CAPITIS M.
SUPERFICIAL TEMPORAL VESSELS
INT. CAROTID A.
STYLOID PROCESS
INT. JUGULAR V.
INT. JUGULAR V.
OCCIPITAL BONE
MASTOID AIR CELLS
RECTUS CAPITIS ANT. M.
POST. BELLY OF DIGASTRIC M.
ATLAS
STERNOCLEIDOMASTOID M.
VERTEBRAL A.
RECTUS CAPITIS LATERALIS M.
INT. CAROTID A. (OCCLUDED)
LONGISSIMUS CAPITIS M.
RECTUS CAPITIS POST. MAJOR & MINOR M.
OBLIQUUS CAPITIS SUP. M.
SPLENIUS CAPITIS M.
CRANIAL N. IX, XI, X
TRAPEZIUS M.
DURA MATER
SEMISPINALIS CAPITIS M.
MEDULLA OBLONGATA
INT. & EXT. VERTEBRAL PLEXUS OF V.

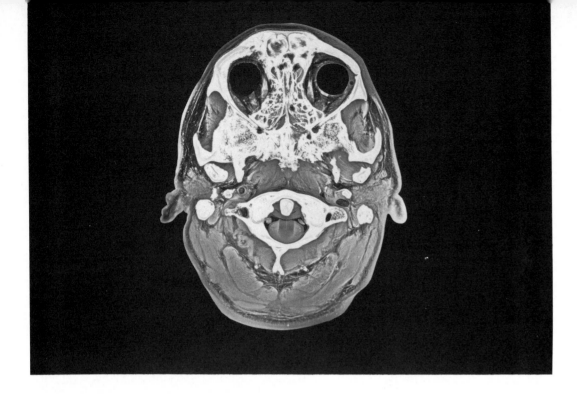

mandible and assists in protrusion of the jaw; acting alternately, the medial pterygoids produce a grinding movement. All of these muscles are innervated by the mandibular branch of the trigeminal nerve. The mandibular nerve can be seen in Sections 1–16 to 1–19.

Clinical Considerations

Apart from previous structures annotated, the dens and its relationship to the atlas are most clearly shown in this section, and it can readily be seen why injuries to the dens will affect the brain stem and spinal cord at this level. The space between the anterior tubercle of the atlas and the dens is measured clinically and should not exceed 3 mm in the adult or 5 mm in the child or an abnormality concerned with either resorption of bone, infection, or trauma must be seriously entertained. This is called the atlanto-tubercular distance.

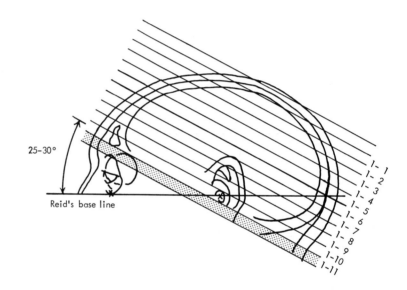

25–30°

Reid's base line

SECTION

1–11

Through the skull, 1 cm below the preceding section

Anatomic Considerations

The four muscles of mastication are the masseter, temporalis, and lateral and medial pterygoid. The masseter is the most superficial of the muscles and can be seen in Sections 1–11 and 1–16 to 1–22. It raises the mandible, and its superficial fibers protract the mandible. The temporalis, because of its large fan-shaped origin, can be observed in Sections 1–5 to 1–19. It raises the mandible, and the horizontal fibers retract it after protraction. The lateral pterygoid is present in Sections 1–10, 1–11, and 1–16 to 1–19. Because of the attachment to the articular disc, the muscles protrude the mandible by moving the head of the mandible and the disc forward. The medial pterygoid is present in this section and in Sections 1–18 to 1–22. It raises the

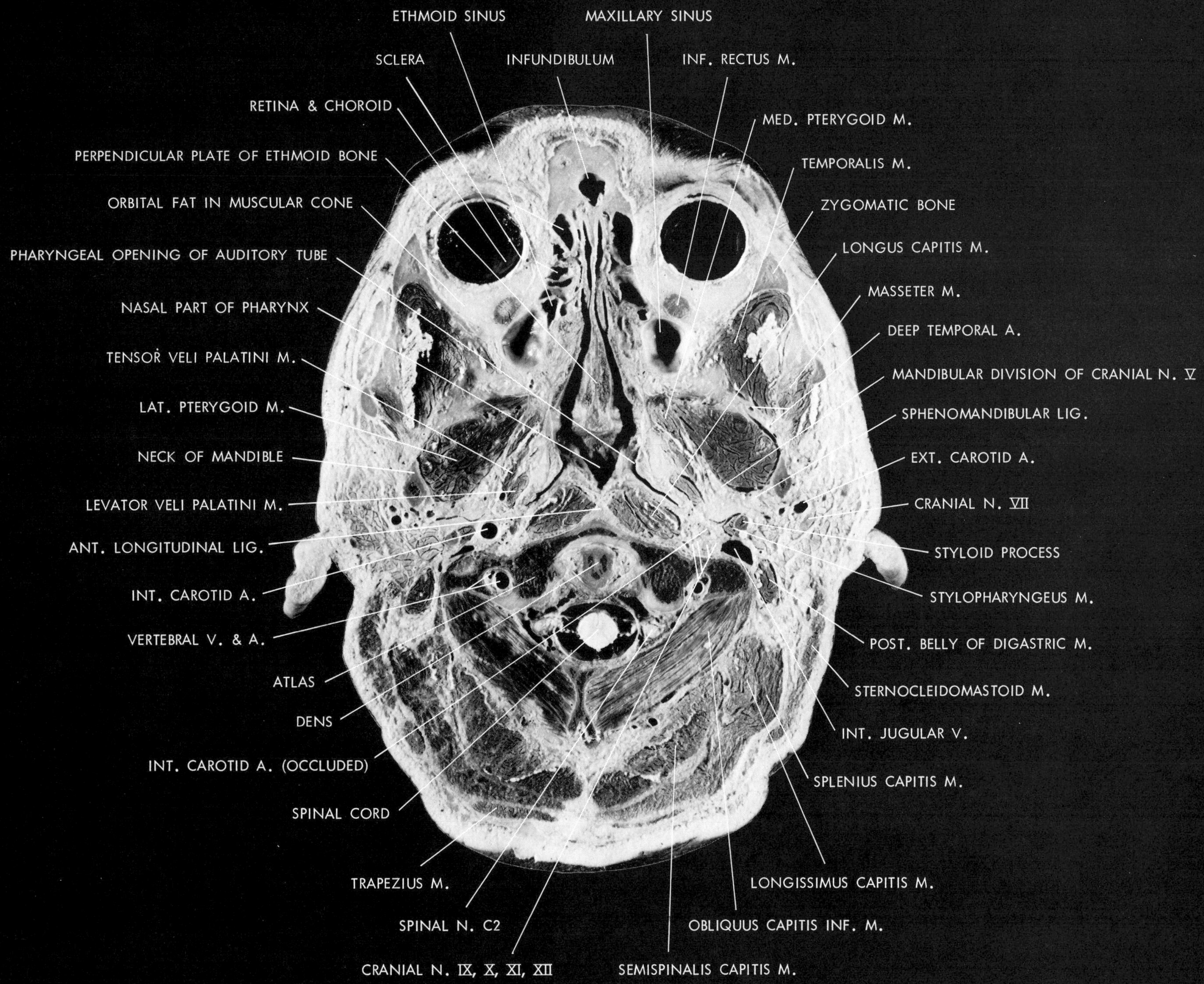

ETHMOID SINUS

MAXILLARY SINUS

SCLERA

INFUNDIBULUM

INF. RECTUS M.

RETINA & CHOROID

MED. PTERYGOID M.

PERPENDICULAR PLATE OF ETHMOID BONE

TEMPORALIS M.

ORBITAL FAT IN MUSCULAR CONE

ZYGOMATIC BONE

PHARYNGEAL OPENING OF AUDITORY TUBE

LONGUS CAPITIS M.

NASAL PART OF PHARYNX

MASSETER M.

TENSOR VELI PALATINI M.

DEEP TEMPORAL A.

MANDIBULAR DIVISION OF CRANIAL N. V

LAT. PTERYGOID M.

SPHENOMANDIBULAR LIG.

NECK OF MANDIBLE

EXT. CAROTID A.

LEVATOR VELI PALATINI M.

CRANIAL N. VII

ANT. LONGITUDINAL LIG.

STYLOID PROCESS

INT. CAROTID A.

STYLOPHARYNGEUS M.

VERTEBRAL V. & A.

POST. BELLY OF DIGASTRIC M.

ATLAS

STERNOCLEIDOMASTOID M.

DENS

INT. JUGULAR V.

INT. CAROTID A. (OCCLUDED)

SPLENIUS CAPITIS M.

SPINAL CORD

TRAPEZIUS M.

LONGISSIMUS CAPITIS M.

SPINAL N. C2

OBLIQUUS CAPITIS INF. M.

CRANIAL N. IX, X, XI, XII

SEMISPINALIS CAPITIS M.

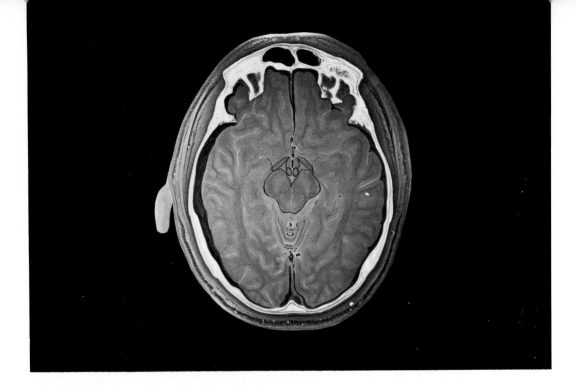

Clinical Considerations

The sections that are taken parallel to Reid's base line, through the orbit and posterior fossa, are those particularly concerned with pathology involving these two major areas, since the prior sections are largely concerned with those of the brain and its contiguous structures.

As indicated in the anatomic description, the bones of the orbit are very thin, and in the so-called "blow-out" fractures there is an increased pressure within the orbit that fractures one or another of these thin bony plates, without necessarily producing a fracture of the infraorbital or supraorbital ridge. It is most frequently, under these circumstances, a fracture involving the thin bone of the ethmoids or the floor of the orbit. Free air may enter the orbit from the ethmoids, or the globe of the eye may become depressed downward to the region of the maxillary antrum, producing double vision. If injuries to these areas are not promptly corrected, these visual disturbances may persist and plastic repair of these healed injuries may become a major surgical problem.

In these views, which are parallel to Reid's base line, it will be noted that one obtains another perspective of the third ventricle, the interpeduncular cistern, the midbrain, the superior cistern, a small portion of the cerebellum, and the occipital lobes.

All of these visualizations have clinical bearing, as has been previously described, but this additional perspective reinforces a clinical opinion.

SECTION
1–12

Through the superior margin of the orbit at a plane parallel to and 2.5 cm above Reid's base line

Anatomic Considerations

Portions of the bony orbits and the structures contained therein can be seen in this illustration and through section 1–17. Each orbit is a pyramid-shaped space with four walls and an apex. As can be seen in the illustrations, the medial walls of the two orbits are nearly parallel to each other, with the ethmoidal air cells and sphenoid sinuses occupying the area between these walls. The lateral walls diverge at 45-degree angles from the medial walls and are therefore oriented at a 90 degree angle to each other. As can be visualized in Section 1–14, if the lateral walls of the orbital cavities were projected posteriorly, they would intersect close to the region of the pituitary gland. The bones that compose the walls of the orbit are quite thin in this region of the skull (especially the medial wall); however, the margins of the orbital aperture are strong. The superior margin (shown in this illustration) and the upper portions of the medial and lateral margins are formed by the frontal bone. The zygomatic bone forms the rest of the lateral margin and most of the inferior one. The maxilla forms the inferomedial angle of the orbital margin.

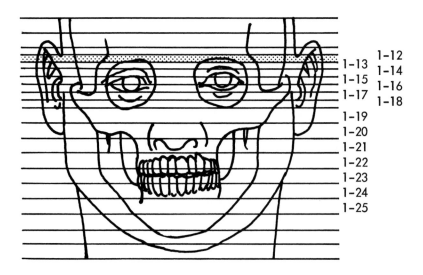

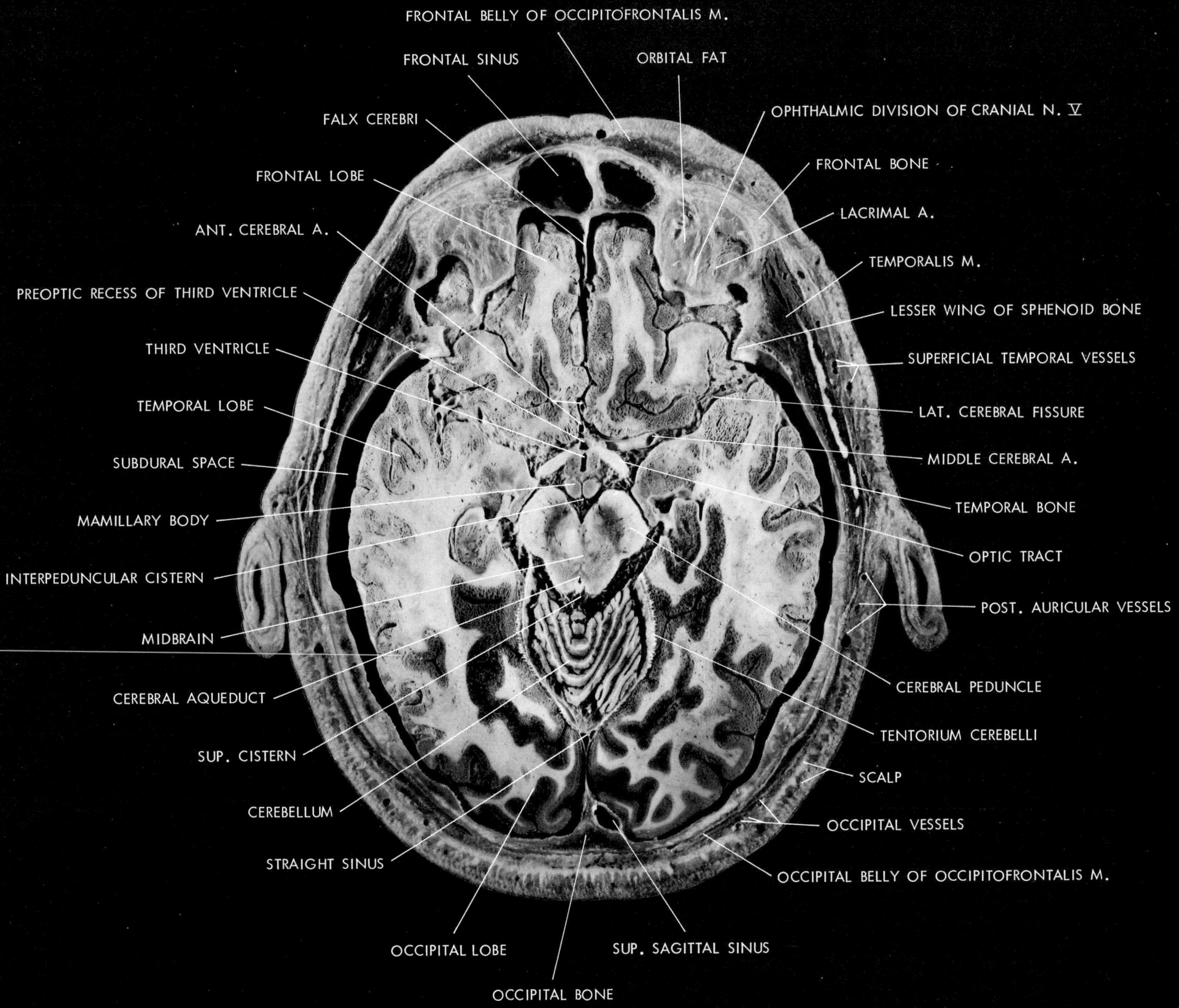

FRONTAL BELLY OF OCCIPITOFRONTALIS M.

FRONTAL SINUS

ORBITAL FAT

FALX CEREBRI

OPHTHALMIC DIVISION OF CRANIAL N. V

FRONTAL LOBE

FRONTAL BONE

ANT. CEREBRAL A.

LACRIMAL A.

PREOPTIC RECESS OF THIRD VENTRICLE

TEMPORALIS M.

LESSER WING OF SPHENOID BONE

THIRD VENTRICLE

SUPERFICIAL TEMPORAL VESSELS

TEMPORAL LOBE

LAT. CEREBRAL FISSURE

SUBDURAL SPACE

MIDDLE CEREBRAL A.

MAMILLARY BODY

TEMPORAL BONE

INTERPEDUNCULAR CISTERN

OPTIC TRACT

MIDBRAIN

POST. AURICULAR VESSELS

CEREBRAL AQUEDUCT

CEREBRAL PEDUNCLE

SUP. CISTERN

TENTORIUM CEREBELLI

CEREBELLUM

SCALP

STRAIGHT SINUS

OCCIPITAL VESSELS

OCCIPITAL BELLY OF OCCIPITOFRONTALIS M.

OCCIPITAL LOBE

SUP. SAGITTAL SINUS

OCCIPITAL BONE

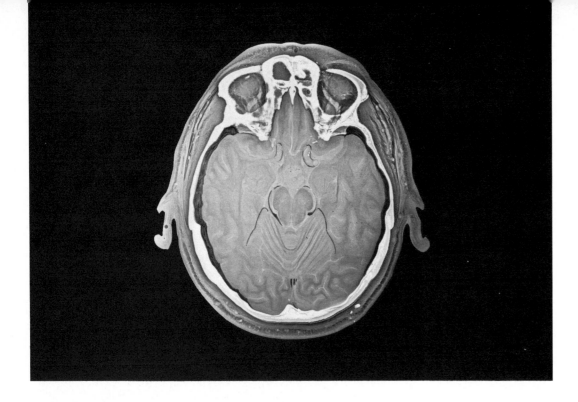

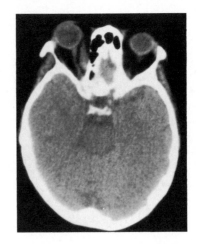

retro-orbital fat is very considerable and allows one to visualize the eyeball and its contents with appreciable clarity because of its very low absorption coefficient. Note that in this section one begins to see the superior oblique muscle and the lacrimal glands of the orbit. In the series of sections that will be shown for the orbit, virtually every muscle, as well as the major arterial supply and nerve content, can be demonstrated; these have very considerable clinical importance.

In this section also one sees the structures adjoining the olfactory apparatus. When a meningioma involves this area, disorders of smell may occur. The additional views of the sellar and parasellar structures, the midbrain, the cerebellum, as well as the occipital lobes, have the same pertinence, as has been previously indicated.

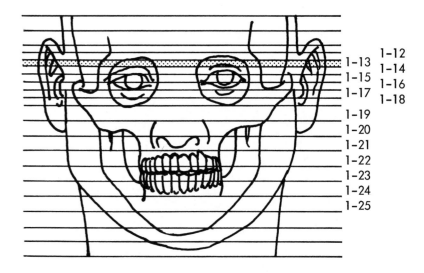

SECTION
1–13

Through the orbit, 0.5 cm below the preceding section

Anatomic Considerations

The superior ophthalmic vein can be seen in this section. This vein communicates anteriorly with the angular vein, which is a tributary of the facial vein. The superior ophthalmic vein has a course similar to that of the ophthalmic artery and receives tributaries that correspond to the branches of the artery. The superior ophthalmic vein ends in the cavernous sinus. The orbit thus serves as a pathway in connecting veins on the anterior aspect of the face with the dural sinuses.

Most of the eyeball can be seen in this illustration and in the next one. These sections show that the eyeball occupies only a portion of the orbit, being limited to the anterior half. An abundant amount of orbital fat is present posterior to the eyeball.

Clinical Considerations

The CT scan shows the orbits of a patient who had thyrotoxicosis. Note the thickened medial rectus muscle (arrow) and right orbital proptosis. There is mild thickening of the left lateral rectus muscle. (Courtesy of Dr. George Flouty and Dr. Sadek Hilal).

This cadaveric section is particularly helpful in demonstrating the orbit and more of the midbrain and cerebellum, as well as in presenting the occipital lobes in a perspective different from that previously shown. The

ETHMOID BONE
FRONTAL BELLY OF OCCIPITOFRONTALIS M.
CRISTA GALLI
FRONTAL SINUS
SUP. OBLIQUE M.
ETHMOID SINUS
ETHMOIDAL A.
SCLERA
CONJUNCTIVAL SAC
SUP. OBLIQUE M.
RETINA & CHOROID
LACRIMAL GLAND
LACRIMAL GLAND
SUP. OPHTHALMIC V.
FRONTAL BONE
ORBITAL FAT
SUP. OPHTHALMIC V.
FRONTAL LOBE
TEMPORALIS M.
OLFACTORY TRACT
SPHENOID BONE
ANT. CEREBRAL A.
SUPERFICIAL TEMPORAL VESSELS
MIDDLE CEREBRAL A.
LEVATOR PALPEBRAE SUPERIORIS M.
OPTIC CHIASMA
SQUAMOUS PORTION OF TEMPORAL BONE
INFUNDIBULUM
TEMPORAL LOBE
CRANIAL N. II
SUBDURAL SPACE
POST. AURICULAR VESSELS
POST. COMMUNICATING A.
DORSUM SELLAE
POST. CEREBRAL A.
BASILAR A.
CRANIAL N. III
MIDBRAIN
TENTORIUM CEREBELLI
LEFT TRANSVERSE SINUS
CEREBELLUM
OCCIPITAL VESSELS
OCCIPITAL BELLY OF OCCIPITOFRONTALIS M.
OCCIPITAL LOBE
OCCIPITAL BONE
SCALP
CEREBRAL AQUEDUCT
STRAIGHT SINUS

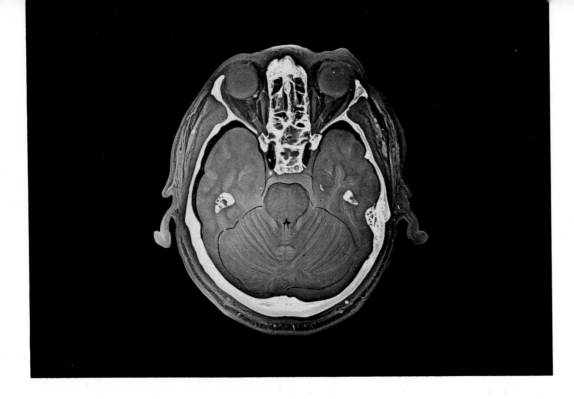

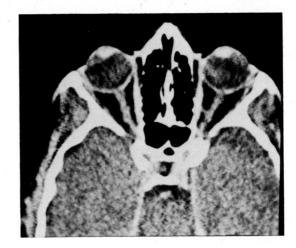

tionships of the lens of the eye to the rest of the eyeball, as well as those of the eyeball to the other orbital structures. Note the excellent visualization of the optic nerve surrounded by the periorbital fat; the lateral rectus muscle and even the sixth cranial nerve are in view, since this section is slightly askew. The medial rectus muscle of the eyeball may be visualized simultaneously with the lateral rectus muscle, as is shown here.

This view is also of some value in demonstrating the pituitary and space-occupying lesions such as small adenomata that become of clinical significance in relation to this great "band-master" of the human endocrine system. The appearance of the pons (as well as the cistern immediately anterior to it) and its relationship to the fourth ventricle are clearly shown herein. These structures are anterior to and somewhat surrounded by the cerebellum and the tentorium cerebelli, as shown. In this view one may visualize the basilar artery and, sometimes, considerable portions of the circle of Willis. At times, the entire circle is visualized on the single section.

SECTION

1–14

Through the orbit, 0.5 cm below the preceding section

Anatomic Considerations

This section passes through the orbital portion of cranial nerve II (optic nerve) as it courses from the retina to the optic canal. Since the optic nerve is really an extension of the central nervous system, it is invested with sheaths from the three meningeal layers. The cranial course of the optic nerves and the optic chiasma can be seen in the preceding section. The optic tracts can be observed in Section 1–12.

Two of the ocular muscles can be seen in this section: the lateral rectus and medial rectus muscles. The superior oblique muscles can be seen in Section 1–13 and the inferior rectus and inferior oblique muscles in Sections 1–15 and 1–17, respectively. (The superior rectus muscle is not shown.) The levator palpebrae superioris raises the eyelid; the recti and oblique muscles move the eyeball. The exclusive function of two of the cranial nerves is to supply two of these ocular muscles: cranial nerve IV (trochlear) innervates the superior oblique muscle, and cranial nerve VI (abducens) innervates the lateral rectus muscle. The other muscles receive their innervation from cranial nerve III (oculomotor).

Clinical Considerations

The CT scan of the orbit shows clearly the optic nerves, extraocular muscles, and the lenses of the eyes (with an increased absorption coefficient). The ophthalmic arteries are crossing both optic nerves. (Courtesy of Dr. George Flouty and Dr. Sadek Hilal.)

In this cadaveric specimen we are fortunate in showing clearly the rela-

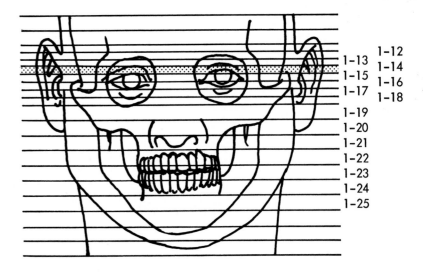

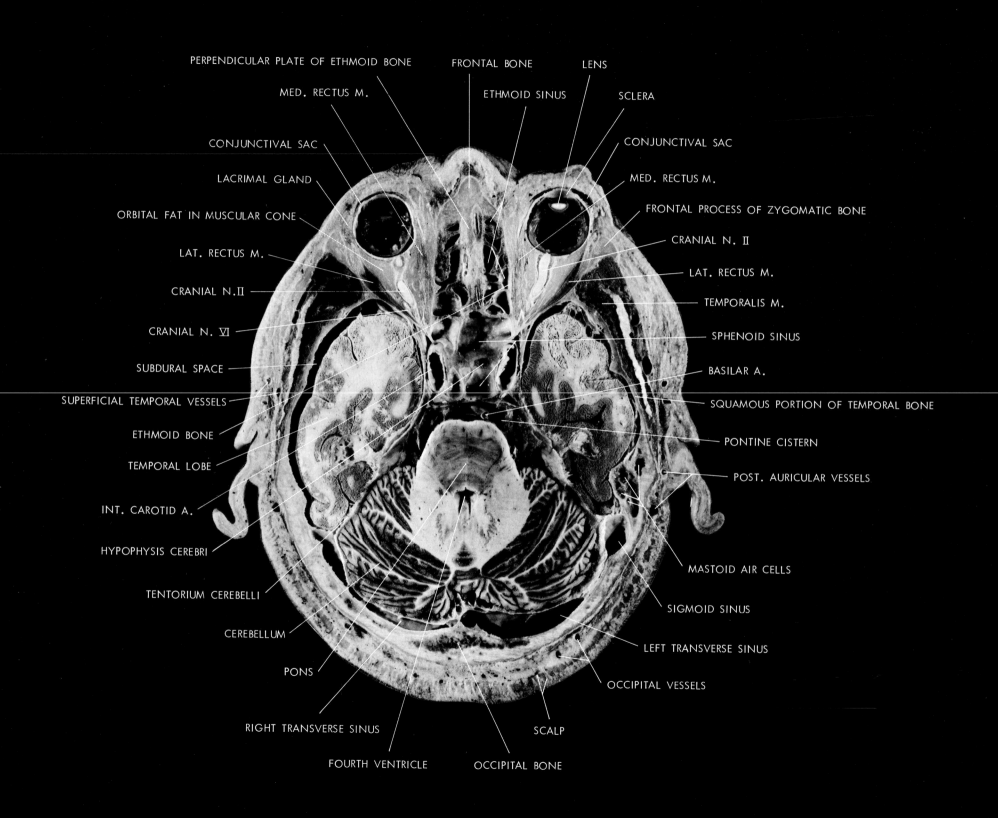

PERPENDICULAR PLATE OF ETHMOID BONE

MED. RECTUS M.

CONJUNCTIVAL SAC

LACRIMAL GLAND

ORBITAL FAT IN MUSCULAR CONE

LAT. RECTUS M.

CRANIAL N. II

CRANIAL N. VI

SUBDURAL SPACE

SUPERFICIAL TEMPORAL VESSELS

ETHMOID BONE

TEMPORAL LOBE

INT. CAROTID A.

HYPOPHYSIS CEREBRI

TENTORIUM CEREBELLI

CEREBELLUM

PONS

RIGHT TRANSVERSE SINUS

FOURTH VENTRICLE

FRONTAL BONE

ETHMOID SINUS

LENS

SCLERA

CONJUNCTIVAL SAC

MED. RECTUS M.

FRONTAL PROCESS OF ZYGOMATIC BONE

CRANIAL N. II

LAT. RECTUS M.

TEMPORALIS M.

SPHENOID SINUS

BASILAR A.

SQUAMOUS PORTION OF TEMPORAL BONE

PONTINE CISTERN

POST. AURICULAR VESSELS

MASTOID AIR CELLS

SIGMOID SINUS

LEFT TRANSVERSE SINUS

OCCIPITAL VESSELS

SCALP

OCCIPITAL BONE

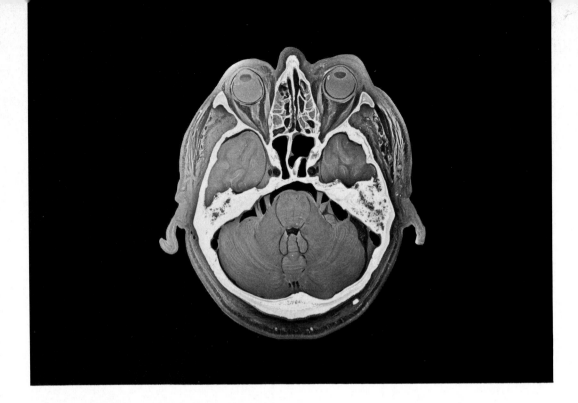

auditory meatus. After entering the skull, the facial nerve travels in the facial canal within the petrous portion of the temporal bone. The facial nerve exits the skull at the stylomastoid foramen (Section 1–18).

Clinical Considerations

Much that has been said about the previous section applies here with further visualization of the periocular muscular structures, the orbital fat, and the paranasal sinuses and with greater detail in respect to the pons and the cerebellum.

One obtains another perspective of the mastoid air cells and contiguous structures, such as the fifth and the seventh cranial nerves. Comments previously made regarding the petrous portion of the temporal bone have application herein as well.

It should be noted that this view is particularly good for demonstrating the very tip of the temporal lobe, which is difficult to visualize under ordinary circumstances in other perspectives.

With contrast enhancement, an excellent visualization of the internal carotid arteries may be obtained just anterior and lateral to the basilar artery. The demonstrations of calcium plaques in these vascular structures are very important with respect to vascular insufficiency of the brain.

SECTION
1–15

Through the orbit, 0.5 cm below the preceding section

Anatomic Considerations

Portions of both cranial nerve V (trigeminal) and cranial nerve VII (facial) can be seen in this illustration. The trigeminal nerve is the major sensory nerve of the face; it innervates the structures that are derived from the first branchial (pharyngeal) arch. The facial nerve supplies the structures of the second branchial arch; it therefore innervates all of the muscles of facial expression. As is indicated by its name, the trigeminal nerve has three components. The ophthalmic division, which can be seen in Section 1–12, is exclusively sensory, as is the maxillary division, which can be observed in the following illustration. The mandibular division of the trigeminal nerve, however, is both sensory and motor; this division can be seen in Section 1–16. The mandibular division is motor to the muscles of mastication and to the other muscles (anterior belly of the digastric, mylohyoid, tensor tympani, and tensor veli palatini) that are also derived from the first branchial arch.

Both the seventh and eighth (vestibulocochlear) cranial nerves exit the cranial cavity *via* the internal auditory meatus. Here, on the specimen's left, the plane of section passed between these two nerves at the internal

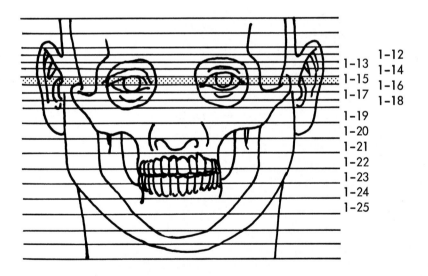

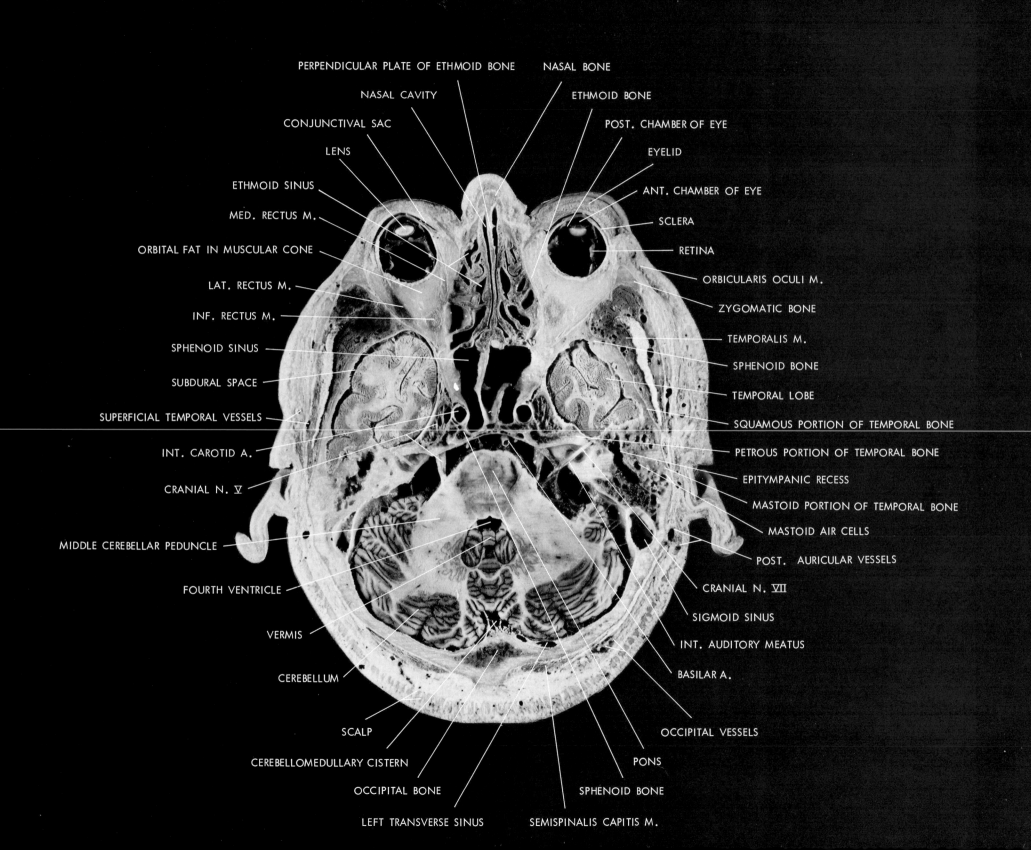

PERPENDICULAR PLATE OF ETHMOID BONE

NASAL BONE

NASAL CAVITY

ETHMOID BONE

CONJUNCTIVAL SAC

POST. CHAMBER OF EYE

LENS

EYELID

ETHMOID SINUS

ANT. CHAMBER OF EYE

MED. RECTUS M.

SCLERA

ORBITAL FAT IN MUSCULAR CONE

RETINA

LAT. RECTUS M.

ORBICULARIS OCULI M.

INF. RECTUS M.

ZYGOMATIC BONE

SPHENOID SINUS

TEMPORALIS M.

SUBDURAL SPACE

SPHENOID BONE

SUPERFICIAL TEMPORAL VESSELS

TEMPORAL LOBE

INT. CAROTID A.

SQUAMOUS PORTION OF TEMPORAL BONE

CRANIAL N. V

PETROUS PORTION OF TEMPORAL BONE

EPITYMPANIC RECESS

MIDDLE CEREBELLAR PEDUNCLE

MASTOID PORTION OF TEMPORAL BONE

MASTOID AIR CELLS

FOURTH VENTRICLE

POST. AURICULAR VESSELS

VERMIS

CRANIAL N. VII

SIGMOID SINUS

CEREBELLUM

INT. AUDITORY MEATUS

BASILAR A.

SCALP

OCCIPITAL VESSELS

CEREBELLOMEDULLARY CISTERN

PONS

OCCIPITAL BONE

SPHENOID BONE

LEFT TRANSVERSE SINUS

SEMISPINALIS CAPITIS M.

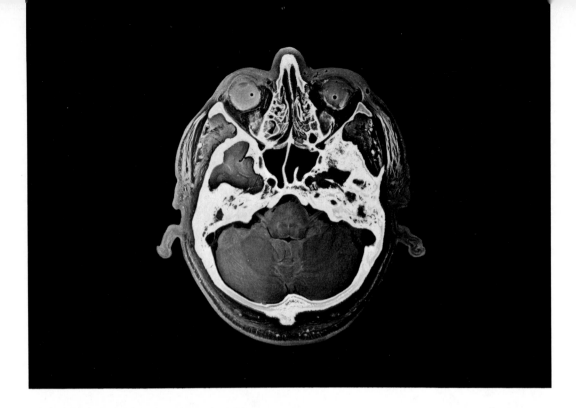

position of the internal carotid artery in this illustration should be compared with its positions in Sections 1–15 and 1–17.

Clinical Considerations

Much that has already been implicated in respect to the orbit applies to this section. Obtaining the sections at 0.4- or 0.5-cm intervals in computed tomography allows one to visualize virtually every anatomic component of the orbit.

The different perspective of the posterior fossa and the adjoining midbrain or pontine structures likewise has very considerable pertinence. These, then, in summary, are the main values that may be attributed to these special views, which are obtained parallel to Reid's base line in this small volume of the head.

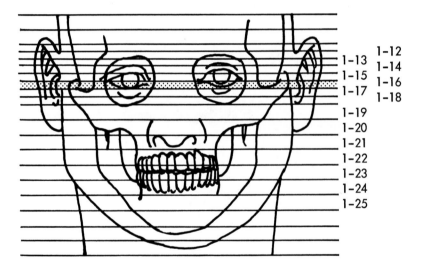

SECTION
1–16

Through the orbit, 0.5 cm below the preceding section

Anatomic Considerations

The common carotid artery (Section 1–25) bifurcates to form the external and internal carotid arteries (Section 1–24). The entire course of the internal carotid artery can be followed by progressing from its origin (Section 1–24) through to where it participates in the formation of the circle of Willis (Section 1–13). At the level shown here, the internal carotid artery is seen entering the cranial cavity. As the internal carotid artery reaches the petrous part of the temporal bone, it enters the carotid canal and then curves to run horizontally, medially, and anteriorly towards the foramen lacerum. The artery then courses superiorly to enter the middle cranial fossa. The

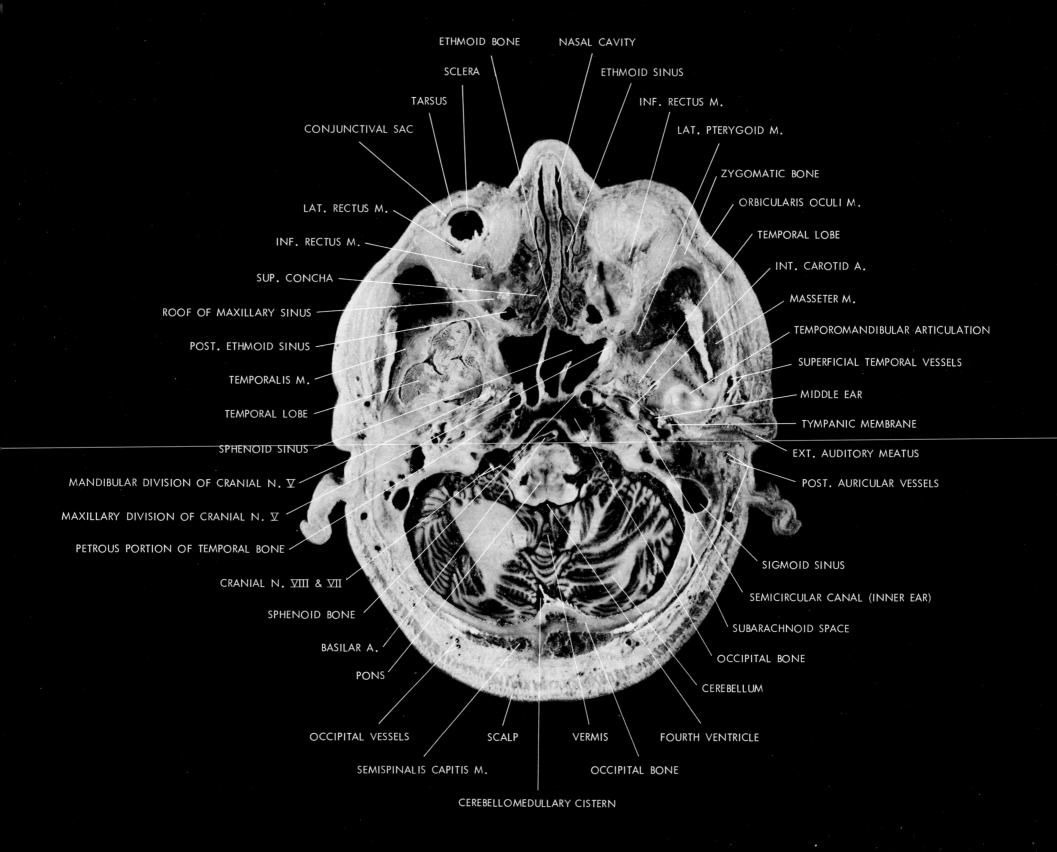

ETHMOID BONE
NASAL CAVITY
SCLERA
ETHMOID SINUS
TARSUS
INF. RECTUS M.
CONJUNCTIVAL SAC
LAT. PTERYGOID M.
ZYGOMATIC BONE
ORBICULARIS OCULI M.
LAT. RECTUS M.
TEMPORAL LOBE
INF. RECTUS M.
INT. CAROTID A.
SUP. CONCHA
MASSETER M.
ROOF OF MAXILLARY SINUS
TEMPOROMANDIBULAR ARTICULATION
POST. ETHMOID SINUS
SUPERFICIAL TEMPORAL VESSELS
TEMPORALIS M.
MIDDLE EAR
TEMPORAL LOBE
TYMPANIC MEMBRANE
SPHENOID SINUS
EXT. AUDITORY MEATUS
MANDIBULAR DIVISION OF CRANIAL N. V
POST. AURICULAR VESSELS
MAXILLARY DIVISION OF CRANIAL N. V
PETROUS PORTION OF TEMPORAL BONE
SIGMOID SINUS
CRANIAL N. VIII & VII
SEMICIRCULAR CANAL (INNER EAR)
SPHENOID BONE
SUBARACHNOID SPACE
BASILAR A.
OCCIPITAL BONE
PONS
CEREBELLUM
OCCIPITAL VESSELS
VERMIS
FOURTH VENTRICLE
SCALP
SEMISPINALIS CAPITIS M.
OCCIPITAL BONE
CEREBELLOMEDULLARY CISTERN

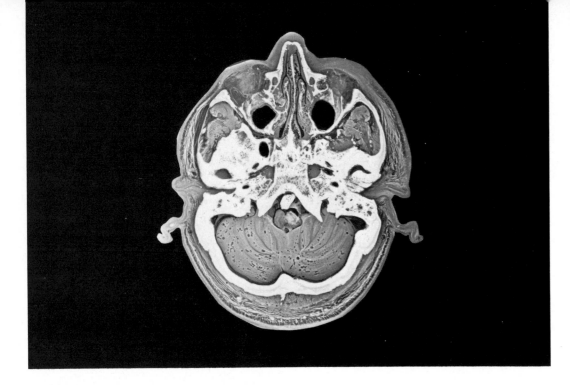

tween the articular disc and temporal bone in the upper compartment of the joint.

Clinical Considerations

This section is virtually the lowermost section of the orbit and, as shown here, allows a minimal visualization of the inferior oblique muscle of the eyeball and the orbicularis oculi muscle.

The maxillary antra are becoming visible, and with them a final visualization of the medulla oblongata and the cerebellar hemispheres. Note the roof of the jugular foramen, which is often extremely difficult to visualize by conventional roentgen means.

The external auditory meatus and the auditory canal are partly visible in this section.

With carotid enhancement, the more lateral placement of the internal carotid arteries is apparent.

At times, it is extremely difficult to obtain detailed concepts regarding the temporomandibular joint by conventional radiography; in this section, however, the intricacies of this double-chambered joint are readily apparent.

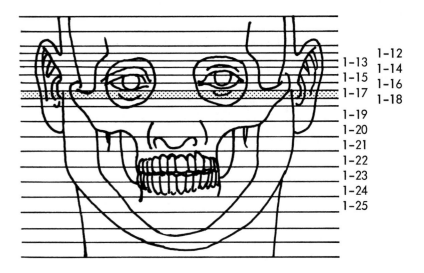

SECTION
1-17

Through Reid's base line, 0.5 cm below the preceding section

Anatomic Considerations

In this illustration and the one preceding, portions of the temporomandibular joint can be observed. The bones involved consist of the head of the mandible articulating with the mandibular fossa and the articular tubercle of the temporal bone. The articular cavity is divided into two synovial joints by the articular disc. The capsule of the joint is attached above to the circumference of the mandibular fossa and the articular tubercle and below to the neck of the mandible. The articular disc is attached to the inner aspect of the capsule. The capsule is strengthened laterally by the lateral ligament. Two separate accessory ligaments, the sphenomandibular and the stylomandibular, are located medially. The morphology of the articulating surfaces allows a hinge-type movement between the articular disc and the mandibular condyle in the lower compartment of the joint and a gliding action be-

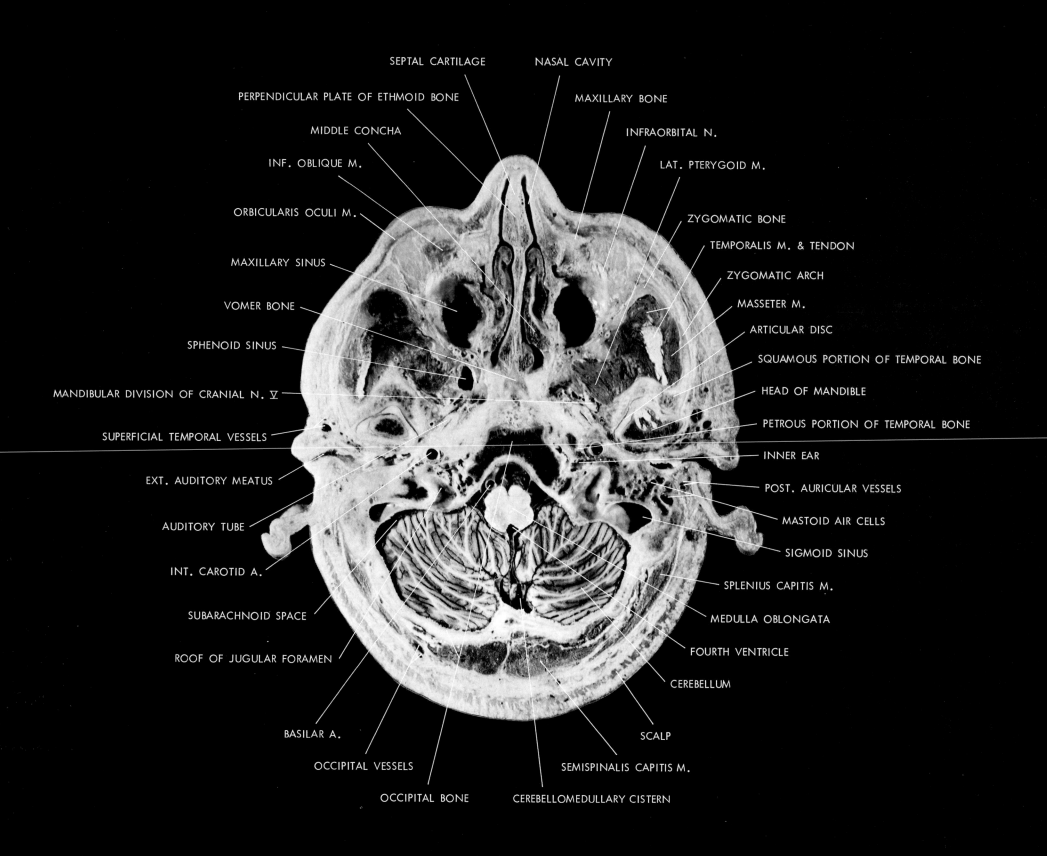

SEPTAL CARTILAGE

NASAL CAVITY

PERPENDICULAR PLATE OF ETHMOID BONE

MAXILLARY BONE

MIDDLE CONCHA

INFRAORBITAL N.

INF. OBLIQUE M.

LAT. PTERYGOID M.

ORBICULARIS OCULI M.

ZYGOMATIC BONE

TEMPORALIS M. & TENDON

MAXILLARY SINUS

ZYGOMATIC ARCH

VOMER BONE

MASSETER M.

ARTICULAR DISC

SPHENOID SINUS

SQUAMOUS PORTION OF TEMPORAL BONE

MANDIBULAR DIVISION OF CRANIAL N. V

HEAD OF MANDIBLE

PETROUS PORTION OF TEMPORAL BONE

SUPERFICIAL TEMPORAL VESSELS

INNER EAR

POST. AURICULAR VESSELS

EXT. AUDITORY MEATUS

MASTOID AIR CELLS

AUDITORY TUBE

SIGMOID SINUS

INT. CAROTID A.

SPLENIUS CAPITIS M.

SUBARACHNOID SPACE

MEDULLA OBLONGATA

ROOF OF JUGULAR FORAMEN

FOURTH VENTRICLE

CEREBELLUM

BASILAR A.

SCALP

OCCIPITAL VESSELS

SEMISPINALIS CAPITIS M.

OCCIPITAL BONE

CEREBELLOMEDULLARY CISTERN

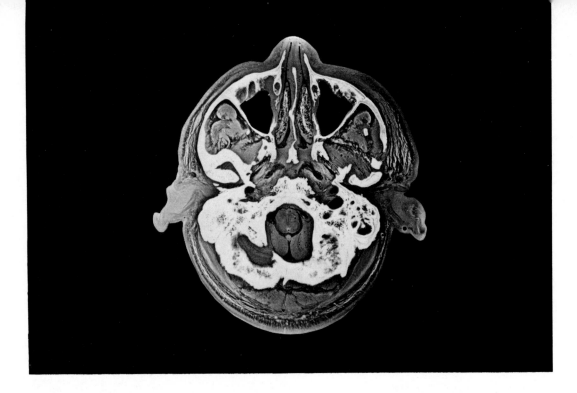

Clinical Considerations

In this section, as well as in Section 1–19, the nasal cavities are in excellent view. The bony and cartilaginous nasal septa are readily seen and would help significantly in the corroboration of pathologic changes affecting nasal cavities, which may be seen by conventional radiography. These would include (1) foreign bodies (rhinoliths); (2) bony and cartilaginous destruction such as might be caused by a caseous condition known as "rhinitis caseosa"; and (3) midline granulomatous lesions involving these areas, such as (a) Wegener's necrotizing granulomatosis; (b) tuberculosis; and, more rarely at this point, (c) syphilis.

Among the noninflammatory lesions involving the nasal cavities are (1) hypertrophy of the turbinate bones; (2) polypi; (3) sarcoid; (4) dermoid cyst; and (5) encephalomeningoceles, which may be transmitted from the cranial cavity *via* the sphenoid, ethmoid, or spheno-orbital route.

Papillomas and angiomas, as well as malignant tumors, may also involve these areas of the nasal cavity.

Even fractures are sometimes very difficult to delineate on conventional radiography, and these too can be either diagnosed primarily or corroborated to excellent advantage by the sagittal route.

The parotid gland comes into view here. Although not seen except in small part, it is often involved by highly invasive locally malignant tumors, which may extend in all directions and thus be manifest particularly in relation to the spread of tumors in these axial projections.

SECTION
1–18

Through the skull, 0.5 cm below the preceding section

Anatomic Considerations

As seen in this section and in several of the adjacent illustrations, the nasal cavity extends from the nostrils in front to the choanae behind and is bounded by medial and lateral walls, a roof, and a floor. The components of the medial wall, or nasal septum, can be seen in this section; from anterior to posterior, the nasal septum is formed by the septal cartilage, the perpendicular plate of the ethmoid bone, and the vomer bone. The lateral wall is characterized by the projections of the nasal conchae and their underlying meatuses. The inferior concha, seen in this illustration, is a separate bone. The superior concha (Section 1–16) and middle concha (Section 1–17) are portions of the ethmoid bone.

The relationships of the nasal cavities to surrounding structures are readily apparent in these cross-sections. Superiorly, the nasal cavity is related to the frontal sinus and anterior cranial fossa and the sphenoid sinus and middle cranial fossa. Laterally, the nasal cavity is related to the ethmoid and maxillary sinuses and the orbit.

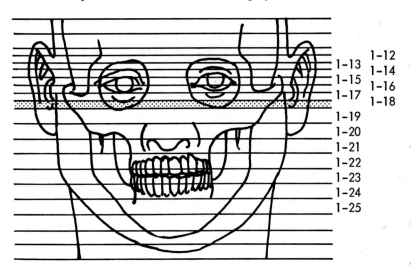

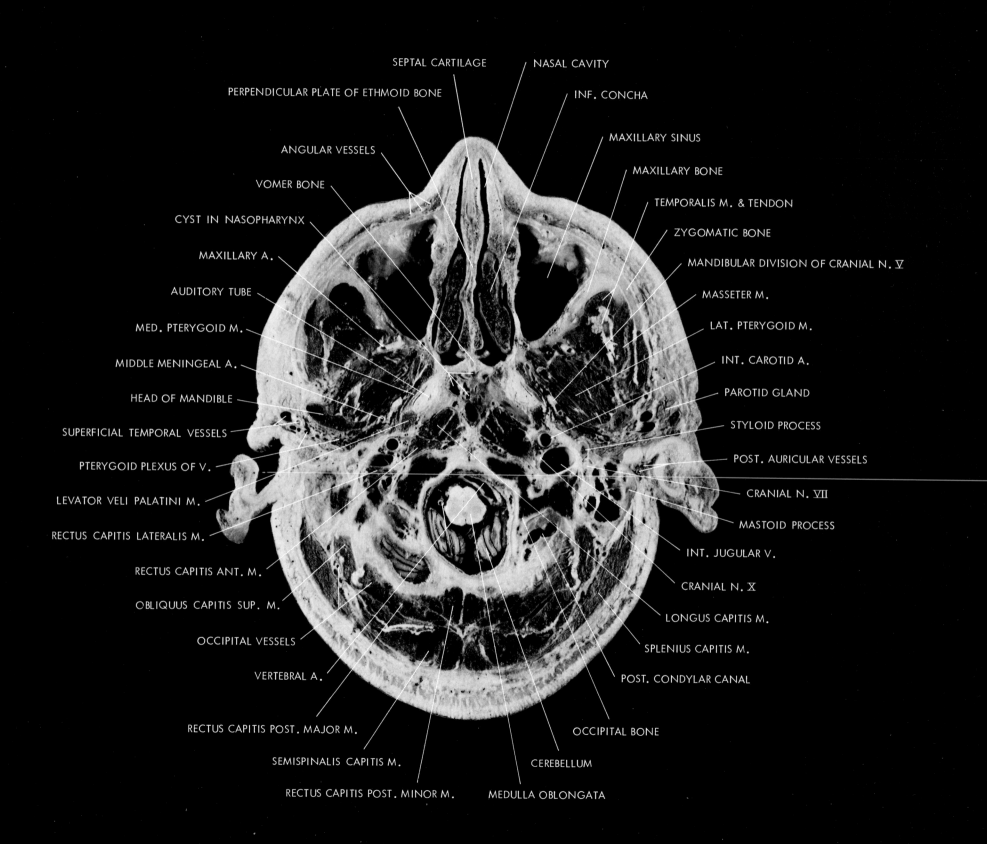

SEPTAL CARTILAGE

NASAL CAVITY

PERPENDICULAR PLATE OF ETHMOID BONE

INF. CONCHA

MAXILLARY SINUS

MAXILLARY BONE

ANGULAR VESSELS

TEMPORALIS M. & TENDON

VOMER BONE

ZYGOMATIC BONE

CYST IN NASOPHARYNX

MANDIBULAR DIVISION OF CRANIAL N. V

MAXILLARY A.

MASSETER M.

AUDITORY TUBE

LAT. PTERYGOID M.

MED. PTERYGOID M.

INT. CAROTID A.

MIDDLE MENINGEAL A.

PAROTID GLAND

HEAD OF MANDIBLE

STYLOID PROCESS

SUPERFICIAL TEMPORAL VESSELS

POST. AURICULAR VESSELS

PTERYGOID PLEXUS OF V.

CRANIAL N. VII

LEVATOR VELI PALATINI M.

MASTOID PROCESS

RECTUS CAPITIS LATERALIS M.

INT. JUGULAR V.

RECTUS CAPITIS ANT. M.

CRANIAL N. X

OBLIQUUS CAPITIS SUP. M.

LONGUS CAPITIS M.

OCCIPITAL VESSELS

SPLENIUS CAPITIS M.

VERTEBRAL A.

POST. CONDYLAR CANAL

RECTUS CAPITIS POST. MAJOR M.

OCCIPITAL BONE

SEMISPINALIS CAPITIS M.

CEREBELLUM

RECTUS CAPITIS POST. MINOR M.

MEDULLA OBLONGATA

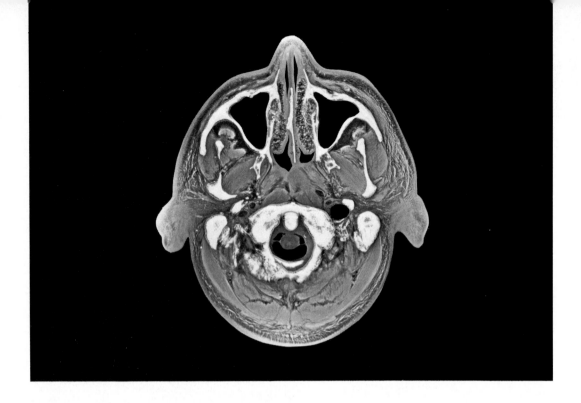

considerably, particularly since attenuation coefficients may vary in several of these lesions, being lesser in mucoceles, for example, than in carcinomata, and thereby be substantiated.

Osteomyelitis may occur in any of the bony walls of the paranasal sinuses; although seen to good advantage in conventional radiography, the full extent of the involvement can be readily distinguished by this means. The so-called "sphenoidal fissure syndrome" (Kretzschmar and Jacot, 1939) represents an osteoperiostitis extending from the sphenoid sinus and ultimately producing pressure upon all of the structures that pass through the sphenoidal fissure.

One cannot overemphasize the importance of the transverse section to an understanding of the full extent of the benign tumors, as well as of the various other cysts and malignant tumors that may involve the paranasal sinuses. Although well demonstrated in conventional radiography, the transverse section is playing an increasing role in planning therapy for, and carrying out cures of, these various lesions. It is not unusual, for example, to have the pterygoid space invaded by a large malignant tumor involving one or the other of the maxillary antra, and this certainly is well demonstrated by the transverse section modality.

Kretzschmar S and Jacot P: Des symptômes précoces et d'une étiologie souvant méconnue du syndrome de la fente sphénoïdale. Schwiz med Schnschr 69:1103–1107, 1939.

SECTION
1-19

Through the atlas and dens, 1 cm below the preceding section

Anatomic Considerations

In this illustration the articulation between the atlas and axis can be observed. The synovial cavities of the pivot joint between the anterior surface of the dens and the anterior arch of the atlas and between the dens and the transverse ligament of the atlas can be seen clearly. Another articulation between the articular processes of the atlas and axis is an arthrodial, or gliding, joint.

Clinical Considerations

Much of the textual material referring to Section 1-18 also pertains to Section 1-19. We will therefore take this opportunity to present some of the inflammatory and allergic states, particularly those affecting the paranasal sinuses and the maxillary antra, that may be verified or more clearly visible in this axial projection. Mucoceles, solitary mucus polyps, retention cysts, and dental cysts all play a part in this area. The diagnosis may be helped

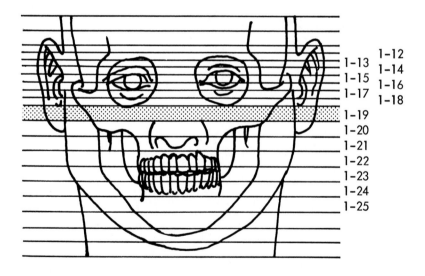

SEPTAL CARTILAGE

PERPENDICULAR PLATE OF ETHMOID BONE

LEVATOR VELI PALATINI M.

INF. CONCHA

VOMER BONE

MAXILLARY BONE

CYST

MAXILLARY SINUS

ANGULAR VESSELS

TENSOR VELI PALATINI M.

NASAL PART OF PHARYNX

BUCCAL FAT PAD

MED. PTERYGOID M.

ZYGOMATIC BONE

CORONOID PROCESS OF MANDIBLE

TEMPORALIS M. & TENDON

LAT. PTERYGOID M.

MASSETER M.

INF. ALVEOLAR A.

STYLOPHARYNGEUS M.

MANDIBULAR DIVISON OF CRANIAL N. V

TRIBUTARY OF SUPERFICIAL TEMPORAL V.

MASSETERIC VESSELS

STYLOID PROCESS

MAXILLARY A.

INT. JUGULAR V.

PAROTID GLAND

CRANIAL N. VII

SUPERFICIAL TEMPORAL A. & V.

POST. BELLY OF DIGASTRIC M.

ANT. LONGITUDINAL LIG.

STERNOCLEIDOMASTOID M.

CRANIAL N. X

MASTOID PROCESS

LONGUS CAPITIS M.

RECTUS CAPITIS LATERALIS M.

OBLIQUUS CAPITIS SUP. M.

LONGISSIMUS CAPITIS M.

DENS

SPLENIUS CAPITIS M.

OCCIPITAL VESSELS

INT. CAROTID A.

SPINAL CORD

VERTEBRAL A.

EXT. VERTEBRAL PLEXUS OF V.

SPINAL N. CI

RECTUS CAPITIS
POST. MAJOR M.

RECTUS CAPITIS
POST. MINOR M.

TRAPEZIUS M.

POST. ARCH OF ATLAS

SEMISPINALIS CAPITIS M.

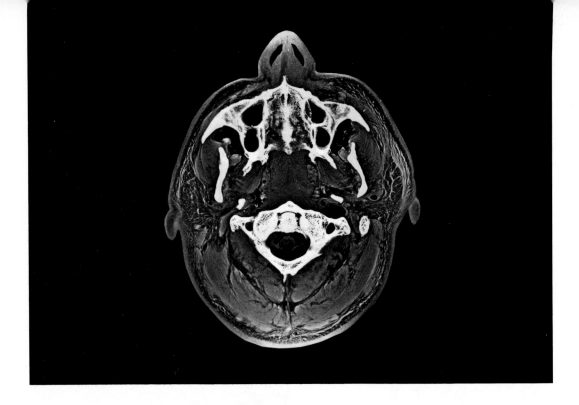

this and adjacent sections, several structures are related to the medial or deep surface of the parotid gland. The posterior belly of the digastric, the muscles that arise from the styloid process, the carotid sheath, and cranial nerves IX through XII are all related to the medial aspect of the parotid gland. The major structures that pass through the substance of the parotid gland are the facial nerve, external carotid artery, and retromandibular vein.

Clinical Considerations

In this section, one notes that the level of the hard palate is shown at the same time as the body of the axis of the second cervical segment. The nasal part of the pharynx becomes visible; this section is thus particularly important for demonstrating invasion from adjoining anatomic areas, such as the sphenoid sinus and sella turcica.

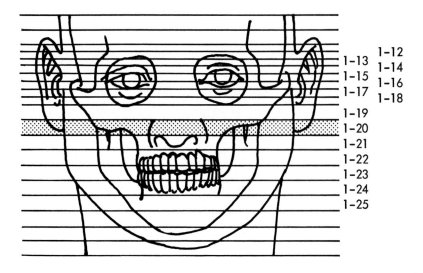

SECTION
1-20

Through the body of C2

Anatomic Considerations

The roof of the mouth is formed by the hard and soft palates, which can be seen in this section. The hard palate is composed of the palatine processes of the maxillary bone anteriorly and the palatine bones posteriorly. The soft palate, which consists of the palatine aponeurosis, muscles, and glands, is attached anteriorly to the posterior aspect of the hard palate and laterally to the wall of the pharynx, as can be seen in the illustration.

The parotid gland, the largest of the salivary glands, can be observed in this section. This gland is located in the depression between the sternocleidomastoid muscle and the ramus of the mandible. As can be seen in

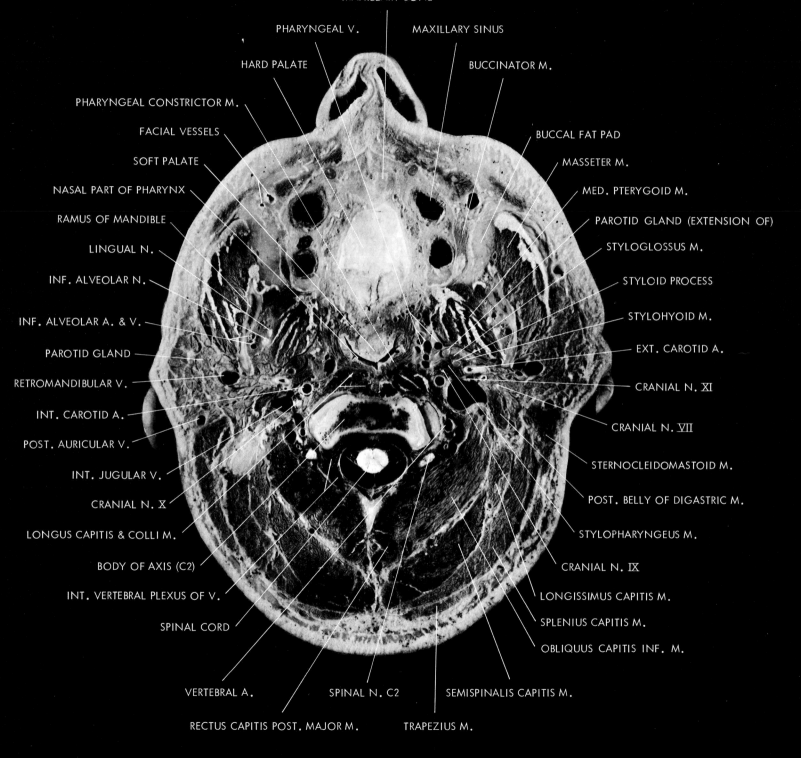

MAXILLARY BONE

PHARYNGEAL V.

MAXILLARY SINUS

HARD PALATE

BUCCINATOR M.

PHARYNGEAL CONSTRICTOR M.

BUCCAL FAT PAD

FACIAL VESSELS

MASSETER M.

SOFT PALATE

MED. PTERYGOID M.

NASAL PART OF PHARYNX

PAROTID GLAND (EXTENSION OF)

RAMUS OF MANDIBLE

STYLOGLOSSUS M.

LINGUAL N.

STYLOID PROCESS

INF. ALVEOLAR N.

STYLOHYOID M.

INF. ALVEOLAR A. & V.

EXT. CAROTID A.

PAROTID GLAND

RETROMANDIBULAR V.

CRANIAL N. XI

INT. CAROTID A.

CRANIAL N. VII

POST. AURICULAR V.

STERNOCLEIDOMASTOID M.

INT. JUGULAR V.

POST. BELLY OF DIGASTRIC M.

CRANIAL N. X

STYLOPHARYNGEUS M.

LONGUS CAPITIS & COLLI M.

CRANIAL N. IX

BODY OF AXIS (C2)

LONGISSIMUS CAPITIS M.

INT. VERTEBRAL PLEXUS OF V.

SPLENIUS CAPITIS M.

SPINAL CORD

OBLIQUUS CAPITIS INF. M.

VERTEBRAL A.

SPINAL N. C2

SEMISPINALIS CAPITIS M.

RECTUS CAPITIS POST. MAJOR M.

TRAPEZIUS M.

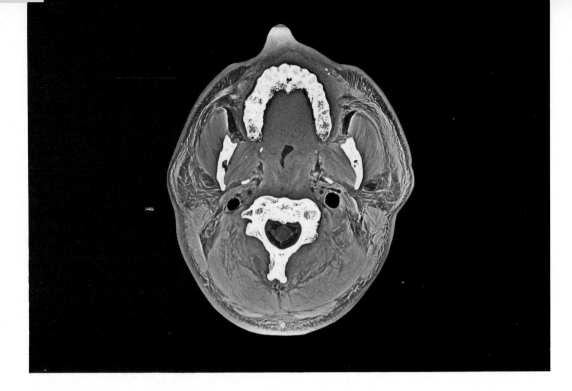

terior and posterior spinal, and posterior inferior cerebellar and medullary arteries in the cranium.

Clinical Considerations

With this section we begin to see the tongue and the oropharynx. Although these areas are readily examined by conventional physical study, this section will be helpful in describing the full extent of inflammation and neoplasia involving this area.

With contrast enhancement, the importance of the relationship of pathology to the large internal carotid arteries, as well as to the jugular veins, also becomes evident.

The parotid gland forms a very significant structure, as seen herein, and extension of neoplasms or inflammatory processes from the parotid gland are of great clinical significance.

SECTION
1-21

Through the body of C3

Anatomic Considerations

The vertebral artery can be observed in Sections 1–18 to 1–28. The vertebral artery arises from the first portion of the subclavian artery and, based on its location, can be divided into four parts. The first part passes to the transverse foramen of the sixth cervical vertebra. The second passes through the transverse foramina of the upper six cervical vertebrae. The third is located in the floor of the suboccipital triangle. The fourth enters the skull through the foramen magnum and at the lower border of the pons joins the vessel of the opposite side to form the basilar artery. The vertebral artery gives off muscular and spinal branches in the neck and gives rise to meningeal, an-

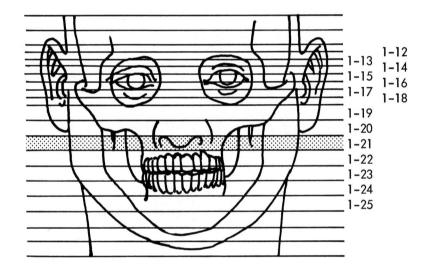

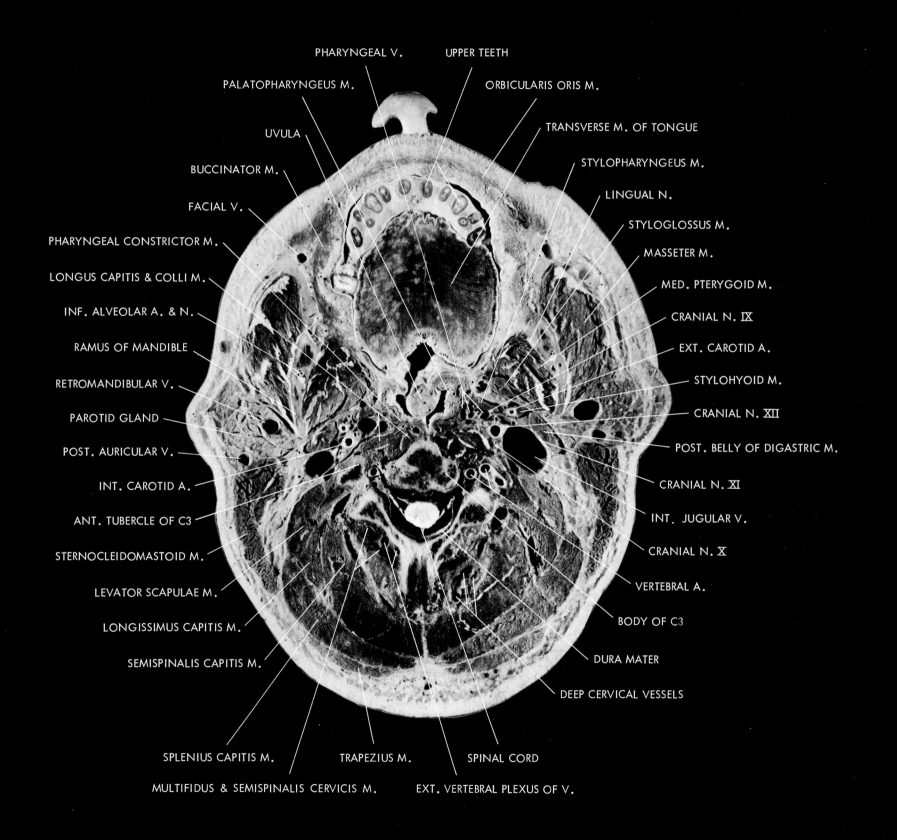

PHARYNGEAL V.   UPPER TEETH

PALATOPHARYNGEUS M.   ORBICULARIS ORIS M.

UVULA   TRANSVERSE M. OF TONGUE

BUCCINATOR M.   STYLOPHARYNGEUS M.

FACIAL V.   LINGUAL N.

PHARYNGEAL CONSTRICTOR M.   STYLOGLOSSUS M.

LONGUS CAPITIS & COLLI M.   MASSETER M.

INF. ALVEOLAR A. & N.   MED. PTERYGOID M.

RAMUS OF MANDIBLE   CRANIAL N. IX

RETROMANDIBULAR V.   EXT. CAROTID A.

PAROTID GLAND   STYLOHYOID M.

POST. AURICULAR V.   CRANIAL N. XII

INT. CAROTID A.   POST. BELLY OF DIGASTRIC M.

ANT. TUBERCLE OF C3   CRANIAL N. XI

STERNOCLEIDOMASTOID M.   INT. JUGULAR V.

LEVATOR SCAPULAE M.   CRANIAL N. X

LONGISSIMUS CAPITIS M.   VERTEBRAL A.

SEMISPINALIS CAPITIS M.   BODY OF C3

DURA MATER

DEEP CERVICAL VESSELS

SPLENIUS CAPITIS M.   TRAPEZIUS M.   SPINAL CORD

MULTIFIDUS & SEMISPINALIS CERVICIS M.   EXT. VERTEBRAL PLEXUS OF V.

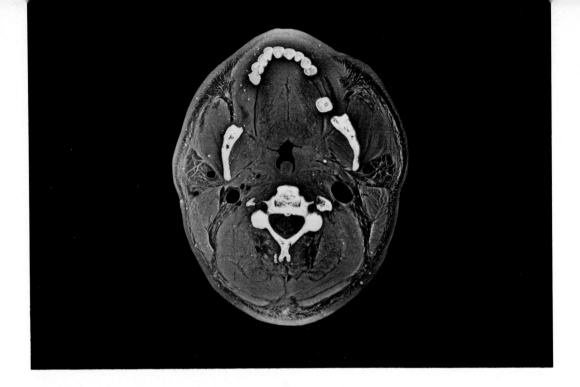

The muscular wall of the pharynx is primarily formed by the three paired constrictor muscles (superior, middle, and inferior). These muscles, which overlap one another, have a major role in constricting the pharynx during swallowing. The arteries to the pharynx are the ascending pharyngeal (from the external carotid) and the ascending palatine (from the facial). The veins form a pharyngeal plexus (in this illustration), which drains into the internal jugular vein and communicates with the pterygoid plexus and cavernous sinus.

Clinical Considerations

Those considerations that have been enumerated for Section 1–21 also have application here. Because of differences in attenuation coefficients, structures such as the ramus of the mandible may be readily differentiated from the muscles and the parotid gland. With contrast enhancement, the internal carotid artery and the blood vessels immediately adjoining it, as well as the jugular vein, likewise become readily apparent.

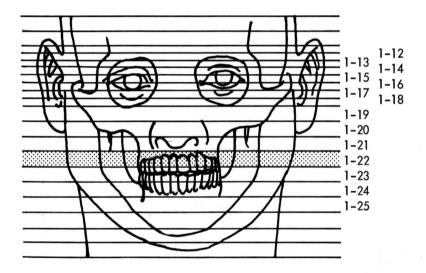

SECTION
1–22

Through the intervertebral disc between C3 and C4

Anatomic Considerations

The pharynx is a muscular tube that extends from the base of the skull to the sixth cervical vertebra, where it becomes continuous with the esophagus. The pharynx is divided into three portions: the nasal (Section 1–19), the oral (in this illustration), and the laryngeal (Section 1–25). The nasal portion is located posterior to the nose and superior to the soft palate. This area always remains patent. The pharyngeal tonsil (adenoids when enlarged) is found in the posterior wall of the nasopharynx, and the termination of the auditory tube is located in the lateral wall. The oral portion of the pharynx extends from the soft palate to the hyoid bone; anteriorly, it communicates with the oral cavity. The laryngeal portion begins at the hyoid bone and extends to the lower border of the cricoid cartilage, where it is continuous with the esophagus.

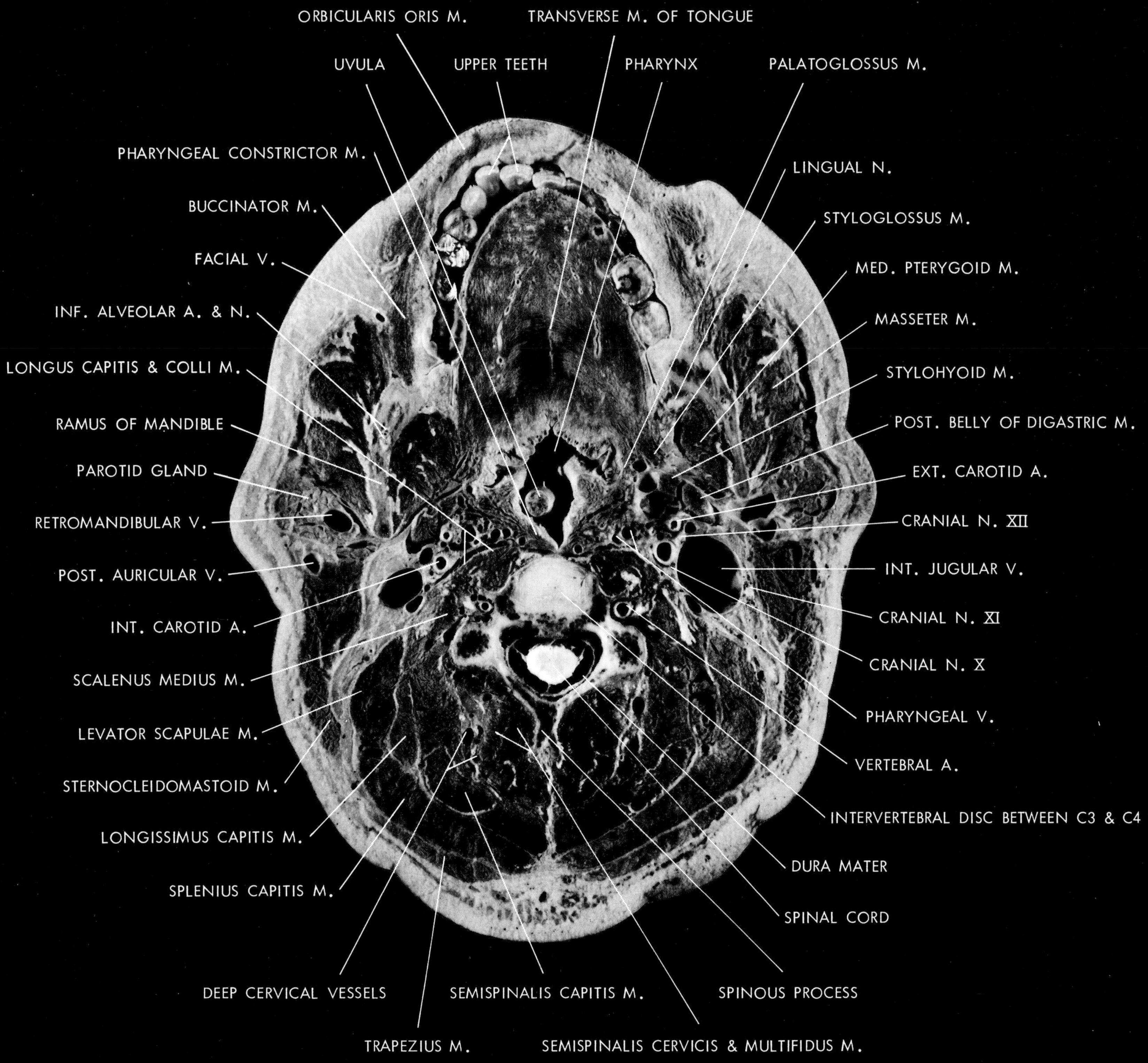

ORBICULARIS ORIS M.　　TRANSVERSE M. OF TONGUE

UVULA　　UPPER TEETH　　PHARYNX　　PALATOGLOSSUS M.

PHARYNGEAL CONSTRICTOR M.

LINGUAL N.

BUCCINATOR M.

STYLOGLOSSUS M.

FACIAL V.

MED. PTERYGOID M.

INF. ALVEOLAR A. & N.

MASSETER M.

LONGUS CAPITIS & COLLI M.

STYLOHYOID M.

RAMUS OF MANDIBLE

POST. BELLY OF DIGASTRIC M.

PAROTID GLAND

EXT. CAROTID A.

RETROMANDIBULAR V.

CRANIAL N. XII

POST. AURICULAR V.

INT. JUGULAR V.

INT. CAROTID A.

CRANIAL N. XI

SCALENUS MEDIUS M.

CRANIAL N. X

LEVATOR SCAPULAE M.

PHARYNGEAL V.

STERNOCLEIDOMASTOID M.

VERTEBRAL A.

LONGISSIMUS CAPITIS M.

INTERVERTEBRAL DISC BETWEEN C3 & C4

SPLENIUS CAPITIS M.

DURA MATER

SPINAL CORD

DEEP CERVICAL VESSELS　　SEMISPINALIS CAPITIS M.　　SPINOUS PROCESS

TRAPEZIUS M.　　SEMISPINALIS CERVICIS & MULTIFIDUS M.

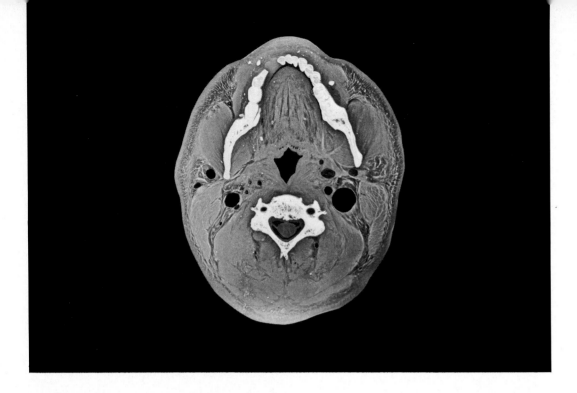

1-20 to 1-23), and palatoglossus (Section 1-22). The nerves to the tongue are the glossopharyngeal, which conveys taste and general sensation to the posterior third of the tongue; the lingual, which is concerned with taste and general sensation to the anterior two thirds of the tongue (the taste fibers carried by the lingual nerve arise from the chorda tympani); and the hypoglossal, which innervates all the muscles of the tongue except the palatoglossus, which is innervated by the cranial portion of the accessory nerve.

Clinical Considerations

Application of computed tomography to cross-sectional anatomy is only beginning to have value in respect to the study of the spinal cord throughout its entire length, but especially the cervical region. The resolution obtainable allows one to distinguish this very important nervous structure as well as its meningeal environment.

The submandibular gland is recognized as almost a direct extension of the mandible posteriorly.

SECTION
1-23

*Through the
body of C4*

Anatomic Considerations

The tongue is first seen in Section 1-21 and continues to Section 1-24. It lies in the floor of the oral cavity, and its posterior portion forms the anterior wall of the oral pharynx. The tongue is covered by a stratified squamous epithelium.

The tongue is divided into two halves by a median fibrous septum; the muscles are divided into two groups: intrinsic and extrinsic. The intrinsic muscles pass in several planes within the tongue and can produce changes in shape. The extrinisic muscles originate outside of the tongue and are responsible for its movements. The extrinsic muscles are the genioglossus (Sections 1-23 and 1-24), hyoglossus (Section 1-24), styloglossus (Sections

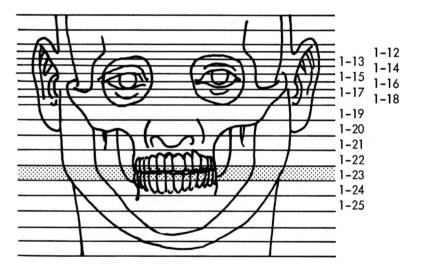

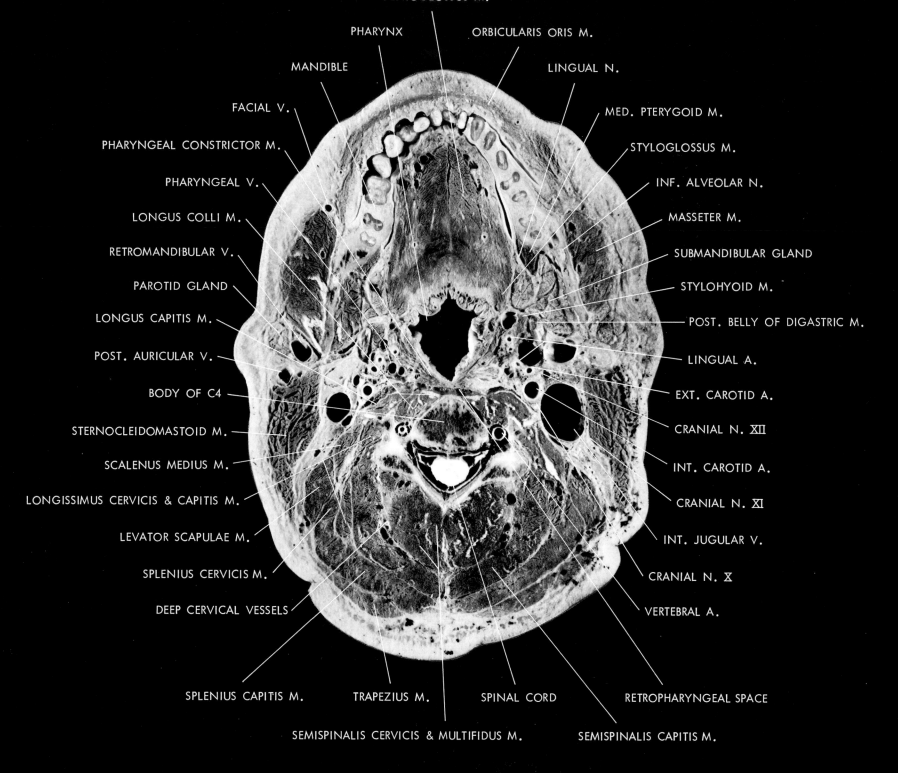

GENIOGLOSSUS M.

PHARYNX

ORBICULARIS ORIS M.

MANDIBLE

LINGUAL N.

FACIAL V.

MED. PTERYGOID M.

PHARYNGEAL CONSTRICTOR M.

STYLOGLOSSUS M.

PHARYNGEAL V.

INF. ALVEOLAR N.

LONGUS COLLI M.

MASSETER M.

RETROMANDIBULAR V.

SUBMANDIBULAR GLAND

PAROTID GLAND

STYLOHYOID M.

LONGUS CAPITIS M.

POST. BELLY OF DIGASTRIC M.

POST. AURICULAR V.

LINGUAL A.

BODY OF C4

EXT. CAROTID A.

STERNOCLEIDOMASTOID M.

CRANIAL N. XII

SCALENUS MEDIUS M.

INT. CAROTID A.

LONGISSIMUS CERVICIS & CAPITIS M.

CRANIAL N. XI

LEVATOR SCAPULAE M.

INT. JUGULAR V.

SPLENIUS CERVICIS M.

CRANIAL N. X

DEEP CERVICAL VESSELS

VERTEBRAL A.

SPLENIUS CAPITIS M.

TRAPEZIUS M.

SPINAL CORD

RETROPHARYNGEAL SPACE

SEMISPINALIS CERVICIS & MULTIFIDUS M.

SEMISPINALIS CAPITIS M.

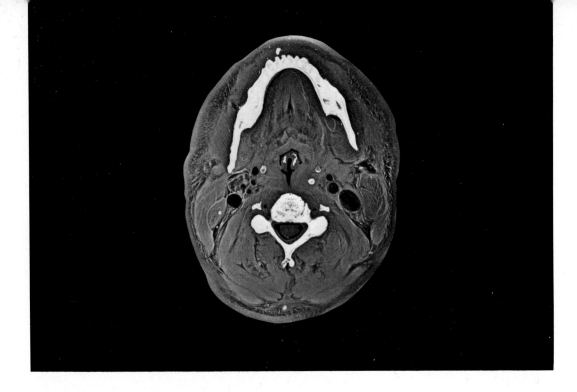

the external carotid has numerous ones. Most of these can be observed in the adjacent illustrations. The external carotid artery terminates in the substance of the parotid gland by dividing into the superficial temporal and maxillary arteries (Section 1–19).

Clinical Considerations

In this section the epiglottis comes into view. It is one of the paralaryngeal structures so often involved by laryngeal tumors, and extension onto the epiglottis is not at all infrequent.

As the mandible becomes less distinct, the submandibular gland, in a location previously identified, becomes even more readily apparent.

With contrast enhancement, the large blood vessels immediately lateral to the projection of the epiglottis can be identified with considerable clarity. It is noteworthy that the internal carotid artery lies medial to the internal jugular vein.

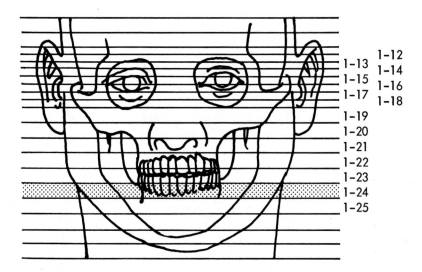

SECTION
1–24

Through the intervertebral disc between C4 and C5

Anatomic Considerations

The proximal or inferior portions of the external and internal carotid arteries can be seen in this section. Both right and left common carotid arteries bifurcate within the substance of the following section. The bifurcation of the common carotid artery usually occurs at the upper end of the thyroid cartilage or at the level of the hyoid bone. The relations of the external carotid and the internal carotid arteries change as these two vessels ascend. Here, at a low level, the external carotid lies anterior and medial to the internal carotid. At a higher level, the external carotid artery is located lateral to the internal carotid (Section 1–20).

Unlike the internal carotid artery, which has no branches in the neck,

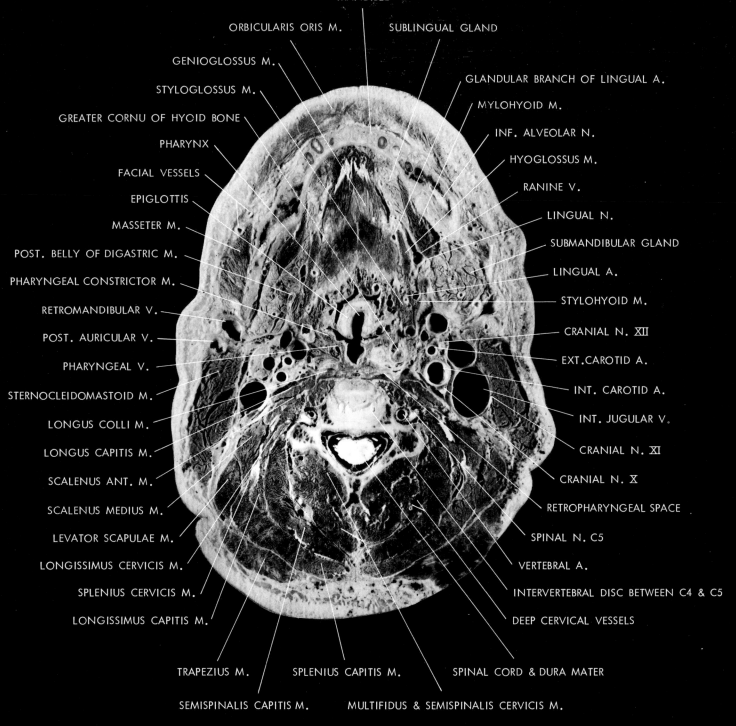

MANDIBLE

ORBICULARIS ORIS M.

SUBLINGUAL GLAND

GENIOGLOSSUS M.

GLANDULAR BRANCH OF LINGUAL A.

STYLOGLOSSUS M.

MYLOHYOID M.

GREATER CORNU OF HYOID BONE

INF. ALVEOLAR N.

PHARYNX

HYOGLOSSUS M.

FACIAL VESSELS

RANINE V.

EPIGLOTTIS

LINGUAL N.

MASSETER M.

SUBMANDIBULAR GLAND

POST. BELLY OF DIGASTRIC M.

LINGUAL A.

PHARYNGEAL CONSTRICTOR M.

STYLOHYOID M.

RETROMANDIBULAR V.

CRANIAL N. XII

POST. AURICULAR V.

EXT. CAROTID A.

PHARYNGEAL V.

INT. CAROTID A.

STERNOCLEIDOMASTOID M.

INT. JUGULAR V.

LONGUS COLLI M.

CRANIAL N. XI

LONGUS CAPITIS M.

CRANIAL N. X

SCALENUS ANT. M.

RETROPHARYNGEAL SPACE

SCALENUS MEDIUS M.

SPINAL N. C5

LEVATOR SCAPULAE M.

VERTEBRAL A.

LONGISSIMUS CERVICIS M.

INTERVERTEBRAL DISC BETWEEN C4 & C5

SPLENIUS CERVICIS M.

DEEP CERVICAL VESSELS

LONGISSIMUS CAPITIS M.

TRAPEZIUS M.

SPLENIUS CAPITIS M.

SPINAL CORD & DURA MATER

SEMISPINALIS CAPITIS M.

MULTIFIDUS & SEMISPINALIS CERVICIS M.

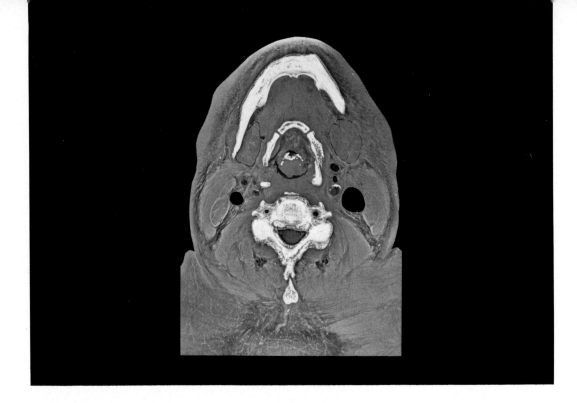

and the genioglossus muscle. It has a series of small ducts that open onto the edge of the sublingual fold.

Clinical Considerations

Although the laryngeal structures are visualized herein, one must recognize that conventional radiography has made great advances in this area of study. Lateral soft tissue roentgenograms of the neck, tomography of a conventional type, and contrast laryngograms, as well as xeroradiography of the larynx, have added tremendously to the dimensions of these studies. It is only the occasional patient who may benefit significantly from a cross-sectional study of this area (Powers et al., 1957; Samuel, 1975).

Powers WE, McGee HH Jr., Seaman WB: Contrast examination of larynx and pharynx. Radiology 68:169–178, 1957.
Samuel E: Xeroradiography or conventional radiography for laryngeal examinations? Can J Otolaryngol 4:59–63, 1975.

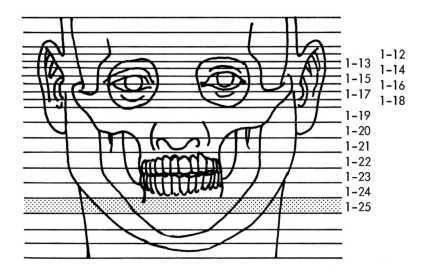

SECTION
1–25

Through the intervertebral disc between C5 and C6

Anatomic Considerations

The two remaining salivary glands, submandibular and sublingual, can be observed in Sections 1–23 to 1–25 and Section 1–24, respectively.

The submandibular gland is divided into a large superficial portion and a small deep portion. The superficial portion is found in the digastric triangle and is covered by skin, the platysma muscle, and the superficial (investing) layer of the cervical fascia. This fascia forms a loose sheath around the gland. The deep surface rests on the mylohyoid, hyoglossus, stylohyoid, and posterior belly of the digastric muscles. The deep portion of the submandibular gland passes around the posterior border of the mylohyoid and comes to lie between the mylohyoid and hyoglossus muscles. The submandibular duct arises from the deep portion, passes between the mylohyoid and genioglossus, and finally opens on the side of the frenulum of the tongue.

The sublingual gland lies in the floor of the mouth between the mandible

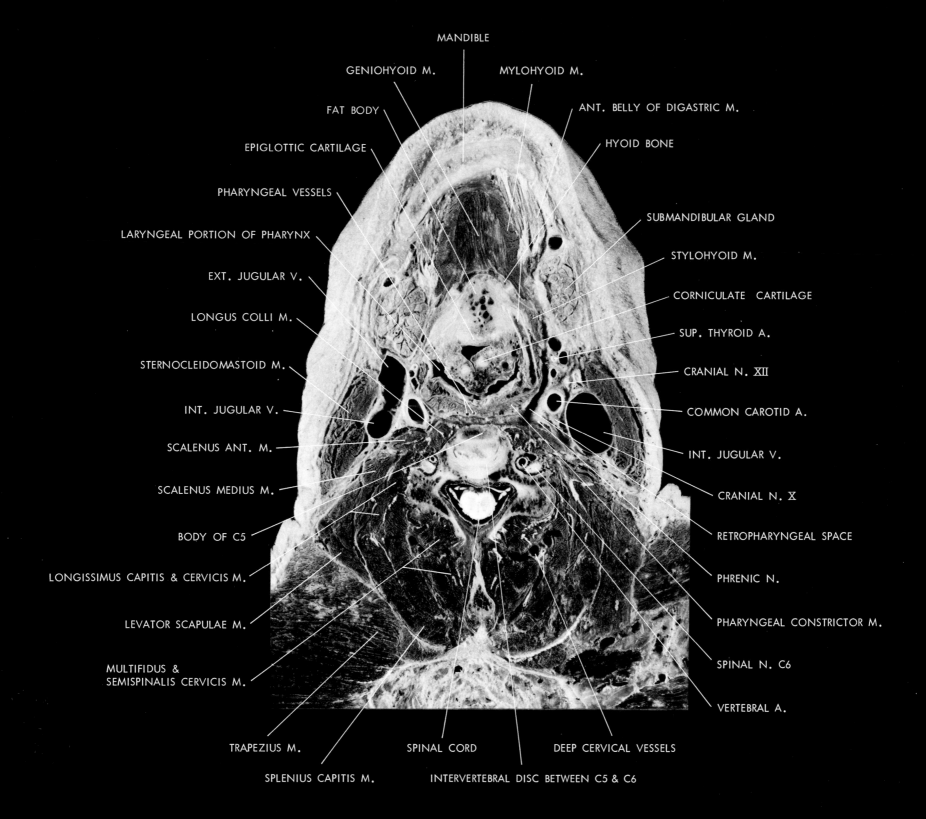

MANDIBLE

GENIOHYOID M.

MYLOHYOID M.

FAT BODY

ANT. BELLY OF DIGASTRIC M.

EPIGLOTTIC CARTILAGE

HYOID BONE

PHARYNGEAL VESSELS

SUBMANDIBULAR GLAND

LARYNGEAL PORTION OF PHARYNX

STYLOHYOID M.

EXT. JUGULAR V.

CORNICULATE CARTILAGE

LONGUS COLLI M.

SUP. THYROID A.

STERNOCLEIDOMASTOID M.

CRANIAL N. XII

INT. JUGULAR V.

COMMON CAROTID A.

SCALENUS ANT. M.

INT. JUGULAR V.

SCALENUS MEDIUS M.

CRANIAL N. X

BODY OF C5

RETROPHARYNGEAL SPACE

LONGISSIMUS CAPITIS & CERVICIS M.

PHRENIC N.

LEVATOR SCAPULAE M.

PHARYNGEAL CONSTRICTOR M.

MULTIFIDUS &
SEMISPINALIS CERVICIS M.

SPINAL N. C6

VERTEBRAL A.

TRAPEZIUS M.

SPINAL CORD

DEEP CERVICAL VESSELS

SPLENIUS CAPITIS M.

INTERVERTEBRAL DISC BETWEEN C5 & C6

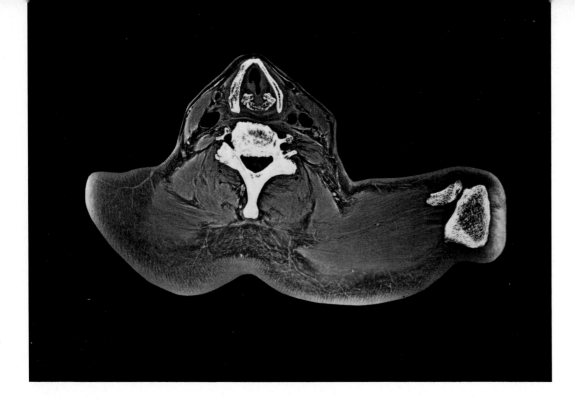

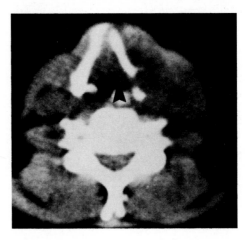

Clinical Considerations

This CT scan demonstrates a patient with moderately differentiated squamous cell carcinoma of the trachea, with extension upward to involve the larynx. Arrow indicates the large soft tissue mass in the left side of the neck invading the larygeal cartilage and extending into the air space, partially obstructing the laryngeal air space. (Courtesy of Dr. Neil Wolfman.)

The points discussed in respect to Section 1–25 are particularly applicable here, where the vocal cords themselves are seen to excellent advantage; furthermore, the cartilages adjoining are identified. Occasionally some of the cartilages may be dislocated; this may be recognized by conventional laryngography as well as tomography (Samuel and Lloyd, 1978).

The commonest sites of abscess formation in the vicinity of the pharynx are the parapharyngeal, peripharyngeal, postvisceral, prevertebral, and peritonsillar. These common sites of infection must be borne in mind whenever one sees cross-sectional studies of this area.

Samuel E and Lloyd GAS: Clinical Radiology of the Ear, Nose and Throat (2nd ed.) W.B. Saunders Co., Philadelphia, 1978, p. 221.

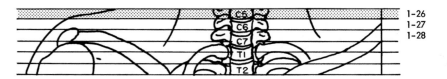

SECTION 1–26

Through the intervertebral disc between C5 and C6 and the upper part of the body of C6

Anatomic Considerations

The specimen in this section is different from that in the preceding one. One of the major structures that can be seen in this section is the larynx. Three of the laryngeal cartilages are present: the unpaired thyroid cartilage, which is seen as two laminae on the anterolateral aspect of the larynx; the cricoid cartilage (also unpaired), which is the only complete cartilaginous ring in the respiratory system; and the paired pyramid-shaped arytenoid cartilages. The epiglottic (unpaired) and paired corniculate cartilages can be seen in the preceding illustration.

This section has passed through the level of the vocal cords. As can be seen on the specimen's left side, each vocal cord is attached anteriorly to the thyroid cartilage and posteriorly to the vocal process of the arytenoid cartilage. The sensory nerve supply to the mucous membrane of the larynx above the level of the vocal cords is from the internal laryngeal branch of the superior laryngeal branch of the vagus. The sensory innervation to the mucous membrane below the level of the vocal cords is from the recurrent laryngeal nerve, also a branch of the vagus.

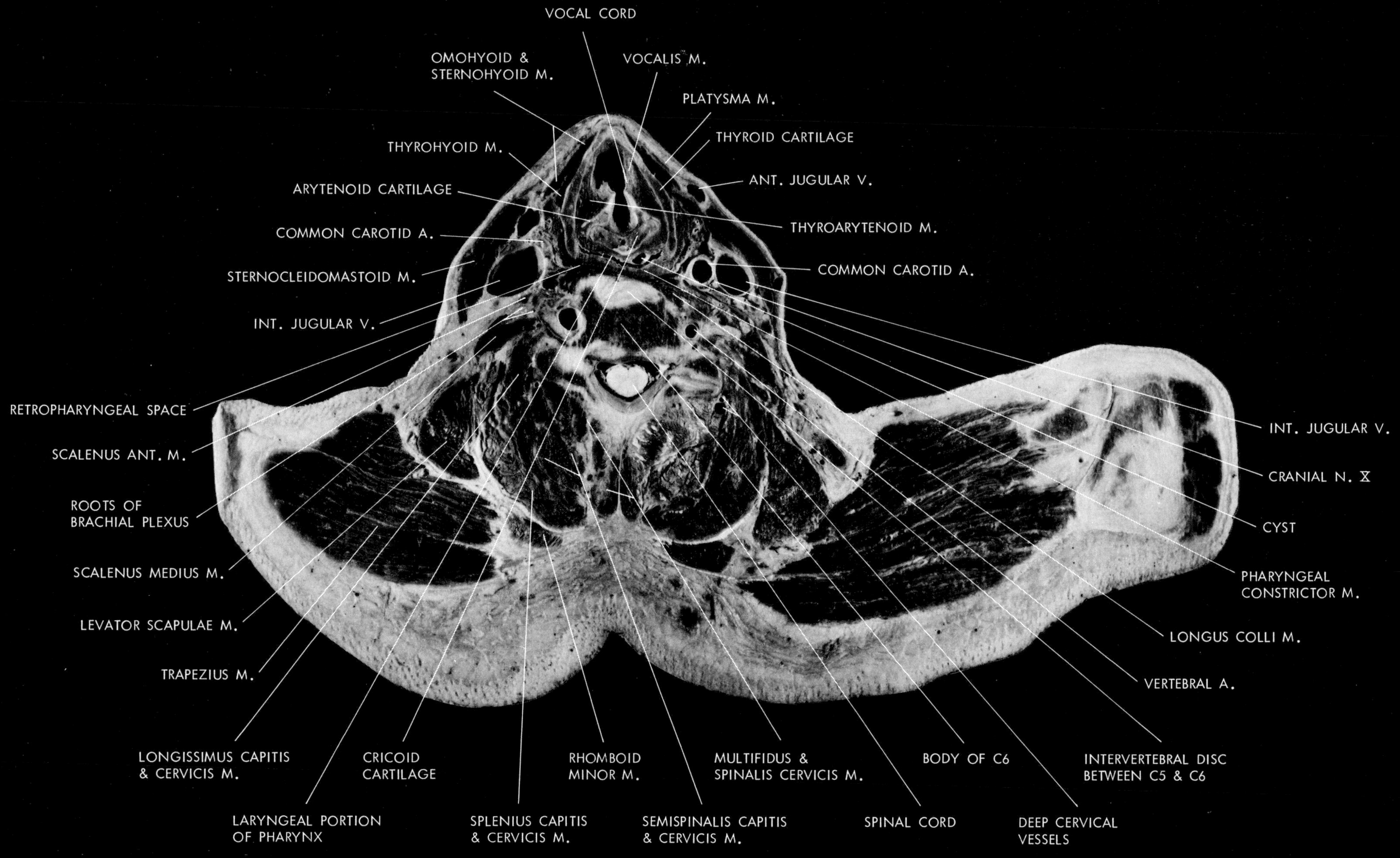

VOCAL CORD

OMOHYOID &
STERNOHYOID M.

VOCALIS M.

PLATYSMA M.

THYROHYOID M.

THYROID CARTILAGE

ARYTENOID CARTILAGE

ANT. JUGULAR V.

COMMON CAROTID A.

THYROARYTENOID M.

STERNOCLEIDOMASTOID M.

COMMON CAROTID A.

INT. JUGULAR V.

RETROPHARYNGEAL SPACE

INT. JUGULAR V.

SCALENUS ANT. M.

CRANIAL N. X

ROOTS OF
BRACHIAL PLEXUS

CYST

SCALENUS MEDIUS M.

PHARYNGEAL
CONSTRICTOR M.

LEVATOR SCAPULAE M.

LONGUS COLLI M.

TRAPEZIUS M.

VERTEBRAL A.

LONGISSIMUS CAPITIS
& CERVICIS M.

CRICOID
CARTILAGE

RHOMBOID
MINOR M.

MULTIFIDUS &
SPINALIS CERVICIS M.

BODY OF C6

INTERVERTEBRAL DISC
BETWEEN C5 & C6

LARYNGEAL PORTION
OF PHARYNX

SPLENIUS CAPITIS
& CERVICIS M.

SEMISPINALIS CAPITIS
& CERVICIS M.

SPINAL CORD

DEEP CERVICAL
VESSELS

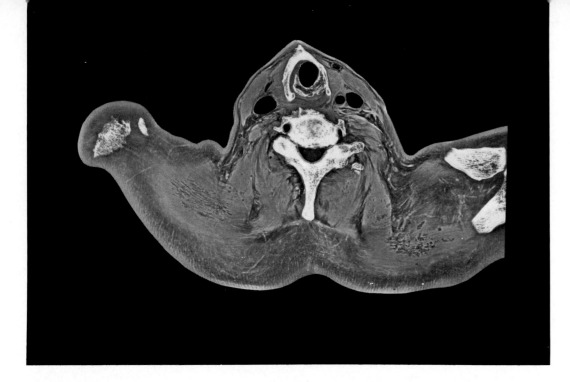

with the other layers of cervical fascia, that is, the investing, pretracheal, and prevertebal.

Clinical Consideratons

The plane of this section passes just above the level of the trachea. Although tumors of the trachea are relatively uncommon, cross-sectional anatomy may be very helpful in such cases, since these may extend or creep along the tracheal mucosa to involve more distal portions of the tracheobronchial tree. The cylindroma occurs most frequently in the cervical portion of the trachea (Clagett et al., 1953). Routine studies are not of great value in respect to the trachea until one employs such special expedients as tomography or contrast agents injected directly into the trachea (tracheograms).

Of course, metastatic tumors are frequently paratracheal and again are readily recognized anywhere along the full length of the trachea.

The thyroid gland is visible in this section. Nuclear medicine makes its greatest inroads with respect to the thyroid gland, but the full extension of enlargements or neoplasms of the thyroid gland, particularly when they are retrotracheal, are significantly helped by cross-sectional studies of this area. This is well demonstrated both in this section and in Section 1-28.

Clagett OT, Moersch HJ, and Grindlay JH: Intrathoracic tracheal tumors: Development of surgical techniques for their removal. Trans Am Surg Ass 70:224, 1953.

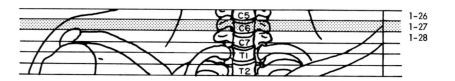

SECTION 1–27

Through the intervertebral disc between C6 and C7

Anatomic Consideratons

The cervical fascia of the neck consists of several layers that communicate with each other, resulting in the formation of spaces or clefts. One of these, the retropharyngeal space, is evident in this illustration. The space is bounded by the buccopharyngeal fascia anteriorly, by the prevertebral fascia posteriorly, and by the carotid sheaths laterally. The space extends from the base of the skull to the posterior mediastinum.

The carotid sheath is the fascial envelope that encloses the common and internal carotid arteries, the internal jugular vein, and the vagus nerve. It extends from the base of the skull to the root of the neck. The sheath blends

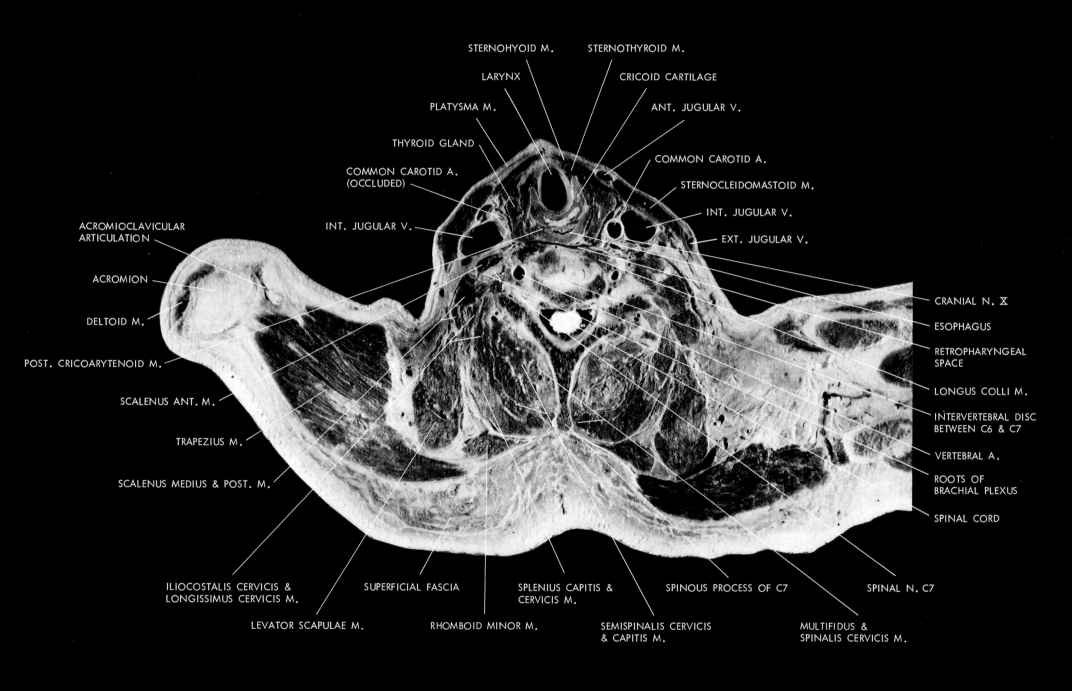

STERNOHYOID M.   STERNOTHYROID M.

LARYNX   CRICOID CARTILAGE

PLATYSMA M.   ANT. JUGULAR V.

THYROID GLAND

COMMON CAROTID A.

COMMON CAROTID A.   STERNOCLEIDOMASTOID M.
(OCCLUDED)

INT. JUGULAR V.   INT. JUGULAR V.

EXT. JUGULAR V.

ACROMIOCLAVICULAR
ARTICULATION

ACROMION

CRANIAL N. X

DELTOID M.

ESOPHAGUS

RETROPHARYNGEAL
SPACE

POST. CRICOARYTENOID M.

LONGUS COLLI M.

SCALENUS ANT. M.

INTERVERTEBRAL DISC
BETWEEN C6 & C7

TRAPEZIUS M.

VERTEBRAL A.

ROOTS OF
BRACHIAL PLEXUS

SCALENUS MEDIUS & POST. M.

SPINAL CORD

ILIOCOSTALIS CERVICIS &
LONGISSIMUS CERVICIS M.   SUPERFICIAL FASCIA   SPLENIUS CAPITIS &
CERVICIS M.   SPINOUS PROCESS OF C7   SPINAL N. C7

LEVATOR SCAPULAE M.   RHOMBOID MINOR M.   SEMISPINALIS CERVICIS
& CAPITIS M.   MULTIFIDUS &
SPINALIS CERVICIS M.

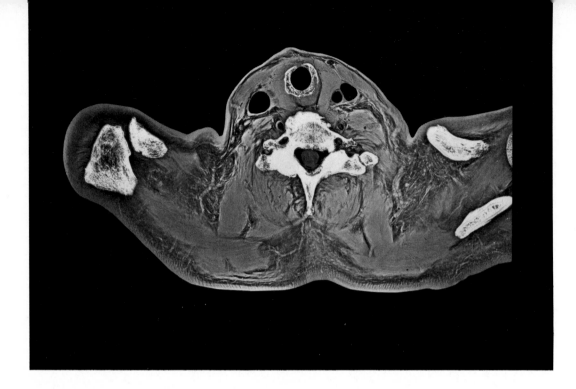

fibroelastic wall that contains a series of U-shaped bars of hyaline cartilage that keep the lumen patent. Anteriorly, the trachea is related from superior to inferior by the isthmus of the thyroid gland (which usually crosses the second, third, and fourth tracheal rings), the sternum, the thymus (if present), the left brachiocephalic vein, the origins of the brachiocephalic and left common carotid arteries, and the arch of the aorta. The esophagus is related posteriorly to the trachea. In the neck, the lateral lobes of the thyroid and the carotid sheath are related laterally to the trachea. In the mediastinum, the trachea is related to the arch of the aorta on the left side, to the azygos vein on the right side, and to the pleura on either side.

Clinical Considerations

Once again the trachea and its adjoining structures are seen in good relationship. One should call attention to some of the unusual sequelae of tracheal intubation, particularly when tubes that cause inflammatory processes within the trachea and subsequent fibrosis and stricture are employed. Present technology has virtually eliminated such complications.

The trachea, the thyroid gland, the esophagus, and the vascular structures on either side, consisting primarily of the internal jugular vein and the common carotid artery, are also identified in their appropriate relationships. One must note that the external jugular vein is lateral to the internal jugular vein and that the common carotid artery is immediately medial to the internal jugular vein.

SECTION
1–28

Through the body of C7

Anatomic Considerations

The trachea begins below the cricoid cartilage at the level of the sixth cervical vertebra and ends in the thorax by dividing into the right and left primary bronchi. Since this section was taken from the same specimen used for the sections of the thorax, the entire course of the trachea can be followed from this secton through Section 2–10, where the trachea bifurcates. In this specimen, the length of the trachea is 12 to 13 cm. The trachea has a

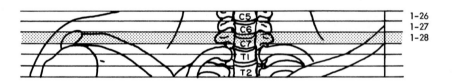

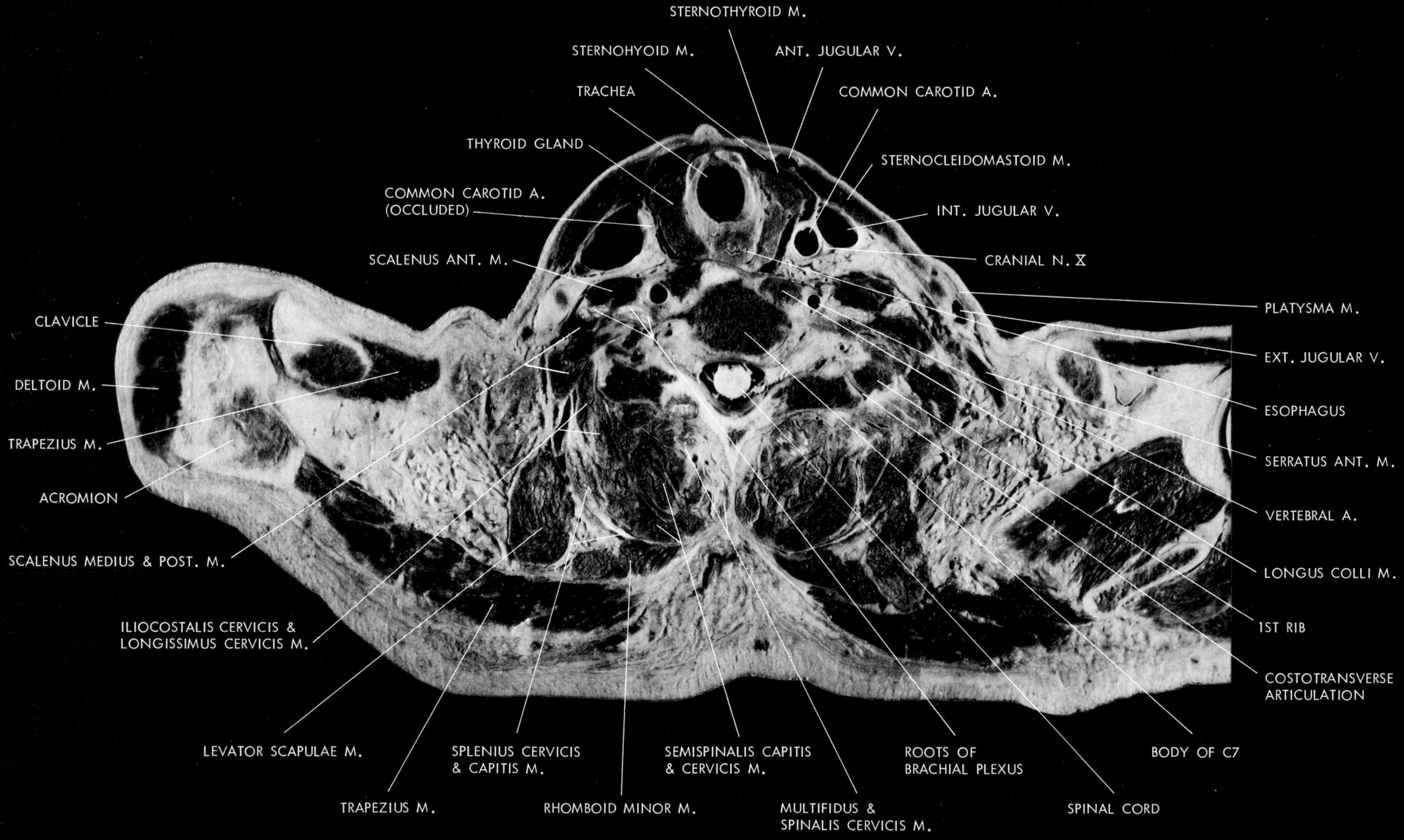

STERNOTHYROID M.

STERNOHYOID M.

ANT. JUGULAR V.

TRACHEA

COMMON CAROTID A.

THYROID GLAND

STERNOCLEIDOMASTOID M.

COMMON CAROTID A.
(OCCLUDED)

INT. JUGULAR V.

SCALENUS ANT. M.

CRANIAL N. X

CLAVICLE

PLATYSMA M.

EXT. JUGULAR V.

DELTOID M.

ESOPHAGUS

TRAPEZIUS M.

SERRATUS ANT. M.

ACROMION

VERTEBRAL A.

SCALENUS MEDIUS & POST. M.

LONGUS COLLI M.

ILIOCOSTALIS CERVICIS &
LONGISSIMUS CERVICIS M.

1ST RIB

COSTOTRANSVERSE
ARTICULATION

LEVATOR SCAPULAE M.

SPLENIUS CERVICIS
& CAPITIS M.

SEMISPINALIS CAPITIS
& CERVICIS M.

ROOTS OF
BRACHIAL PLEXUS

BODY OF C7

TRAPEZIUS M.

RHOMBOID MINOR M.

MULTIFIDUS &
SPINALIS CERVICIS M.

SPINAL CORD

2
Thorax

INTRODUCTION

The accompanying sketch shows that the sections pertaining to the thorax are from vertebral levels T1 to T12; therefore, sections showing structures of the neck, shoulder, and abdomen are present.

The sections of the thorax are from the same specimen as those from the neck (Sections 1–26 to 1–28). Different specimens were used for the thorax and the abdomen.

Because of the pathology of some of the great vessels of the thorax, the walls became separated during the processing of the sections. These artifacts were touched up in Sections 2–1 to 2–14.

Owing to their morphology, some of the structures are not identifiable in all of the sections. The thoracic duct is not seen in all of the presentations because the thin-walled structure was collapsed in most of the sections. Some of the nerves are not seen because they blended in with the surrounding connective tissue.

To reduce the number of labels, the ribs were indicated only in every other section.

A lipoma of the right atrium is present in Sections 2–16 to 2–19. The lipoma was confirmed by the pathologist.

The diagnostic potential of computed tomography of the thorax is in its introductory phase at this writing. Possibly one of the most extensive reviews of this subject (based on approximately 300 examinations) is that offered by Heitzman and associates (1979). They recorded the five general categories for utilization of scanning of the thorax as follows: (1) lung, (2) mediastinum and hilum, (3) pleura and chest, (4) heart and great vessels, and (5) diaphragm and crura.

LUNG. In conventional radiographic studies of the mediastinum, there is considerable overlap of anatomic structures. The heart, for example, overlies shadows immediately contiguous with it, and esophagrams must be used to delineate the left atrium posteriorly or the descending thoracic aorta. Very often image intensification techniques are required to amplify differentiation between a structure that might be vascular in origin and one that is not. This is particularly true where an aneurysm is suspected. Computed axial tomography permits the transverse display of an image, both with and without contrast enhancement, giving us a third-dimensional approach to separate conveniently the various anatomic structures of the mediastinum, including even the chambers of the heart.

Some lesions of the lung, such as small nodules near the lung periphery and nodules contiguous with or involving the pleura, may escape detection with conventional radiography. Computed tomography has been recommended for this purpose.

Putman (1978) estimates that conventional whole-lung tomography will detect additional pulmonary nodules in approximately 10 per cent of patients when compared with conventional chest radiography. This percentage will vary according to the primary malignancy, expertise of the chest radiologist, and technique of the standard x-ray procedures. The detection of nodules does not necessarily mean metastasis, and much more study is necessary before whole-chest computed axial tomography is justifiable.

Since sensors in most apparatus of this type give one a very accurate description of absorption coefficient of tissues enclosed within a certain number of voxels in the computer, the technique offers at least a mechanism of beginning to define the density of tissues and perhaps separating transudate, exudate, cellularity, or even neoplastic processes. Of course, very considerable additional work will be required to establish normal values.

MEDIASTINUM AND HILUM. One of the greatest problems confronting a diagnosis of mediastinal disease is the differentiation of lymphoid tissue from fatty tissue and the latter from vascular and muscular tissues. Since computed tomography is able to determine accurately the absorption coefficient of these various tissues, such processes as fatty structures, malignant lymphomas, or structures connected with the heart and its major vessels become readily distinguishable. The latter can be additionally distinguished with the aid of contrast enhancement.

Moreover, in staging of malignant lymphomatous diseases, it becomes imperative to know the full extent of the disease process within the mediastinum, and computed tomography is ideal for this purpose.

The Questionably Abnormal Hilum. In conventional radiography it is often difficult to distinguish the various anatomic portions of the hilum. The pulmonary artery, particularly, can at times resemble an artery and associated lymph nodes. Recognition of characteristic contrast-enhanced vascular structures with computed tomography makes this differentiation very feasible.

PLEURA AND CHEST WALL. Conventional radiography is known to miss lesions of the pleura and chest wall. A number of instances have been reported in which lesions not seen by conventional means are well demonstrated by computed tomography. Certainly pleural effusions are readily identified from other disease processes.

HEART AND GREAT VESSELS. With two-second and some more rapid scans available, respiratory and cardiac motion, which might interfere significantly with the resolution and definition of anatomic detail, appear to be less important factors than might have been anticipated. Nevertheless, development of a gating mechanism that will allow very rapid exposures at certain phases of the cardiac cycle, together with contrast enhancement, will be a significant advance.

DIAPHRAGM AND CRURA. The diaphragmatic crura are clearly seen by computed tomography, and at times they may even be somewhat nodular rather than fibrillar. No other radiographic means allows us to define these structures so accurately. The association of the crura with enlarged lymph nodes, the aorta, the esophagus, and other contiguous structures makes this a very valuable adjunct in the diagnostic armamentarium.

SUMMARY. The main applications of computed tomography of the chest at this time are as follows:
1. For staging purposes in patients with mediastinal bronchogenic carcinoma or malignant lymphoma.
2. For any assessment of a mediastinal tumor, including its absorption coefficient.
3. To distinguish solid from cystic masses of the mediastinum, especially by their attenuation coefficients.
4. For the diagnosis of fatty tumors of the mediastinum, since they have an absorption coefficient of from minus 50 to minus 150 Hounsfield units.
5. For more accurate detection of pleural implants from metastatic disease than is possible with conventional radiography.

6. For the diagnosis of retrocardiac cysts, such as foregut duplication cysts.
7. For the puncture of such detected cysts under computed tomographic (or indeed ordinary fluoroscopic) controls, so that the aspirated fluid can be analyzed.
8. For the better delineation of vascular structures such as aneurysms, which generally show a coefficient absorption range of plus 50 to plus 60 Hounsfield units before the administration of contrast material and a considerably higher number after the administration of contrast agent.
9. For the detection of mural thrombi, dissecting hematoma, and bleeding into the mediastinum, particularly if contrast enhancement is employed.
10. For demonstration of enlarged pulmonary and systemic arteries and veins, particularly with the aid of contrast enhancement. This is espe-

cially important if conventional radiography does not permit us to determine the cause of a prominent hilum, and in these circumstances it may be either vascular or nonvascular in origin.
11. To detect calcifications in the heart, in the vessels, or in any mass that may be revealed by any other diagnostic modality. Cardiac calcification may be seen in thrombi, in tumors, or in coronary vessels. Areas of mild cardiac damage may at times become calcified, and all of these may be demonstrated by computed tomography.

Heitzman ER, Proto AV, and Goldwin RL: The role of computerized tomography in the diagnosis of diseases of the thorax. JAMA 241:933–936, 1979.
Putman C: Computed Tomographic Scanning of the Thorax: Course 209B Syllabus: Radiology of the Chest, 1978, Radiological Society of North America.

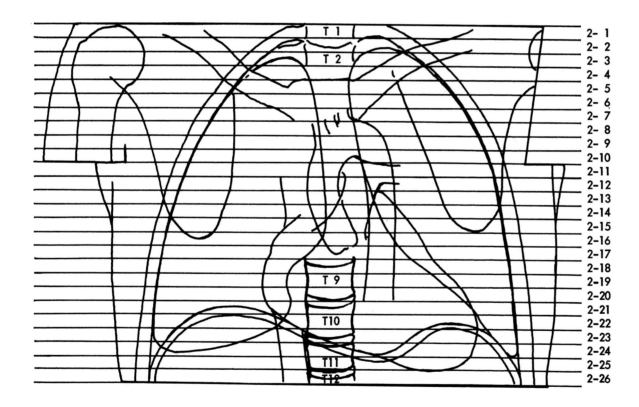

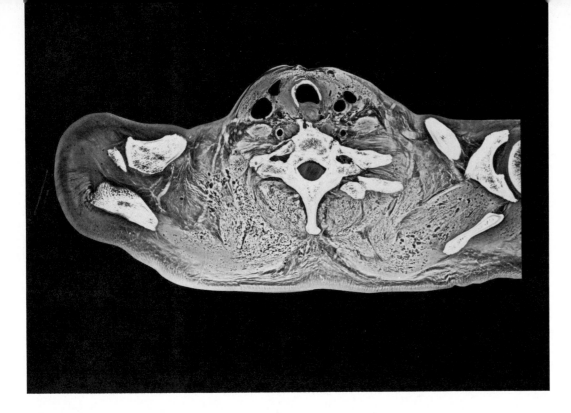

Anatomic Considerations

In this section the relationships of the trachea to the thyroid gland and to the esophagus can be observed. The thyroid is composed of two lateral lobes, which are related to the anterolateral surface of the trachea, and the isthmus, which connects the two lateral lobes. The isthmus is related to the anterior aspect of the second, third, and fourth tracheal cartilages. At this level (upper thorax) and in the neck, the esophagus can be seen to lie directly posterior to the trachea. However, as the esophagus descends in the thorax, it is inclined to the left; therefore, at lower levels, the trachea is related not only anterior to but also to the right of the esophagus. Compare the relations of these structures in this section with Section 2–9.

Clinical Considerations

This section shows transversely the relations of the thyroid, trachea, and esophagus, as well as the roots of the brachial plexus.

The thyroid gland can ordinarily be readily identified, particularly if it is intensified with iodine. In any case, its absorption coefficient is somewhat greater than that of the adjoining structures. It is probable, however, that radioisotopic scans of the thyroid will continue to be the diagnostic method of choice.

At times, clinically, the thyroid gland is retrotracheal but is readily identifiable and differentiated from the esophagus, particularly if the esophagus is enhanced with meglumine diatrizoate preparation (Gastrografin) or a small amount of barium in honey.

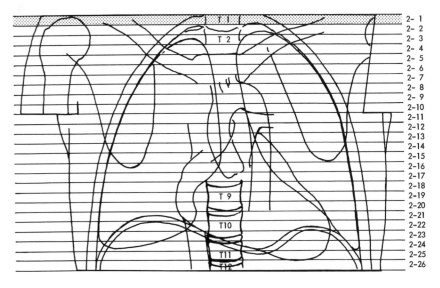

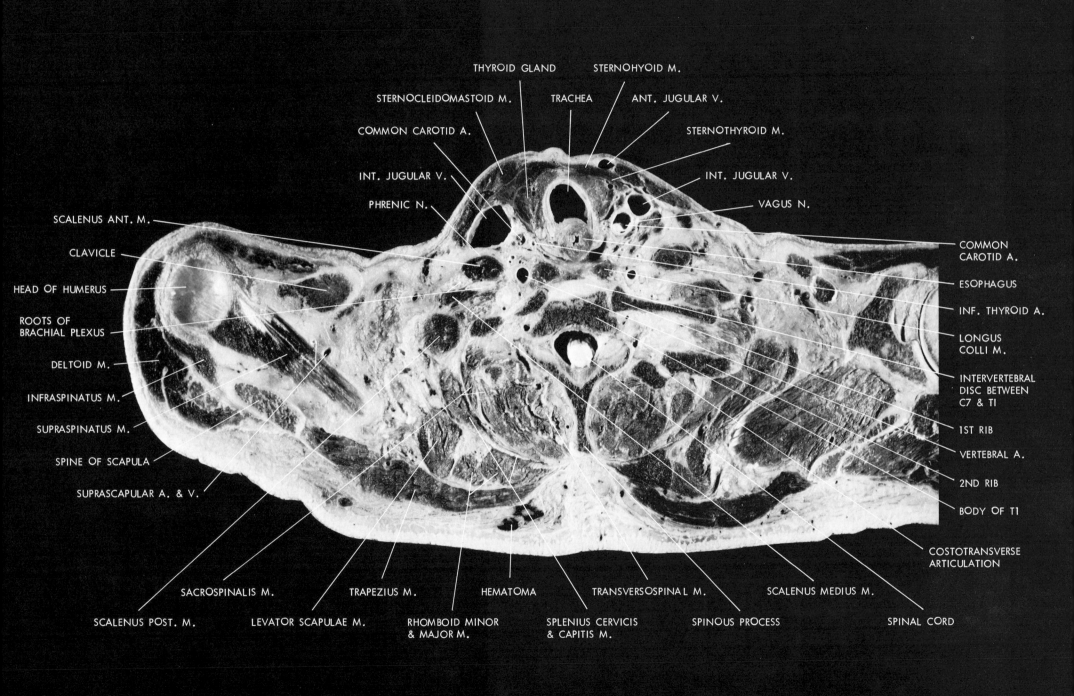

THYROID GLAND   STERNOHYOID M.

STERNOCLEIDOMASTOID M.   TRACHEA   ANT. JUGULAR V.

COMMON CAROTID A.   STERNOTHYROID M.

INT. JUGULAR V.   INT. JUGULAR V.

PHRENIC N.   VAGUS N.

SCALENUS ANT. M.

CLAVICLE   COMMON CAROTID A.

HEAD OF HUMERUS   ESOPHAGUS

INF. THYROID A.

ROOTS OF BRACHIAL PLEXUS   LONGUS COLLI M.

DELTOID M.

INTERVERTEBRAL DISC BETWEEN C7 & T1

INFRASPINATUS M.

SUPRASPINATUS M.   1ST RIB

SPINE OF SCAPULA   VERTEBRAL A.

SUPRASCAPULAR A. & V.   2ND RIB

BODY OF T1

COSTOTRANSVERSE ARTICULATION

SACROSPINALIS M.   TRAPEZIUS M.   HEMATOMA   TRANSVERSOSPINAL M.   SCALENUS MEDIUS M.

SCALENUS POST. M.   LEVATOR SCAPULAE M.   RHOMBOID MINOR & MAJOR M.   SPLENIUS CERVICIS & CAPITIS M.   SPINOUS PROCESS   SPINAL CORD

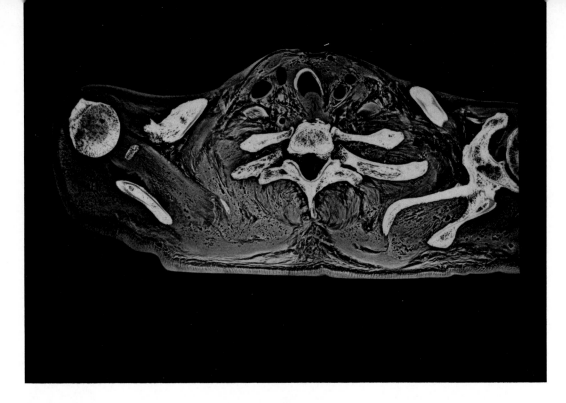

lesions in this location, although we have not had occasion ourselves to demonstrate this. Barrett's epithelium is at times found at this level in the esophagus and is subject to ulceration. Although conventional radiography may help such diagnoses, the rapidity with which the swallowing action occurs would make a cross-sectional study highly advantageous.

It will be noted that in these sections there is a clear, fatty differentiation between the various muscles surrounding the vertebral body. These areas are also prone to invasion by tumor masses, and the differentiation of a tumor mass from a muscle might otherwise be very difficult. This would emphasize the importance of knowing the cross-sectional anatomy of this area in considerable detail. For example, an abnormal lymph node or muscle mass might adjoin the scalene muscle, and differentiation from the muscle might be difficult without biopsy.

Finally, in the case of neck injuries, the soft tissue planes adjoining the vertebral bodies are often distended with blood. Although we have not had occasion to study such an example, it certainly appears feasible to differentiate the fascial planes filled with blood from the normal fascial planes occupying this area. This could help diagnose prevertebral bleeding and other mass lesions.

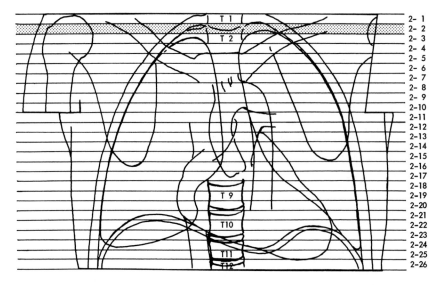

SECTION
2–2

Through the intervertebral disc between T1 and T2

Anatomic Considerations

In this illustration and in the preceding one the important relationship of the roots of the brachial plexus to the scalenus anterior muscle and scalenus medius muscle can be observed. The roots that appear between these muscles consist of anterior primary rami of spinal nerves C5 to T1. The roots have a short course in this area and unite to form the three trunks of the brachial plexus. The upper trunk is formed by spinal nerves C5 and C6, the middle trunk by C7, and the lower trunk by C8 and T1. The brachial plexus will be considered with the upper extremity.

The phrenic nerve can be seen in this illustration on the anterior surface of the scalenus anterior muscle. It is derived mainly from spinal nerve C4 but may receive contributions from C3 and C5. It passes into the thorax and innervates the pleura, pericardium, and diaphragm.

Clinical Considerations

At times this area of the esophagus is subject to either ulceration or neoplasm. The cross-sectional study could readily be used to detect such pathologic

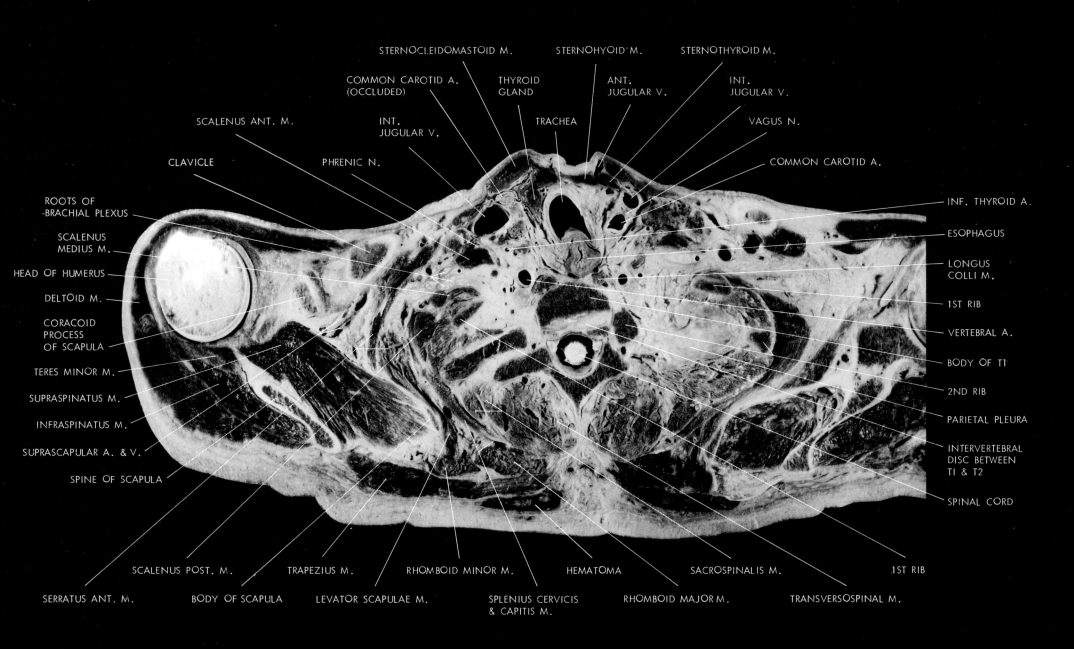

STERNOCLEIDOMASTOID M.   STERNOHYOID M.   STERNOTHYROID M.

COMMON CAROTID A.   THYROID   ANT.   INT.
(OCCLUDED)   GLAND   JUGULAR V.   JUGULAR V.

SCALENUS ANT. M.   INT.   TRACHEA   VAGUS N.
JUGULAR V.

CLAVICLE   PHRENIC N.   COMMON CAROTID A.

ROOTS OF   INF. THYROID A.
BRACHIAL PLEXUS

SCALENUS   ESOPHAGUS
MEDIUS M.

HEAD OF HUMERUS   LONGUS
COLLI M.

DELTOID M.   1ST RIB

CORACOID   VERTEBRAL A.
PROCESS
OF SCAPULA   BODY OF T1

TERES MINOR M.   2ND RIB

SUPRASPINATUS M.   PARIETAL PLEURA

INFRASPINATUS M.   INTERVERTEBRAL
DISC BETWEEN
SUPRASCAPULAR A. & V.   T1 & T2

SPINE OF SCAPULA   SPINAL CORD

SCALENUS POST. M.   TRAPEZIUS M.   RHOMBOID MINOR M.   HEMATOMA   SACROSPINALIS M.   1ST RIB

SERRATUS ANT. M.   BODY OF SCAPULA   LEVATOR SCAPULAE M.   SPLENIUS CERVICIS   RHOMBOID MAJOR M.   TRANSVERSOSPINAL M.
& CAPITIS M.

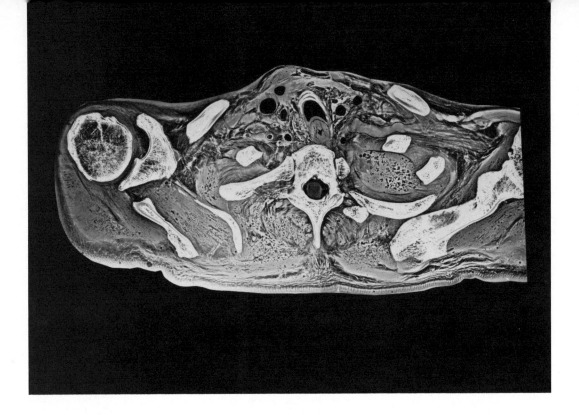

Clinical Considerations

The thyroid gland may extend downward into this section adjoining the trachea and is readily differentiable, as in the case of earlier sections at the base of the neck.

The brachiocephalic and subclavian arteries, differentiable at this level, may be subject to aneurysm formation accompanied with an aneurysm of the ascending aorta, particularly in the presence of syphilis. This section, particularly with contrast enhancement, would be suitable for detecting this condition.

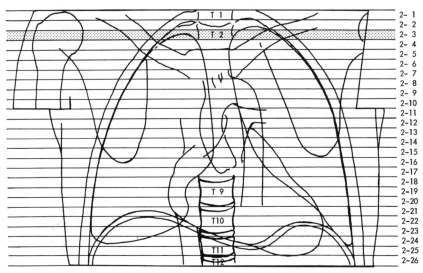

SECTION
2–3

*Through the
body of T2*

Anatomic Considerations

In this illustration and in Section 2–4 the apex of the lung can be observed. It extends into the root of the neck approximately 4 cm above the sternal end of the first rib. The apex of the lung lies posterior and superior to the medial third of the clavicle. It is grooved by the subclavian artery, which is separated from the lung by the cupula of the pleura.

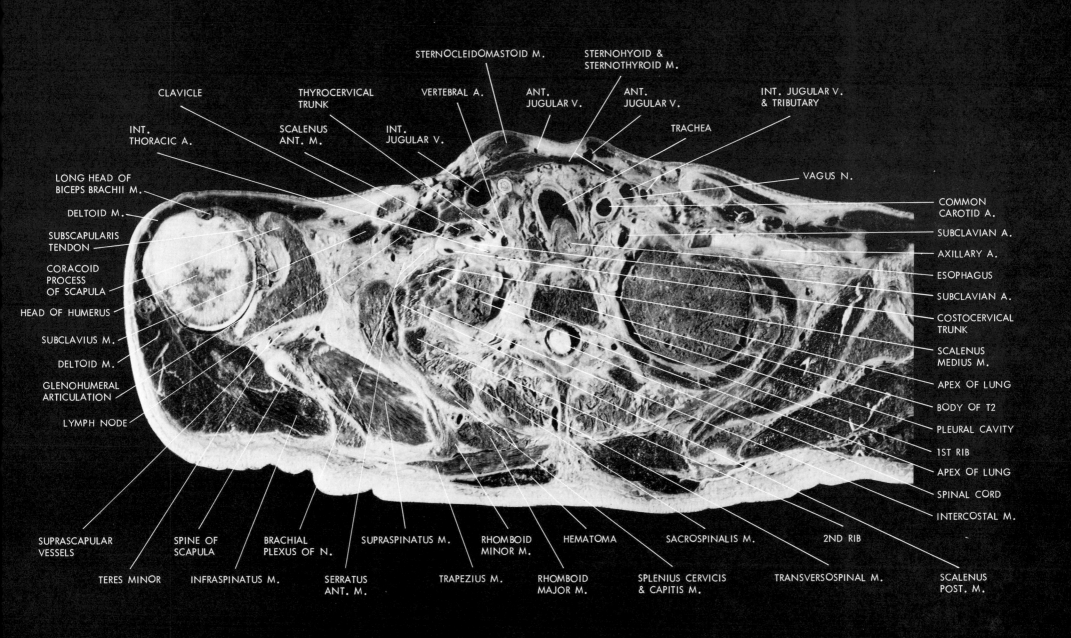

STERNOCLEIDOMASTOID M.

STERNOHYOID & STERNOTHYROID M.

CLAVICLE

THYROCERVICAL TRUNK

VERTEBRAL A.

ANT. JUGULAR V.

ANT. JUGULAR V.

INT. JUGULAR V. & TRIBUTARY

INT. THORACIC A.

SCALENUS ANT. M.

INT. JUGULAR V.

TRACHEA

LONG HEAD OF BICEPS BRACHII M.

VAGUS N.

DELTOID M.

COMMON CAROTID A.

SUBSCAPULARIS TENDON

SUBCLAVIAN A.

AXILLARY A.

CORACOID PROCESS OF SCAPULA

ESOPHAGUS

SUBCLAVIAN A.

HEAD OF HUMERUS

COSTOCERVICAL TRUNK

SUBCLAVIUS M.

SCALENUS MEDIUS M.

DELTOID M.

GLENOHUMERAL ARTICULATION

APEX OF LUNG

BODY OF T2

LYMPH NODE

PLEURAL CAVITY

1ST RIB

APEX OF LUNG

SPINAL CORD

INTERCOSTAL M.

SUPRASCAPULAR VESSELS

SPINE OF SCAPULA

BRACHIAL PLEXUS OF N.

SUPRASPINATUS M.

RHOMBOID MINOR M.

HEMATOMA

SACROSPINALIS M.

2ND RIB

TERES MINOR

INFRASPINATUS M.

SERRATUS ANT. M.

TRAPEZIUS M.

RHOMBOID MAJOR M.

SPLENIUS CERVICIS & CAPITIS M.

TRANSVERSOSPINAL M.

SCALENUS POST. M.

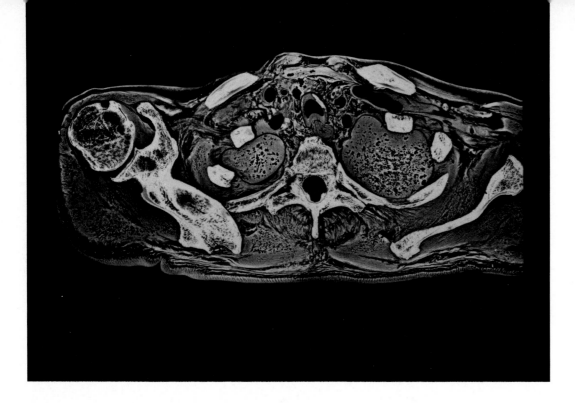

become involved by metastatic neoplasm. This is such a frequent finding that the left nodal area has been called "Virchow's node" and is often biopsied to lend some knowledge regarding the basic disease process in a patient.

A disease process often discussed in this area is a posterior sulcus tumor of bronchogenic origin (Pancoast's tumor). The origin of this tumor was previously believed to be other than bronchogenic, but in recent times its exact relationship has been better defined. One can readily detect how a posterior sulcus tumor of the Pancoast type might involve the apex of the lung, adjoining rib, and even the adjoining intercostal nerve and brachial plexus. One of the first pathologic findings one seeks radiographically with such tumor involvement is destruction of the adjoining rib.

The posterior relationship of the apex of the lung above the level of the clavicle is readily discernible in the left half of this section. Thus, one may say almost unequivocally that a lesion of the lung found to be present posterior to the trachea is almost certainly apical in situation or does not originate in the lung.

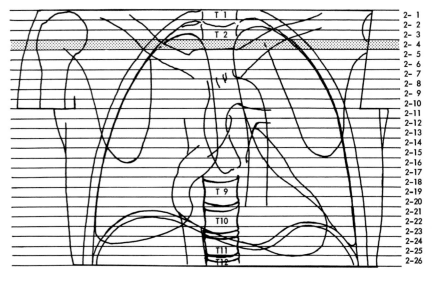

SECTION 2–4

Through the intervertebral disc between T2 and T3

Anatomic Considerations

The thoracic inlet (upper thoracic aperture) is bounded posteriorly by the first thoracic vertebra, laterally by the first rib and its costal cartilage, and anteriorly by the manubrium of the sternum. These structures separate the neck from the thorax. A portion of the thoracic inlet (first rib) can be observed in this illustration. To see the entire thoracic inlet in cross-section, however, several illustrations need to be observed (2–1 to 2–7 in this specimen) because of the slope of the ribs.

Clinical Considerations

The lymph nodes found in this area, particularly to the left of the midline and anteriorly disposed in respect to the brachiocephalic artery, are prone to

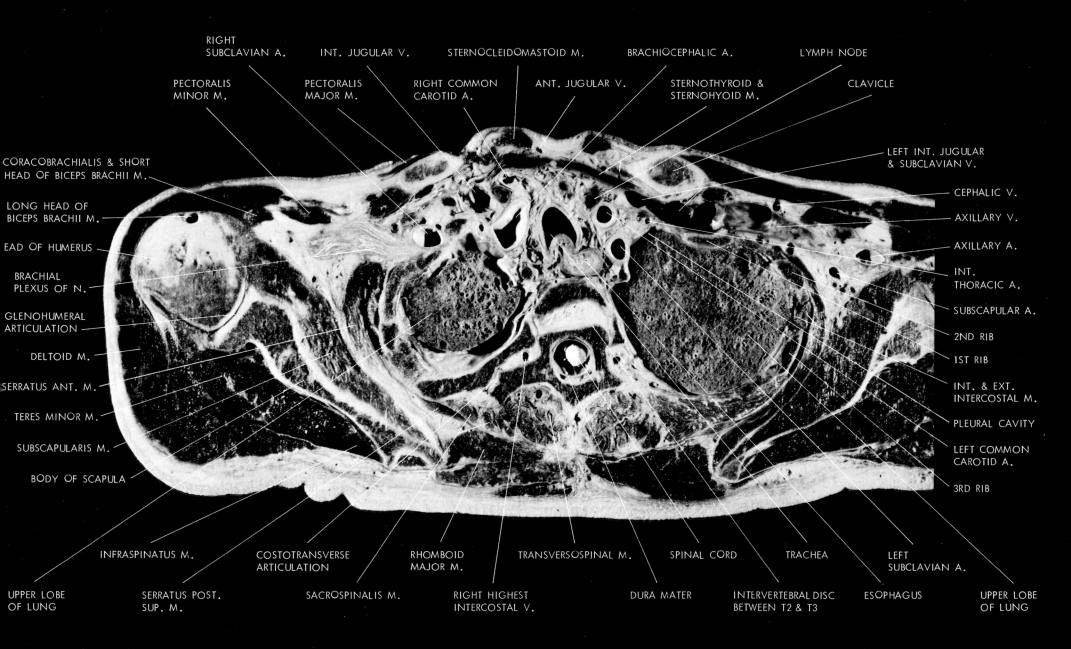

RIGHT SUBCLAVIAN A.

INT. JUGULAR V.

STERNOCLEIDOMASTOID M.

BRACHIOCEPHALIC A.

LYMPH NODE

PECTORALIS MINOR M.

PECTORALIS MAJOR M.

RIGHT COMMON CAROTID A.

ANT. JUGULAR V.

STERNOTHYROID & STERNOHYOID M.

CLAVICLE

CORACOBRACHIALIS & SHORT HEAD OF BICEPS BRACHII M.

LEFT INT. JUGULAR & SUBCLAVIAN V.

LONG HEAD OF BICEPS BRACHII M.

CEPHALIC V.

EAD OF HUMERUS

AXILLARY V.

BRACHIAL PLEXUS OF N.

AXILLARY A.

INT. THORACIC A.

GLENOHUMERAL ARTICULATION

SUBSCAPULAR A.

DELTOID M.

2ND RIB

1ST RIB

SERRATUS ANT. M.

INT. & EXT. INTERCOSTAL M.

TERES MINOR M.

PLEURAL CAVITY

SUBSCAPULARIS M.

LEFT COMMON CAROTID A.

BODY OF SCAPULA

3RD RIB

INFRASPINATUS M.

COSTOTRANSVERSE ARTICULATION

RHOMBOID MAJOR M.

TRANSVERSOSPINAL M.

SPINAL CORD

TRACHEA

LEFT SUBCLAVIAN A.

UPPER LOBE OF LUNG

SERRATUS POST. SUP. M.

SACROSPINALIS M.

RIGHT HIGHEST INTERCOSTAL V.

DURA MATER

INTERVERTEBRAL DISC BETWEEN T2 & T3

ESOPHAGUS

UPPER LOBE OF LUNG

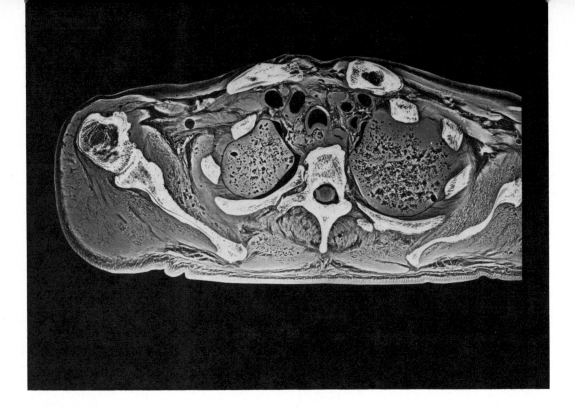

The superior mediastinum can be seen in this section and in several of the following ones. In general, the chief contents of the superior mediastinum are, from anterior to posterior, the large veins, large arteries, trachea, and esophagus. In a young patient the thymus gland would also be present; it would be located anterior to the large veins.

Clinical Considerations

It is important to note in this section that the esophagus is not directly behind the trachea but rather somewhat to its left. This relationship becomes of great importance when dealing with the surgical approach to the esophagus in the treatment of malignancies involving this area.

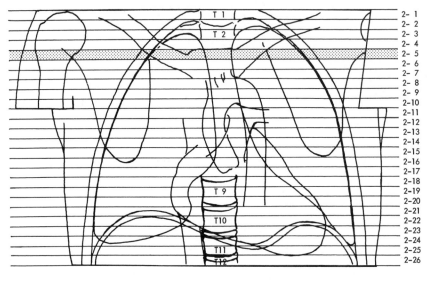

SECTION
2–5

Through the body of T3

Anatomic Considerations

The thoracic cavity can be divided into a median portion (mediastinum) and the laterally located lungs and pleurae. The mediastinum extends superiorly to the thoracic inlet and inferiorly to the diaphragm. The mediastinum is divided into superior and inferior portions by an imaginary plane that extends from the sternal angle (junction of manubrium and body) to the lower portion of the fourth thoracic vertebra. The inferior portion is subdivided into anterior, middle, and posterior mediastina by the pericardium, which forms the middle mediastinum. The anterior mediastinum lies anterior to the pericardium, and the posterior mediastinum lies posterior to the sac of the heart.

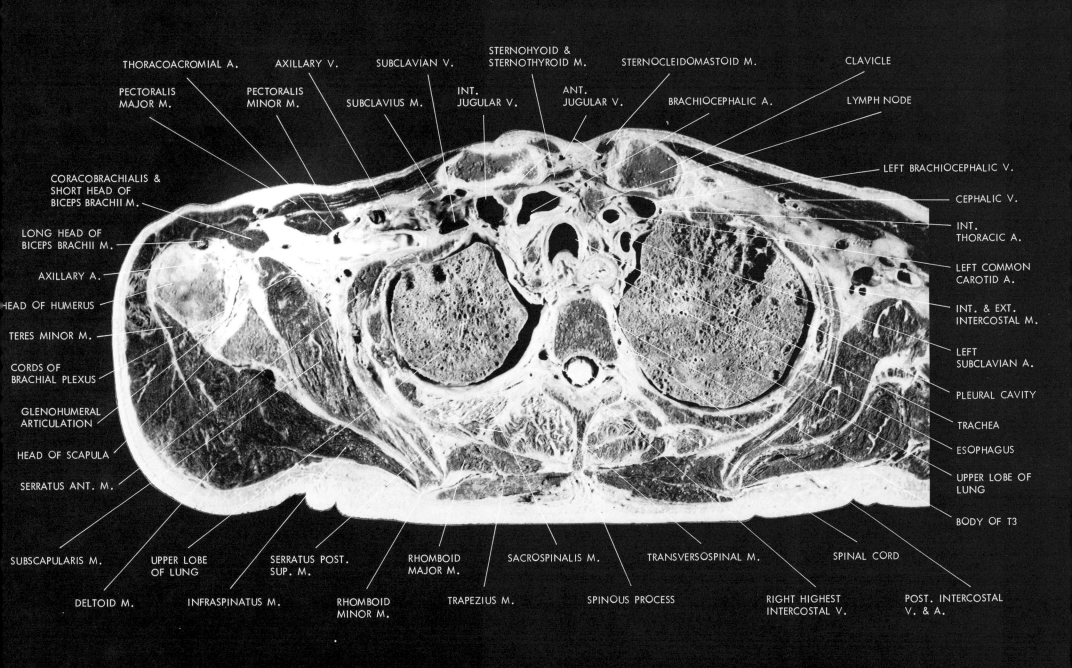

THORACOACROMIAL A.   AXILLARY V.   SUBCLAVIAN V.   STERNOHYOID & STERNOTHYROID M.   STERNOCLEIDOMASTOID M.   CLAVICLE

PECTORALIS MAJOR M.   PECTORALIS MINOR M.   SUBCLAVIUS M.   INT. JUGULAR V.   ANT. JUGULAR V.   BRACHIOCEPHALIC A.   LYMPH NODE

CORACOBRACHIALIS & SHORT HEAD OF BICEPS BRACHII M.

LEFT BRACHIOCEPHALIC V.

CEPHALIC V.

LONG HEAD OF BICEPS BRACHII M.

INT. THORACIC A.

LEFT COMMON CAROTID A.

AXILLARY A.

HEAD OF HUMERUS

INT. & EXT. INTERCOSTAL M.

TERES MINOR M.

LEFT SUBCLAVIAN A.

CORDS OF BRACHIAL PLEXUS

PLEURAL CAVITY

GLENOHUMERAL ARTICULATION

TRACHEA

HEAD OF SCAPULA

ESOPHAGUS

SERRATUS ANT. M.

UPPER LOBE OF LUNG

BODY OF T3

SUBSCAPULARIS M.   UPPER LOBE OF LUNG   SERRATUS POST. SUP. M.   RHOMBOID MAJOR M.   SACROSPINALIS M.   TRANSVERSOSPINAL M.   SPINAL CORD

DELTOID M.   INFRASPINATUS M.   RHOMBOID MINOR M.   TRAPEZIUS M.   SPINOUS PROCESS   RIGHT HIGHEST INTERCOSTAL V.   POST. INTERCOSTAL V. & A.

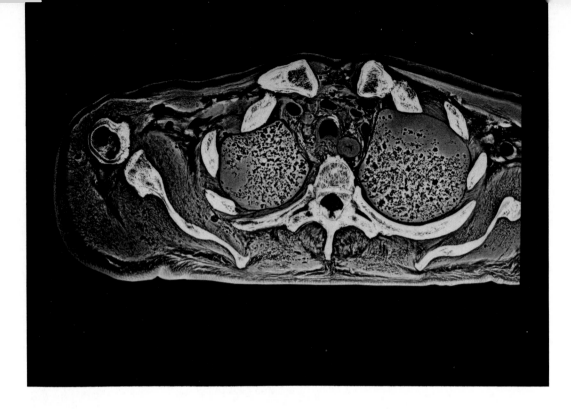

sternoclavicular ligaments. The main attachment of the disc is between the clavicle and the first costal cartilage near the manubrium; this prevents medial displacement of the clavicle onto the sternum.

The costovertebral articulation is divided into two sets of synovial joints. One connects the head of the rib with the vertebral body and intervening intervertebral disc; the other connects the tubercle and neck of the rib with the transverse process. The first set of articulations is observed in all ribs except the 1st, 10th, 11th, and 12th, which articulate with a single vertebra. The second set of articulations is not present in the 11th and 12th ribs.

Clinical Considerations

Paratracheal lymph nodes are frequently involved in the extension of neoplastic processes from the neck downward to the chest, or in bronchogenic carcinomas involving the mediastinum. It is important to establish the normality of size of these nodes and their relationships to contiguous structures whenever these lesions may be encountered.

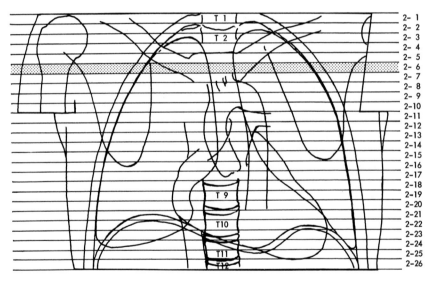

SECTION 2-6

Through the intervertebral disc between T3 and T4

Anatomic Considerations

In this illustration the sternoclavicular and the costovertebral articulations can be observed.

The sternoclavicular articulation is a synovial joint. The medial end of the clavicle articulates with the clavicular notch of the manubrium and the superior surface of the first costal cartilage. This is the only articulation between the upper extremity and the axial skeleton. The wide range of movement at the shoulder joint is due to the position of the clavicle between the shoulder and the manubrium. The articular capsule is thickened anteriorly and posteriorly, forming the anterior and posterior sternoclavicular ligaments. Other ligaments that give support to the joint are the interclavicular and costoclavicular ligaments. The synovial cavity is divided into two parts by an articular disc that is continuous with the anterior and posterior

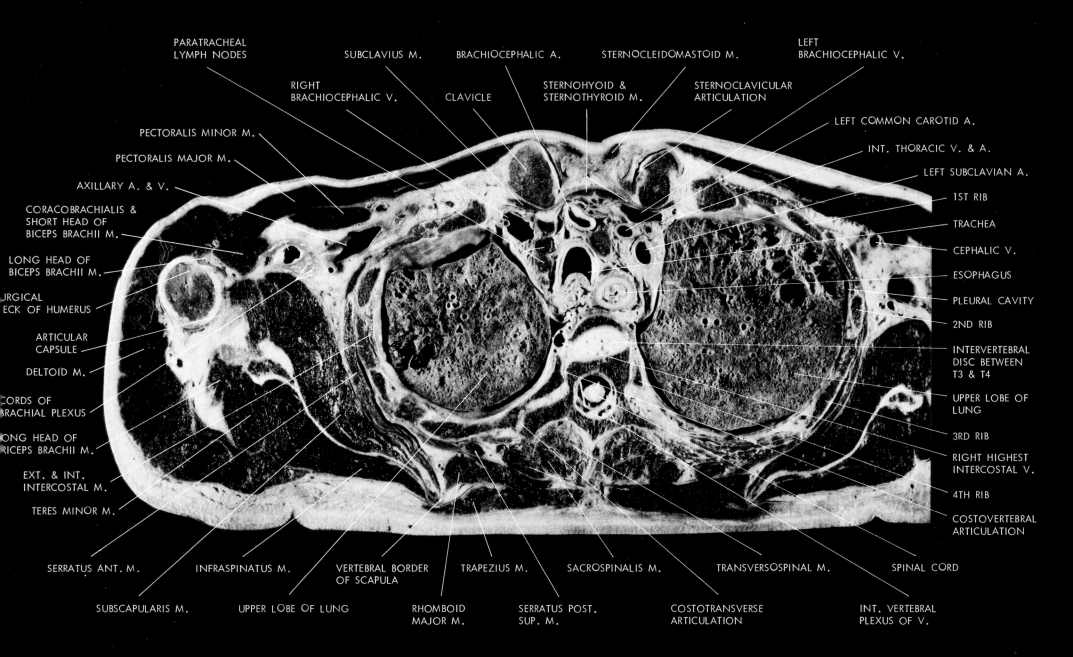

PARATRACHEAL LYMPH NODES

SUBCLAVIUS M.

BRACHIOCEPHALIC A.

STERNOCLEIDOMASTOID M.

LEFT BRACHIOCEPHALIC V.

RIGHT BRACHIOCEPHALIC V.

CLAVICLE

STERNOHYOID & STERNOTHYROID M.

STERNOCLAVICULAR ARTICULATION

LEFT COMMON CAROTID A.

INT. THORACIC V. & A.

PECTORALIS MINOR M.

PECTORALIS MAJOR M.

AXILLARY A. & V.

CORACOBRACHIALIS & SHORT HEAD OF BICEPS BRACHII M.

LONG HEAD OF BICEPS BRACHII M.

URGICAL ECK OF HUMERUS

ARTICULAR CAPSULE

DELTOID M.

CORDS OF BRACHIAL PLEXUS

ONG HEAD OF RICEPS BRACHII M.

EXT. & INT. INTERCOSTAL M.

TERES MINOR M.

LEFT SUBCLAVIAN A.

1ST RIB

TRACHEA

CEPHALIC V.

ESOPHAGUS

PLEURAL CAVITY

2ND RIB

INTERVERTEBRAL DISC BETWEEN T3 & T4

UPPER LOBE OF LUNG

3RD RIB

RIGHT HIGHEST INTERCOSTAL V.

4TH RIB

COSTOVERTEBRAL ARTICULATION

SERRATUS ANT. M.

INFRASPINATUS M.

VERTEBRAL BORDER OF SCAPULA

TRAPEZIUS M.

SACROSPINALIS M.

TRANSVERSOSPINAL M.

SPINAL CORD

SUBSCAPULARIS M.

UPPER LOBE OF LUNG

RHOMBOID MAJOR M.

SERRATUS POST. SUP. M.

COSTOTRANSVERSE ARTICULATION

INT. VERTEBRAL PLEXUS OF V.

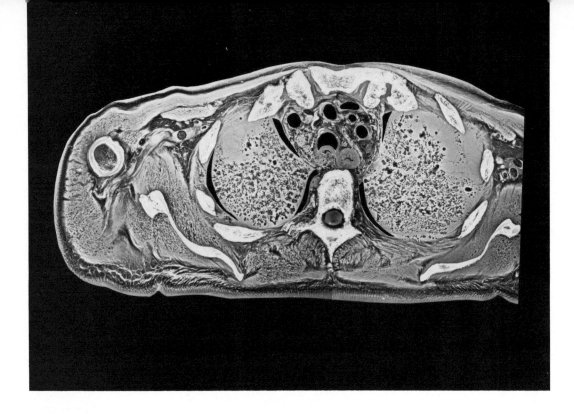

arise from the convexity of the arch of the aorta. These three branches can be observed in this section. The left brachiocephalic vein crosses anterior to these arteries, close to their origins.

Clinical Considerations

The proximity of the pectoralis muscles to the axillary arteries and veins, as well as to the brachial plexus, may serve to explain the difficulties a surgeon at times encounters with radical breast resections, when avoidance of these vital structures is imperative. Removal of the pectoralis muscles is likewise important in an effort to remove the full extent of the carcinomatous disease. These patients not infrequently will develop lymphedema with considerable discomfort. At times defects in component parts of the brachial plexus may also develop.

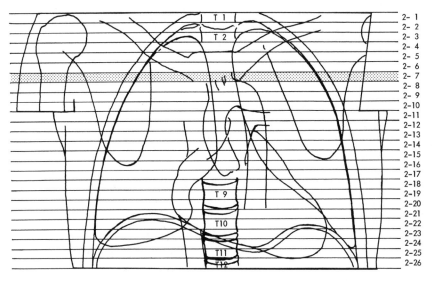

SECTION 2-7

Through the body of T4

Anatomic Considerations

A portion of the wall of the arch of the aorta can be seen in this illustration. The entire arch can be observed in this section through Section 2–9. The arch of the aorta begins at the level of the second sternocostal articulation as a continuation of the ascending aorta (Section 2–10). After a short ascent to the right, the aorta bends to the left around the trachea and then turns inferiorly and posteriorly. As the arch of the aorta reaches the vertebral column, it becomes continuous with the descending aorta. This usually occurs at the level of T4; in this specimen, however, the descending aorta is first seen at T5.

The brachiocephalic, left common carotid, and left subclavian arteries

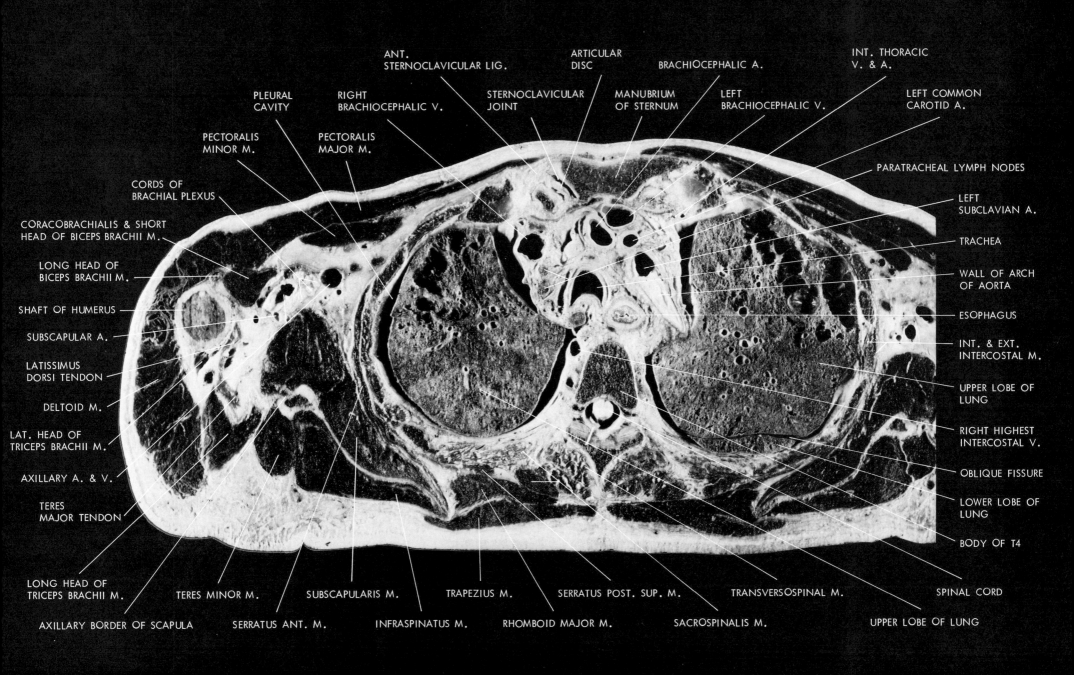

ANT.
STERNOCLAVICULAR LIG.

ARTICULAR
DISC

BRACHIOCEPHALIC A.

INT. THORACIC
V. & A.

PLEURAL
CAVITY

RIGHT
BRACHIOCEPHALIC V.

STERNOCLAVICULAR
JOINT

MANUBRIUM
OF STERNUM

LEFT
BRACHIOCEPHALIC V.

LEFT COMMON
CAROTID A.

PECTORALIS
MINOR M.

PECTORALIS
MAJOR M.

PARATRACHEAL LYMPH NODES

CORDS OF
BRACHIAL PLEXUS

LEFT
SUBCLAVIAN A.

CORACOBRACHIALIS & SHORT
HEAD OF BICEPS BRACHII M.

TRACHEA

LONG HEAD OF
BICEPS BRACHII M.

WALL OF ARCH
OF AORTA

SHAFT OF HUMERUS

ESOPHAGUS

SUBSCAPULAR A.

INT. & EXT.
INTERCOSTAL M.

LATISSIMUS
DORSI TENDON

DELTOID M.

UPPER LOBE OF
LUNG

LAT. HEAD OF
TRICEPS BRACHII M.

RIGHT HIGHEST
INTERCOSTAL V.

AXILLARY A. & V.

OBLIQUE FISSURE

TERES
MAJOR TENDON

LOWER LOBE OF
LUNG

BODY OF T4

LONG HEAD OF
TRICEPS BRACHII M.

TERES MINOR M.

SUBSCAPULARIS M.

TRAPEZIUS M.

SERRATUS POST. SUP. M.

TRANSVERSOSPINAL M.

SPINAL CORD

AXILLARY BORDER OF SCAPULA

SERRATUS ANT. M.

INFRASPINATUS M.

RHOMBOID MAJOR M.

SACROSPINALIS M.

UPPER LOBE OF LUNG

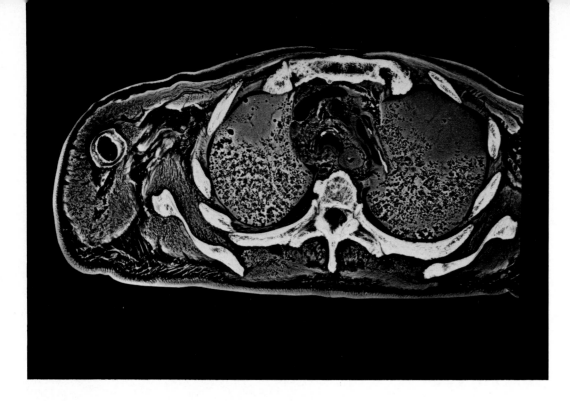

terminates behind the cartilage of the first rib. Posteriorly it is related to the brachiocephalic, left common carotid, and left subclavian arteries.

The right brachiocephalic vein is formed posterior to the sternoclavicular joint and passes inferior to join the left brachiocephalic vein to form the superior vena cava.

The brachiocephalic veins are formed by the union of the internal jugular and subclavian veins.

Clinical Considerations

Even with a 2-second computed tomographic exposure, the arch of the aorta is readily identified as the oblique structure shown herein, when intensified with contrast media. Its contiguity to the esophagus, which is almost in the same sheath as the descending thoracic aorta at lower levels, is shown in good relationship here. The esophagus too can be intensified with a weak barium paste intermixed with honey.

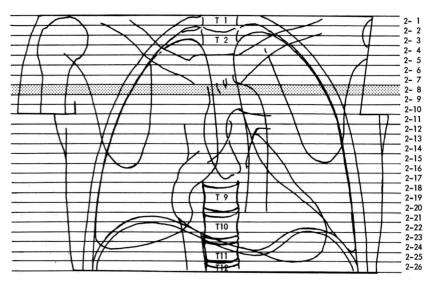

SECTION 2-8

Through the intervertebral disc between T4 and T5

Anatomic Considerations

In this illustration and in Sections 2–9 to 2–16 the superior vena cava can be seen. It is formed by the junction of the right and left brachiocephalic veins. The termination of the left brachiocephalic vein also can be observed. The superior vena cava begins deep to the cartilage of the first rib close to the sternum and terminates in the right atrium at the level of the third right costal cartilage. The inferior portion of the vena cava is within the pericardium. Prior to entering the pericardium, it receives the azygos vein and small mediastinal veins.

The left brachiocephalic vein is longer than the right and begins posterior to the sternal end of the clavicle, passes obliquely behind the manubrium, and

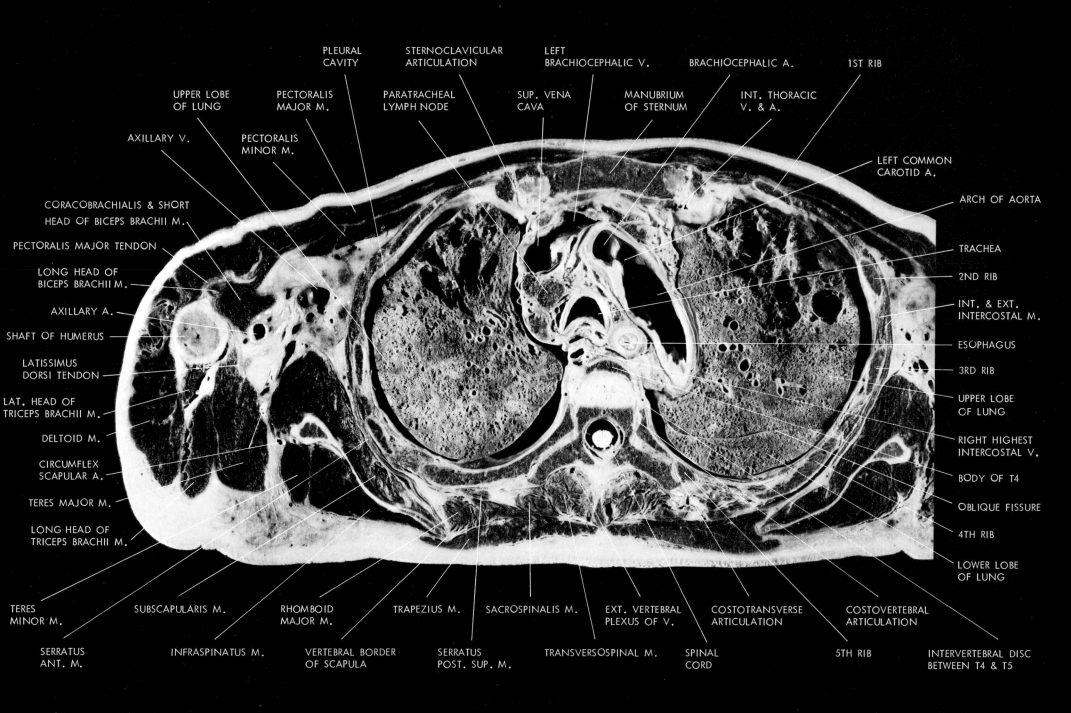

PLEURAL
CAVITY

STERNOCLAVICULAR
ARTICULATION

LEFT
BRACHIOCEPHALIC V.

BRACHIOCEPHALIC A.

1ST RIB

UPPER LOBE
OF LUNG

PECTORALIS
MAJOR M.

PARATRACHEAL
LYMPH NODE

SUP. VENA
CAVA

MANUBRIUM
OF STERNUM

INT. THORACIC
V. & A.

AXILLARY V.

PECTORALIS
MINOR M.

LEFT COMMON
CAROTID A.

CORACOBRACHIALIS & SHORT
HEAD OF BICEPS BRACHII M.

ARCH OF AORTA

PECTORALIS MAJOR TENDON

TRACHEA

LONG HEAD OF
BICEPS BRACHII M.

2ND RIB

AXILLARY A.

INT. & EXT.
INTERCOSTAL M.

SHAFT OF HUMERUS

ESOPHAGUS

LATISSIMUS
DORSI TENDON

3RD RIB

LAT. HEAD OF
TRICEPS BRACHII M.

UPPER LOBE
OF LUNG

DELTOID M.

RIGHT HIGHEST
INTERCOSTAL V.

CIRCUMFLEX
SCAPULAR A.

BODY OF T4

TERES MAJOR M.

OBLIQUE FISSURE

LONG HEAD OF
TRICEPS BRACHII M.

4TH RIB

LOWER LOBE
OF LUNG

TERES
MINOR M.

SUBSCAPULARIS M.

RHOMBOID
MAJOR M.

TRAPEZIUS M.

SACROSPINALIS M.

EXT. VERTEBRAL
PLEXUS OF V.

COSTOTRANSVERSE
ARTICULATION

COSTOVERTEBRAL
ARTICULATION

SERRATUS
ANT. M.

INFRASPINATUS M.

VERTEBRAL BORDER
OF SCAPULA

SERRATUS
POST. SUP. M.

TRANSVERSOSPINAL M.

SPINAL
CORD

5TH RIB

INTERVERTEBRAL DISC
BETWEEN T4 & T5

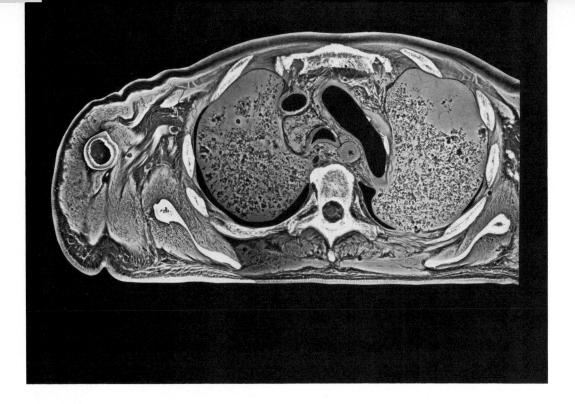

reflections of areas of the parietal pleura with adjacent areas constitute the lines of pleural reflection.

Clinical Considerations

The close proximity of paratracheal lymph nodes to the superior vena cava, as shown in this section, is often related to the superior vena caval block syndrome. In this condition a neoplastic or inflammatory process may produce an obstruction of the superior vena cava, with considerable swelling of the structures cephalad to this. The proximity of these lymph nodes to the superior vena cava can be readily identified with appropriate contrast enhancement.

This section also is valuable in the staging of lymphomatous involvement, since involvement of the paratracheal lymph nodes is readily detected and important for inclusion in treatment by the radiotherapist.

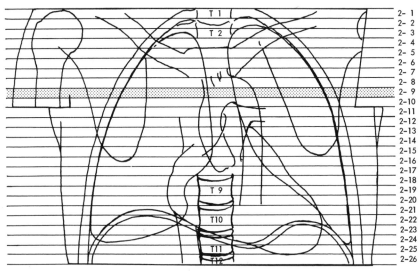

SECTION 2–9

Through the body of T5

Anatomic Considerations

The pleura consists of two layers of serous membranes that form a closed sac around a lung. The outer layer of serous membrane is the parietal pleura, which lines the thoracic cavity and is adjacent to the deep fascia of the thoracic wall (endothoracic fascia). The inner layer, which is adherent to the lung tissue, is the visceral one. The pleural cavity is the space between the two layers of serous membranes. The parietal pleura is divided into costal, mediastinal, cervical, and diaphragmatic portions, on the basis of the relationships of the pleura to surrounding structures. In this illustration both the costal and the mediastinal portions of the pleura can be observed. The

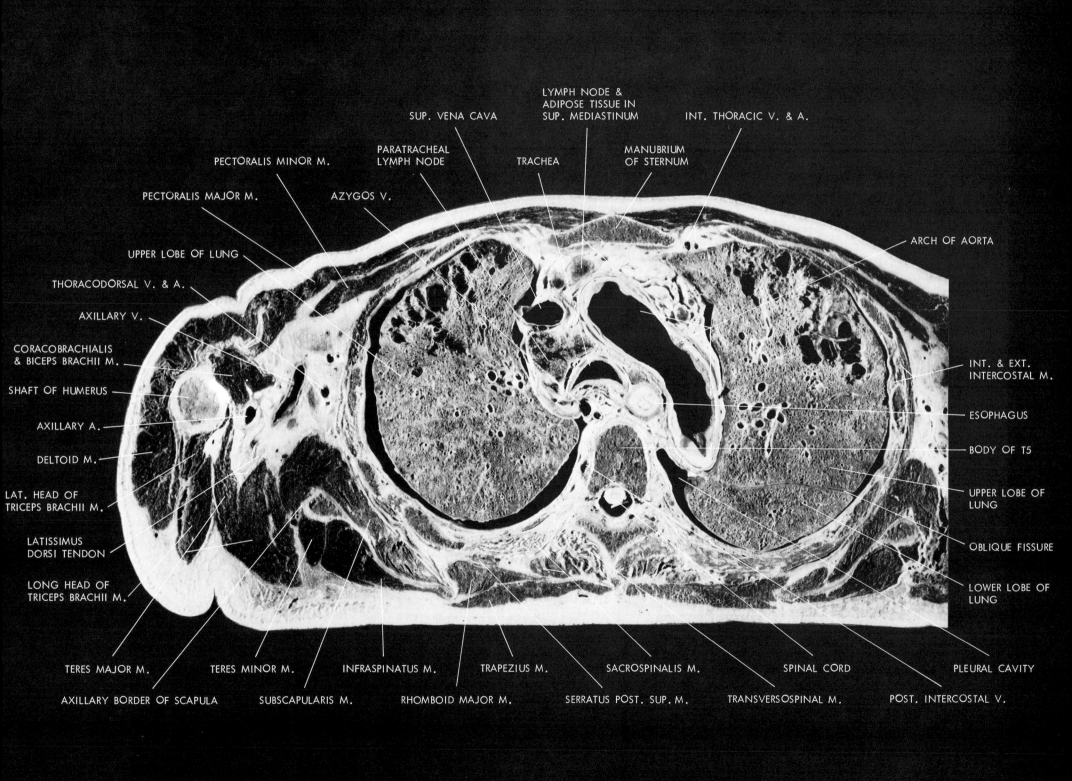

LYMPH NODE &
ADIPOSE TISSUE IN
SUP. MEDIASTINUM

SUP. VENA CAVA

INT. THORACIC V. & A.

PECTORALIS MINOR M.

PARATRACHEAL
LYMPH NODE

TRACHEA

MANUBRIUM
OF STERNUM

PECTORALIS MAJOR M.

AZYGOS V.

ARCH OF AORTA

UPPER LOBE OF LUNG

THORACODORSAL V. & A.

AXILLARY V.

CORACOBRACHIALIS
& BICEPS BRACHII M.

INT. & EXT.
INTERCOSTAL M.

SHAFT OF HUMERUS

ESOPHAGUS

AXILLARY A.

BODY OF T5

DELTOID M.

UPPER LOBE OF
LUNG

LAT. HEAD OF
TRICEPS BRACHII M.

LATISSIMUS
DORSI TENDON

OBLIQUE FISSURE

LONG HEAD OF
TRICEPS BRACHII M.

LOWER LOBE OF
LUNG

TERES MAJOR M.

TERES MINOR M.

INFRASPINATUS M.

TRAPEZIUS M.

SACROSPINALIS M.

SPINAL CORD

PLEURAL CAVITY

AXILLARY BORDER OF SCAPULA

SUBSCAPULARIS M.

RHOMBOID MAJOR M.

SERRATUS POST. SUP. M.

TRANSVERSOSPINAL M.

POST. INTERCOSTAL V.

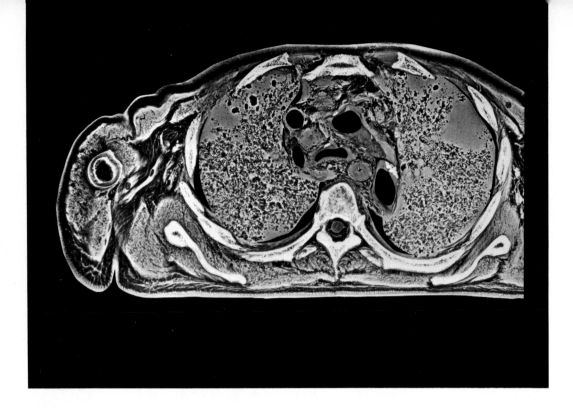

Anterior to the ascending aorta is a considerable amount of adipose tissue, which may undergo neoplastic alteration, giving rise to lipomas of the mediastinum.

Aneurysms of the ascending aorta ordinarily enlarge to the right and anteriorly, encroaching upon the adipose tissue and enlarging to the right of the superior vena cava anteriorly. Aneurysms of the aorta may become so large that they even erode the sternum.

The level of the bifurcation of the trachea is particularly important clinically in patients who have undergone tracheal intubation. Ordinarily, the ideal position for the distal end of the intratracheal tube is approximately 4 cm above this level, since further extension may lead to obstruction, particularly of the left bronchus.

Measurements have been made of this portion of the azygos vein (sometimes referred to as the azygos arch), and in the erect, fully expanded lung the distance between the right main stem bronchus and the outermost margin of the azygos vein ordinarily does not exceed 6 or 8 mm. Certainly a measurement beyond 10 mm must be taken as an indicator of possible "venous back-up" into the azygos system, suggesting right-sided heart failure or enlargement of the azygos lymph node.

This lung is abnormal in that it contains numerous cysts or cavity-like structures and is probably emphysematous.

The close relationship between the descending thoracic aorta and esophagus has considerable radiologic importance when one studies frontal radiographs with the esophagus outlined by barium, which also outlines the posterior margin of the left atrium.

SECTION 2–10

Through the intervertebral disc between T5 and T6

Anatomic Considerations

The azygos vein begins in the abdomen opposite vertebra L1 or L2 either by an extension of the ascending lumbar vein or from a branch of the renal vein or from a branch of the inferior vena cava. Usually entering the thorax through the right side of the aortic hiatus, it passes superiorly along the right side of the vertebral column and arches forward over the root of the lung to join the superior vena cava, which can be seen in this illustration. The azygos vein has many tributaries: (1) the right superior intercostal vein, (2) the right lower posterior intercostal and right subcostal veins, (3) the hemiazygos and frequently the accessory hemiazygos veins, (4) bronchial veins, and (5) occasionally esophageal and pericardial veins.

Because of the extensive communication of the azygos and hemiazygos veins, they have a vital role in collateral circulation in the event the venae cavae are obstructed.

Clinical Considerations

Between the ascending aorta and bifurcation of the trachea are lymph nodes of considerable importance, since these lymph nodes are so frequently involved with malignant lymphomas and bronchogenic carcinoma.

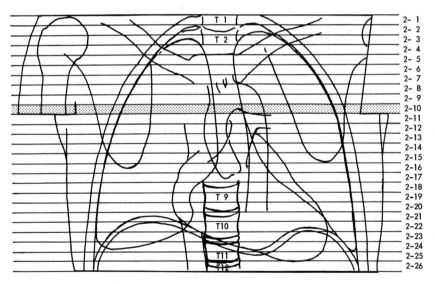

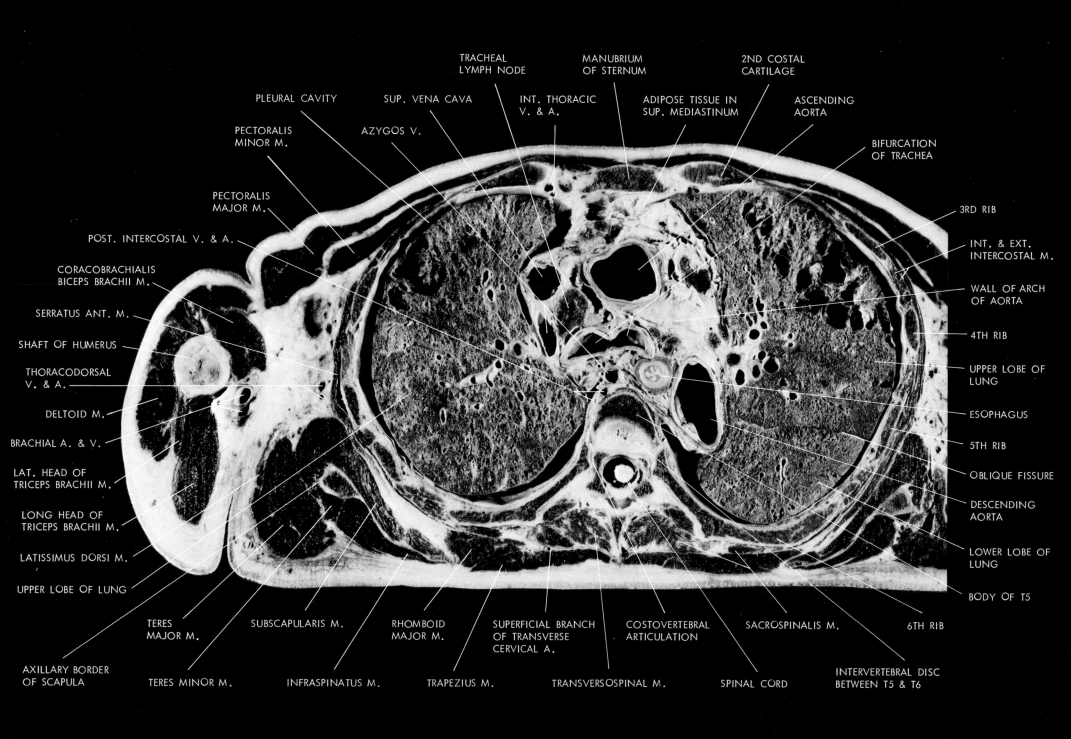

TRACHEAL
LYMPH NODE

MANUBRIUM
OF STERNUM

2ND COSTAL
CARTILAGE

PLEURAL CAVITY

SUP. VENA CAVA

INT. THORACIC
V. & A.

ADIPOSE TISSUE IN
SUP. MEDIASTINUM

ASCENDING
AORTA

PECTORALIS
MINOR M.

AZYGOS V.

BIFURCATION
OF TRACHEA

PECTORALIS
MAJOR M.

3RD RIB

POST. INTERCOSTAL V. & A.

INT. & EXT.
INTERCOSTAL M.

CORACOBRACHIALIS
BICEPS BRACHII M.

WALL OF ARCH
OF AORTA

SERRATUS ANT. M.

4TH RIB

SHAFT OF HUMERUS

UPPER LOBE OF
LUNG

THORACODORSAL
V. & A.

ESOPHAGUS

DELTOID M.

5TH RIB

BRACHIAL A. & V.

OBLIQUE FISSURE

LAT. HEAD OF
TRICEPS BRACHII M.

DESCENDING
AORTA

LONG HEAD OF
TRICEPS BRACHII M.

LOWER LOBE OF
LUNG

LATISSIMUS DORSI M.

UPPER LOBE OF LUNG

BODY OF T5

TERES
MAJOR M.

SUBSCAPULARIS M.

RHOMBOID
MAJOR M.

SUPERFICIAL BRANCH
OF TRANSVERSE
CERVICAL A.

COSTOVERTEBRAL
ARTICULATION

SACROSPINALIS M.

6TH RIB

AXILLARY BORDER
OF SCAPULA

TERES MINOR M.

INFRASPINATUS M.

TRAPEZIUS M.

TRANSVERSOSPINAL M.

SPINAL CORD

INTERVERTEBRAL DISC
BETWEEN T5 & T6

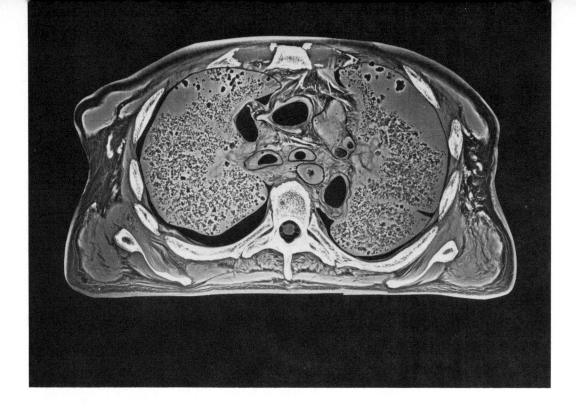

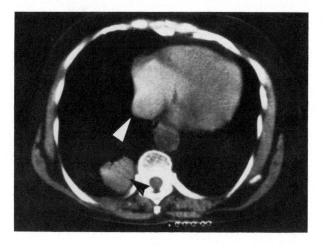

ance, since it is closely attached at this level with the base of the heart and the visceral pericardium. With the accumulation of fluid, the space between the parietal and visceral pericardia becomes increased by a substance of fluid density detectable not only by ultrasound but also by computed tomography. The azygos in this section is seen in axial plane since it is coming from left to right to join the superior vena cava. It lies just anterior to the vertebral body (T6) at this level. This is part of the arch of the azygos mentioned in connection with Section 2–10.

One must note that, although the bronchi and even the pulmonary arteries are beginning to make their appearance at this level, the pulmonary veins enter the thoracic cage much more caudad, to empty into the left atrium.

SECTION 2–11

Through the upper portion of the body of T6

Anatomic Considerations

The right lung has three lobes that are separated by an oblique and a horizontal fissure. The left lung is divided into two lobes by an oblique fissure. Each lung has a base, apex, costal surface, and mediastinal surface. The structures entering the hilum of the lung can be seen in this illustration and in several of the adjacent sections. The primary or principal bronchi, one for each lung, arise from the bifurcation of the trachea. In this specimen, the trachea bifurcates at the body of the fifth thoracic vertebra (see Section 2–10).

Clinical Considerations

The CT scan of the thorax shows lung carcinoma, primary in the right hilus (white arrow), and metastases in the lungs — right more than left. The 5 cm sphere is in the right posterior medial lung (black arrow); metastases are in the right upper lobe.

The position of lymph nodes in the mediastinum is extremely important clinically; lymph nodes are ordinarily designated by the structure contiguous with them. For example, the lymph nodes adjoining the trachea are "paratracheal"; those lying between the trachea and bronchus, "tracheobronchial"; those lying around a bronchus and juxtaposed, "peribronchial." On occasion there may also be very small lymph nodes in the lung substance *per se*; these are called "intrapulmonary."

In the cadaveric section the parietal pericardium also makes its appear-

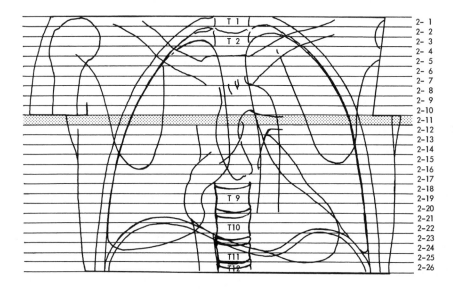

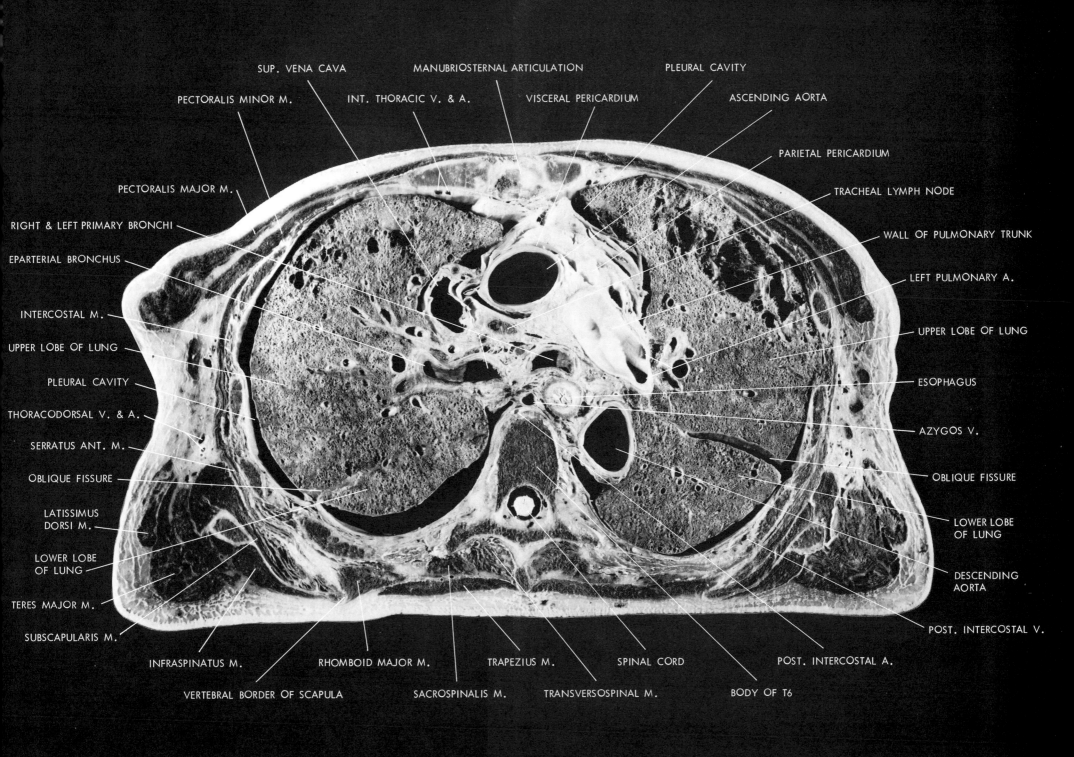

SUP. VENA CAVA

MANUBRIOSTERNAL ARTICULATION

PLEURAL CAVITY

PECTORALIS MINOR M.

INT. THORACIC V. & A.

VISCERAL PERICARDIUM

ASCENDING AORTA

PARIETAL PERICARDIUM

PECTORALIS MAJOR M.

TRACHEAL LYMPH NODE

RIGHT & LEFT PRIMARY BRONCHI

WALL OF PULMONARY TRUNK

EPARTERIAL BRONCHUS

LEFT PULMONARY A.

INTERCOSTAL M.

UPPER LOBE OF LUNG

UPPER LOBE OF LUNG

ESOPHAGUS

PLEURAL CAVITY

THORACODORSAL V. & A.

AZYGOS V.

SERRATUS ANT. M.

OBLIQUE FISSURE

OBLIQUE FISSURE

LATISSIMUS DORSI M.

LOWER LOBE OF LUNG

LOWER LOBE OF LUNG

DESCENDING AORTA

TERES MAJOR M.

POST. INTERCOSTAL V.

SUBSCAPULARIS M.

INFRASPINATUS M.

RHOMBOID MAJOR M.

TRAPEZIUS M.

SPINAL CORD

POST. INTERCOSTAL A.

VERTEBRAL BORDER OF SCAPULA

SACROSPINALIS M.

TRANSVERSOSPINAL M.

BODY OF T6

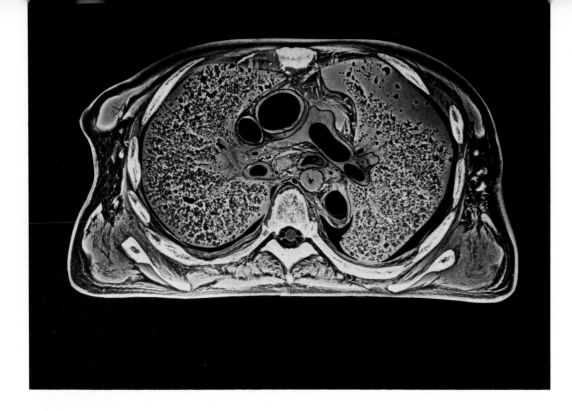

the pulmonary artery may be visualized in 4 to 6 seconds, whereas the aorta is not visualized until 2 to 4 seconds later. Thus there is a place for very rapid bolus injection in cross-sectional contrast enhancement.

The pericardial cavity as shown here is actually a potential cavity with the parietal and visceral pericardia being closely adherent during life. The cavity becomes most apparent when filled with fluid or air, which can readily be detected by computed tomography (or by conventional radiography if a gaseous medium is involved).

The left and right bronchi can be visualized herein, with the right bronchus slightly posterior to the left. These can be readily differentiated from vascular structures when contrast enhancement is employed.

Although thymic structure is not shown in this section, it could easily be visualized at this level if the thymus were enlarged (Mink et al., 1978). Discovery of a thymoma in a patient with myasthenia gravis makes surgical intervention mandatory, since often an etiologic relationship exists between the two. Most mediastinal thymomas lie anterior to or just below the aortic arch in the anterior mediastinum.

Note the curvilinear shape of the oblique fissure of the left lung. In lateral radiography, this shadow may become thickened or intensified by fluid and appear plaquelike.

Mink JH, Bein ME, Sukov R, Herrmann C Jr, Winter J, Sample WF, and Mulder D: Computed tomography of the anterior mediastinum in patients with myasthenia gravis and suspected thymoma. AJR 130:239–246, 1978.

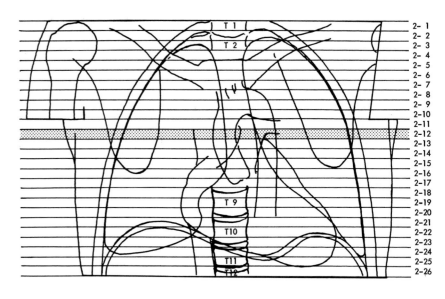

SECTION
2–12

Through the lower portion of the body of T6

Anatomic Considerations

The internal thoracic artery arises from the first part of the subclavian artery and passes through the thoracic inlet posterior to the clavicle and first costal cartilage. It passes posterior to the upper six costal cartilages 1 cm from the edge of the sternum. The artery ends at the sixth intercostal space by dividing into the superior epigastric and musculophrenic arteries. In addition to branches to the mediastinum, it gives off the anterior intercostal and perforating arteries.

The internal thoracic veins drain the areas supplied by the arteries and terminate in the corresponding brachiocephalic veins.

Clinical Considerations

The relative relationships of the right pulmonary artery, superior vena cava, and ascending aorta are particularly noteworthy in the right anterior mediastinum. The pulmonary artery may be intensified with contrast enhancement, as are the superior vena cava and ascending aorta; with rapid bolus injection,

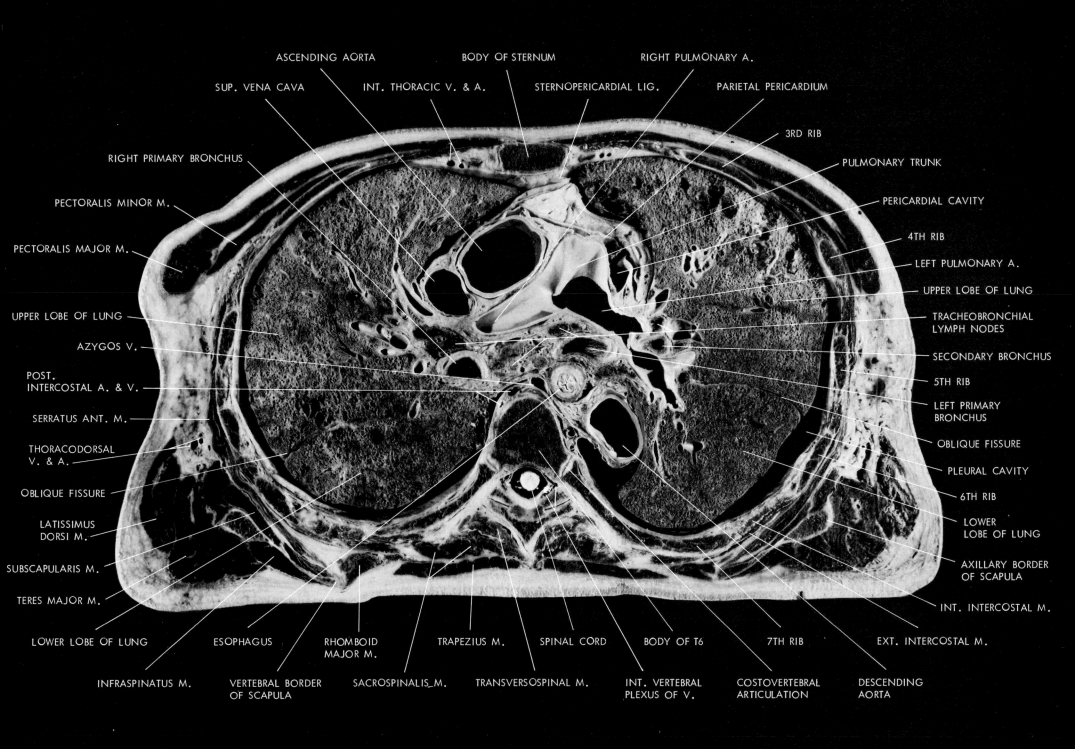

ASCENDING AORTA

BODY OF STERNUM

RIGHT PULMONARY A.

SUP. VENA CAVA

INT. THORACIC V. & A.

STERNOPERICARDIAL LIG.

PARIETAL PERICARDIUM

3RD RIB

PULMONARY TRUNK

RIGHT PRIMARY BRONCHUS

PERICARDIAL CAVITY

PECTORALIS MINOR M.

4TH RIB

PECTORALIS MAJOR M.

LEFT PULMONARY A.

UPPER LOBE OF LUNG

UPPER LOBE OF LUNG

TRACHEOBRONCHIAL
LYMPH NODES

AZYGOS V.

SECONDARY BRONCHUS

POST.
INTERCOSTAL A. & V.

5TH RIB

LEFT PRIMARY
BRONCHUS

SERRATUS ANT. M.

THORACODORSAL
V. & A.

OBLIQUE FISSURE

OBLIQUE FISSURE

PLEURAL CAVITY

LATISSIMUS
DORSI M.

6TH RIB

SUBSCAPULARIS M.

LOWER
LOBE OF LUNG

AXILLARY BORDER
OF SCAPULA

TERES MAJOR M.

INT. INTERCOSTAL M.

LOWER LOBE OF LUNG

ESOPHAGUS

RHOMBOID
MAJOR M.

TRAPEZIUS M.

SPINAL CORD

BODY OF T6

7TH RIB

EXT. INTERCOSTAL M.

DESCENDING
AORTA

INFRASPINATUS M.

VERTEBRAL BORDER
OF SCAPULA

SACROSPINALIS_M.

TRANSVERSOSPINAL M.

INT. VERTEBRAL
PLEXUS OF V.

COSTOVERTEBRAL
ARTICULATION

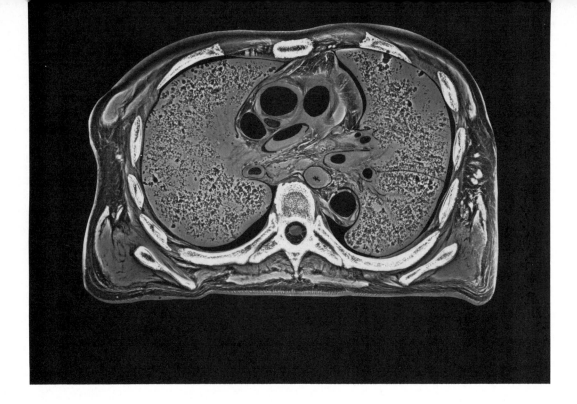

Clinical Considerations

It sometimes might not be best to study nodular lesions within the lung parenchyma by this cross-sectional mode. Scholten and Kreel (1977) have examined the axial distribution of lung metastases as seen radiologically at autopsy. Generally, spherical metastases with well-defined edges could be distinguished from metastases with more irregular edges. Some metastases contained cavitation (the latter was seen in three cases of adenocarcinoma). In general the investigators concluded that metastases were found at the lung periphery in most instances, regardless of their size or whether they had either the well- or ill-defined margins and regardless of the origin of the tumor. Although occasional metastases may be seen with computed tomography that are not detected otherwise, the exact role of computed tomography has not as yet been determined in this study. The metastases most apt to be missed by conventional radiography are those that are juxtapleural.

Scholten ET and Kreel L: Distribution of lung metastases in the axial plane: A combined radiologic–pathologic study. Radiol Clin (Basel) 46:248–265, 1977.

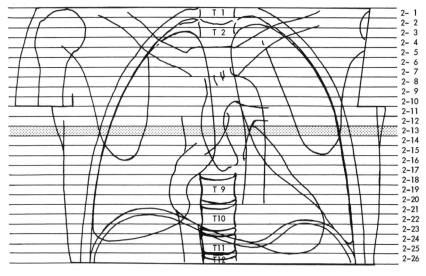

SECTION 2–13

Through the upper portion of the body of T7

Anatomic Considerations

The esophagus, which is approximately 22 to 25 cm long, can be followed in Sections 2–1 to 2–25. It begins at the level of the cricoid cartilage; passes through the neck, the superior and posterior mediastina, the diaphragm at vertebral level T10; and 1.5 cm inferior to that point enters the cardiac orifice of the stomach.

In the illustrations it can be observed that the esophagus has numerous relations throughout its course. Some of these will be considered at this time. The trachea (Sections 2–1 to 2–4), left bronchus (Sections 2–10 to 2–13), and left atrium (Sections 2–14 to 2–19) are anterior. The arch of the aorta is to the left (Sections 2–7 to 2–9). In Sections 2–10 to 2–25, the relation of the thoracic aorta to the esophagus can be seen; the aorta is at first to the left and then gradually passes posteriorly. Other posterior relations are the longus colli muscles (Sections 2–1 to 2–2), the bodies of the thoracic vertebrae (Sections 2–3 to 2–23), and the azygos vein (Sections 2–5 to 2–24). In Sections 2–9 to 2–14 the azygos vein is to the right of the esophagus. The trachea is to the right of the esophagus (Section 2–5) to its bifurcation (Section 2–9). The narrowest parts of the esophagus are at its origin, where the left bronchus crosses it, and at its termination.

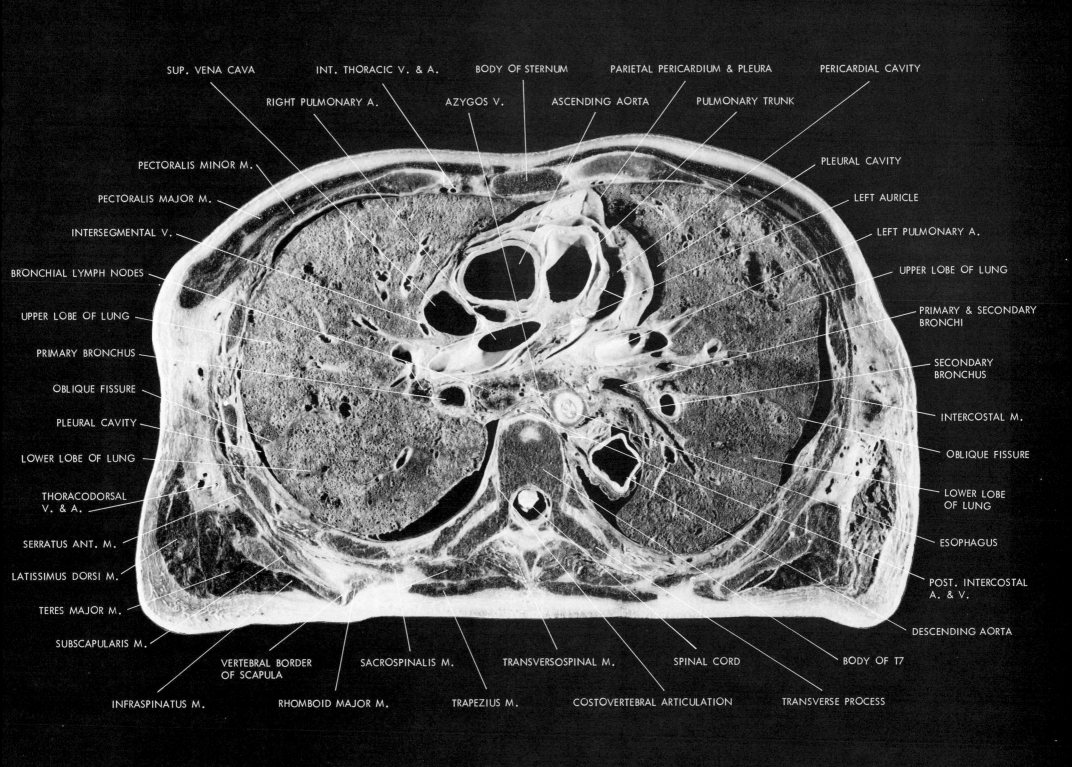

SUP. VENA CAVA

INT. THORACIC V. & A.

BODY OF STERNUM

PARIETAL PERICARDIUM & PLEURA

PERICARDIAL CAVITY

RIGHT PULMONARY A.

AZYGOS V.

ASCENDING AORTA

PULMONARY TRUNK

PECTORALIS MINOR M.

PLEURAL CAVITY

PECTORALIS MAJOR M.

LEFT AURICLE

INTERSEGMENTAL V.

LEFT PULMONARY A.

BRONCHIAL LYMPH NODES

UPPER LOBE OF LUNG

UPPER LOBE OF LUNG

PRIMARY & SECONDARY BRONCHI

PRIMARY BRONCHUS

SECONDARY BRONCHUS

OBLIQUE FISSURE

PLEURAL CAVITY

INTERCOSTAL M.

LOWER LOBE OF LUNG

OBLIQUE FISSURE

THORACODORSAL V. & A.

LOWER LOBE OF LUNG

SERRATUS ANT. M.

ESOPHAGUS

LATISSIMUS DORSI M.

POST. INTERCOSTAL A. & V.

TERES MAJOR M.

DESCENDING AORTA

SUBSCAPULARIS M.

VERTEBRAL BORDER OF SCAPULA

SACROSPINALIS M.

TRANSVERSOSPINAL M.

SPINAL CORD

BODY OF T7

INFRASPINATUS M.

RHOMBOID MAJOR M.

TRAPEZIUS M.

COSTOVERTEBRAL ARTICULATION

TRANSVERSE PROCESS

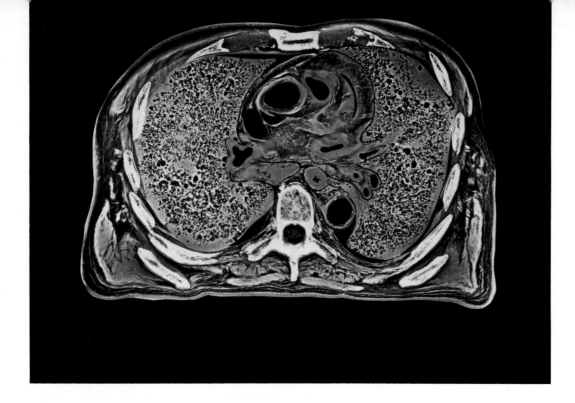

Clinical Considerations

In this section the left auricle is seen to excellent advantage. Its close relationship to the left atrium is likewise visualized and it will be noted that it is actually an appendage of the left atrium. The close proximity of the esophagus to the left atrium is likewise important, the esophagus lying virtually midway between the left atrium and the descending thoracic aorta. As the left atrium becomes enlarged, as in patients with mitral valvular disease, the esophagus is displaced posteriorly toward the descending aorta. It is this displacement that allows us to differentiate enlargement of the left atrium and mitral valvular disease.

The relationship between the ascending aorta and pulmonary trunk must be borne in mind constantly. The two are almost at the same level, but generally the pulmonary artery courses slightly anterior and to the left of the ascending aorta.

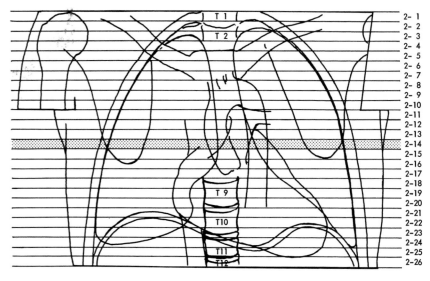

SECTION
2-14

Through the lower portion of the body of T7

Anatomic Considerations

The pericardium is the sac that encloses the heart and great vessels. It consists of an outer fibrous layer and a serous component. The serous layer directly adjacent to the heart is the visceral pericardium (epicardium); the serous layer of the fibrous sac is the parietal pericardium. The pericardial cavity is the space between the two serous layers. This cavity normally contains a small amount of fluid that acts as a lubricant to facilitate movement of the heart.

This cadaveric section shows the transverse sinus, which is a passage that lies between the reflection of serous pericardium around the aorta and pulmonary trunk and the reflection around the large veins.

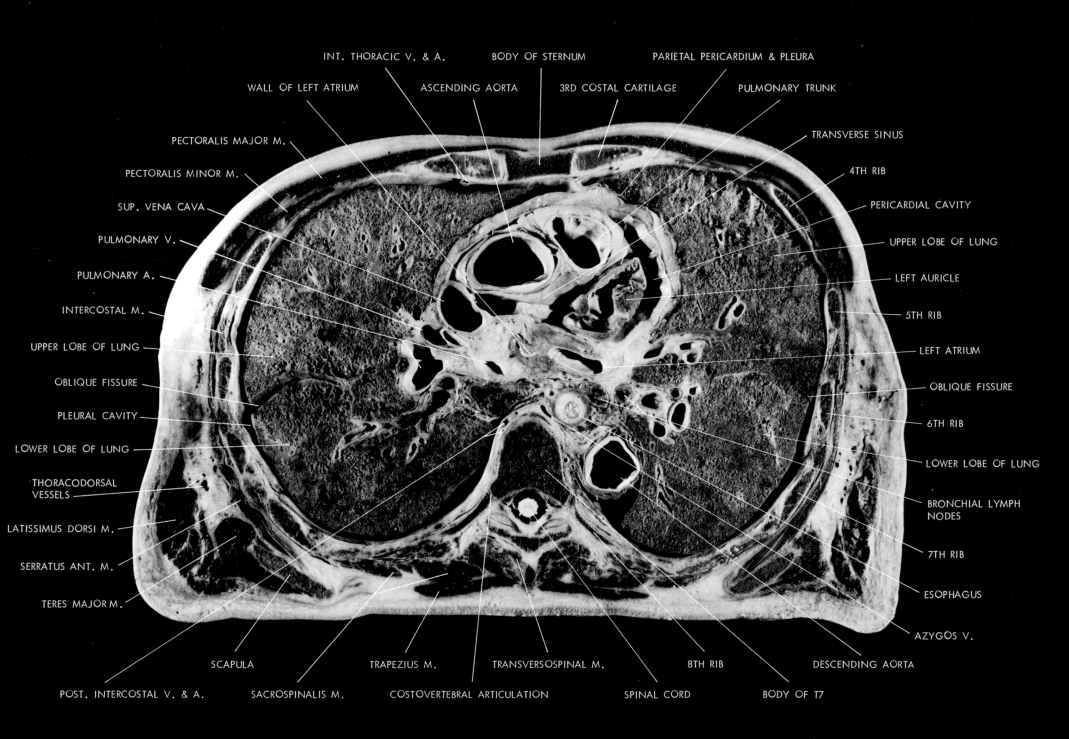

INT. THORACIC V. & A.

BODY OF STERNUM

PARIETAL PERICARDIUM & PLEURA

WALL OF LEFT ATRIUM

ASCENDING AORTA

3RD COSTAL CARTILAGE

PULMONARY TRUNK

PECTORALIS MAJOR M.

TRANSVERSE SINUS

PECTORALIS MINOR M.

4TH RIB

SUP. VENA CAVA

PERICARDIAL CAVITY

PULMONARY V.

UPPER LOBE OF LUNG

PULMONARY A.

LEFT AURICLE

INTERCOSTAL M.

5TH RIB

UPPER LOBE OF LUNG

LEFT ATRIUM

OBLIQUE FISSURE

OBLIQUE FISSURE

PLEURAL CAVITY

6TH RIB

LOWER LOBE OF LUNG

LOWER LOBE OF LUNG

THORACODORSAL
VESSELS

BRONCHIAL LYMPH
NODES

LATISSIMUS DORSI M.

7TH RIB

SERRATUS ANT. M.

ESOPHAGUS

TERES MAJOR M.

AZYGOS V.

SCAPULA

TRAPEZIUS M.

TRANSVERSOSPINAL M.

8TH RIB

DESCENDING AORTA

POST. INTERCOSTAL V. & A.

SACROSPINALIS M.

COSTOVERTEBRAL ARTICULATION

SPINAL CORD

BODY OF T7

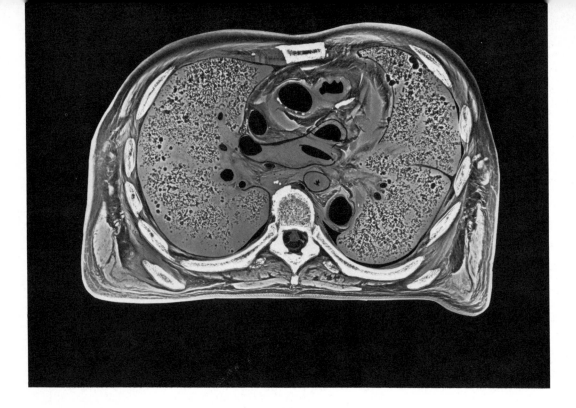

Clinical Considerations

In this section the pulmonary veins are coming into better view as they empty into the left atrium. No longer are the pulmonary arteries and their larger branches visualized. The pulmonary trunk, however, is actually slightly anterior to and to the left of the ascending aorta.

The student must bear in mind constantly the important relationship of all the vascular structures as visualized herein: the superior vena cava, the ascending aorta, the pulmonary trunk, the left atrium, the pulmonary veins, and the descending thoracic aorta, with the azygos vein just anterior and medial to the esophagus. Since the esophagus is so closely adjacent to the left atrium, it can readily be understood why enlargements of the left atrium affect the esophagus more readily than do elongations or tortuosities of the aorta.

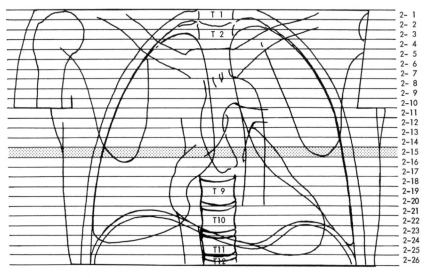

SECTION
2–15

Through the intervertebral disc between T7 and T8

Anatomic Considerations

The base of the heart (Sections 2–14 to 2–19) is formed primarily by the left atrium, some of the right atrium, and the proximal portions of the pulmonary veins and arteries. It is bounded by the bifurcation of the pulmonary trunk superiorly, the coronary sinus inferiorly, the sulcus terminalis on the right, and the oblique vein of the atrium on the left. In this specimen the base is separated from the bodies of the vertebrae by the esophagus and partly by the azygos vein. The thoracic aorta, which is considered a posterior relation of the base, is located more to the left of the bodies of the vertebrae. The four pulmonary veins and the superior and inferior venae cavae enter the base of the heart.

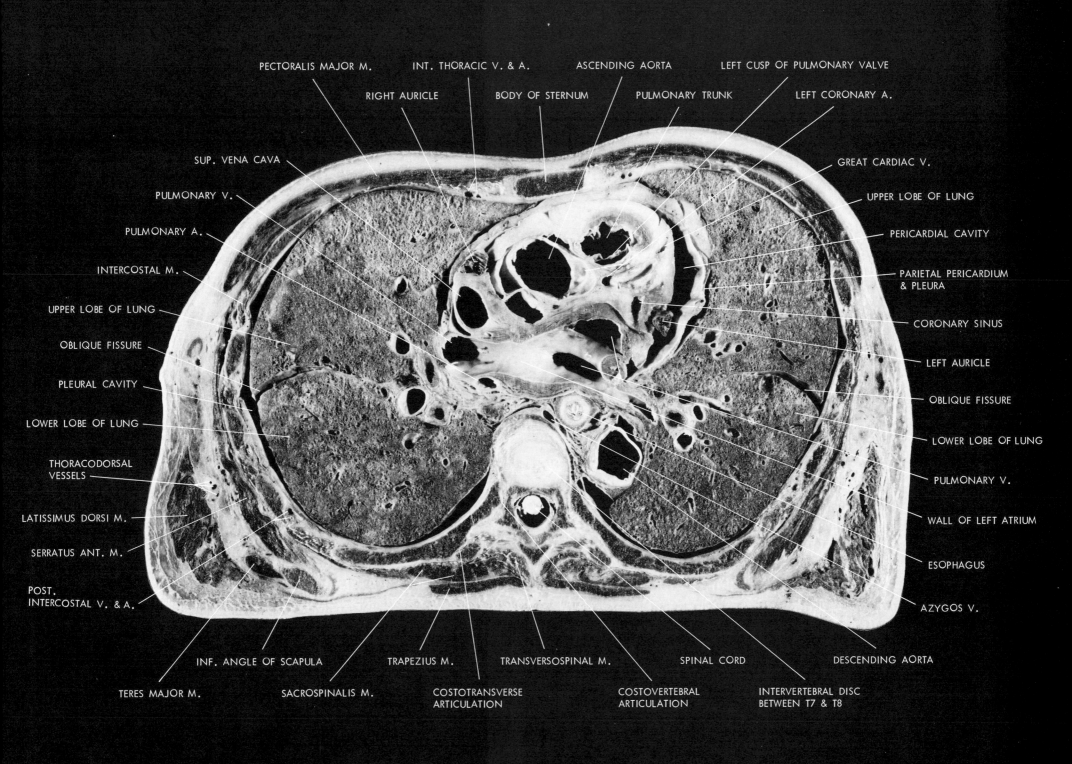

PECTORALIS MAJOR M.   INT. THORACIC V. & A.   ASCENDING AORTA   LEFT CUSP OF PULMONARY VALVE

RIGHT AURICLE   BODY OF STERNUM   PULMONARY TRUNK   LEFT CORONARY A.

SUP. VENA CAVA

GREAT CARDIAC V.

PULMONARY V.

UPPER LOBE OF LUNG

PULMONARY A.

PERICARDIAL CAVITY

INTERCOSTAL M.

PARIETAL PERICARDIUM & PLEURA

UPPER LOBE OF LUNG

CORONARY SINUS

OBLIQUE FISSURE

LEFT AURICLE

PLEURAL CAVITY

OBLIQUE FISSURE

LOWER LOBE OF LUNG

LOWER LOBE OF LUNG

THORACODORSAL VESSELS

PULMONARY V.

LATISSIMUS DORSI M.

WALL OF LEFT ATRIUM

SERRATUS ANT. M.

ESOPHAGUS

POST. INTERCOSTAL V. & A.

AZYGOS V.

INF. ANGLE OF SCAPULA   TRAPEZIUS M.   TRANSVERSOSPINAL M.   SPINAL CORD   DESCENDING AORTA

TERES MAJOR M.   SACROSPINALIS M.   COSTOTRANSVERSE ARTICULATION   COSTOVERTEBRAL ARTICULATION   INTERVERTEBRAL DISC BETWEEN T7 & T8

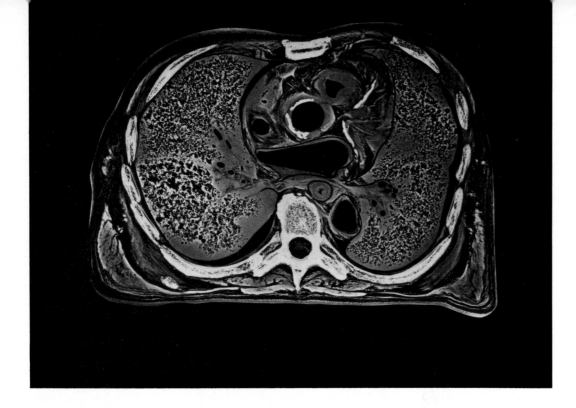

anterior descending interventricular branch and a circumflex one. The right coronary artery supplies the right atrium and right ventricle. The left coronary artery supplies the left atrium and both ventricles.

Clinical Considerations

In this section the right ventricle first makes its appearance. The wall of the left ventricle can be identified, but its cavity is not yet in evidence. Hence contrast enhancement can differentiate the two.

Note the coronary sinus and its close proximity to the branches of the pulmonary veins as they proceed anteriorly to empty into the left atrium.

In this section one begins to see the uppermost portion of the right atrium just anterior to the superior vena cava.

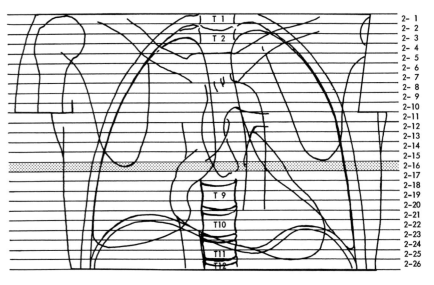

SECTION
2–16

Through the body of T8

Anatomic Considerations

The blood supply to the heart is provided by the right and left coronary arteries. These arteries and some of their branches can be seen in several of the following sections. The right and left coronary arteries arise from the aorta just superior to the aortic valve. The right coronary artery runs forward between the pulmonary trunk and right auricle and then descends in the right atrioventricular groove; the artery then courses to the left on the diaphragmatic surface of the heart and ends beyond the interventricular groove. The left coronary artery courses under the left auricle and then bifurcates into an

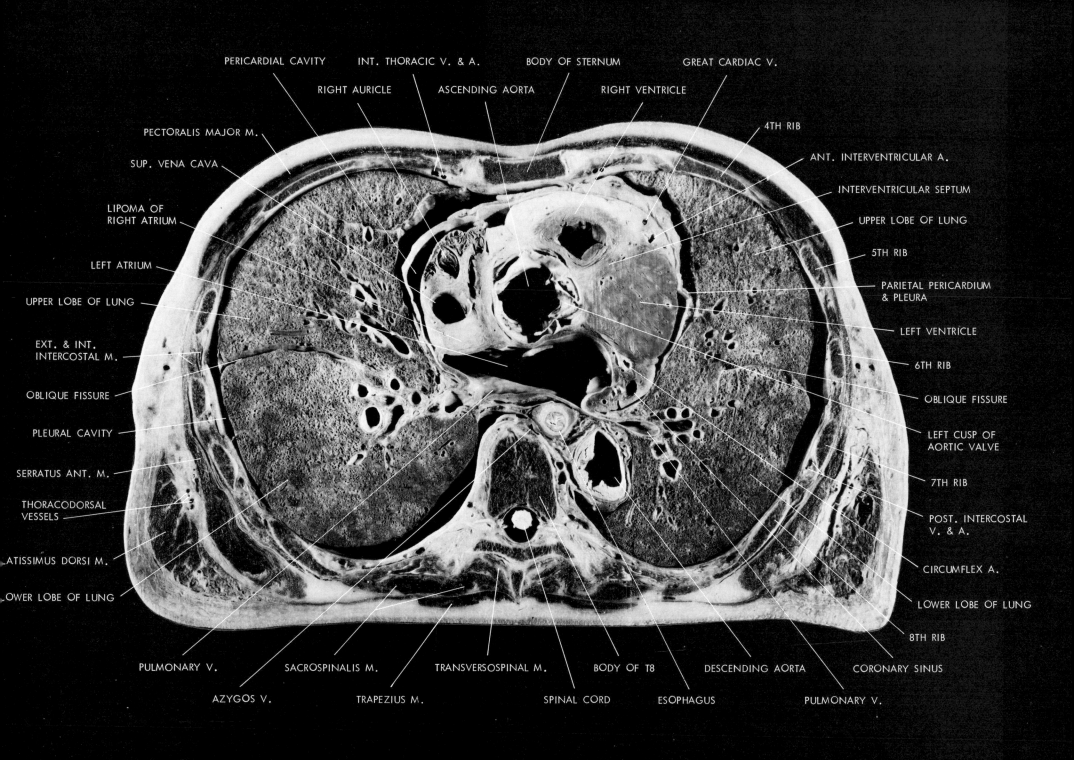

PERICARDIAL CAVITY INT. THORACIC V. & A. BODY OF STERNUM GREAT CARDIAC V.

RIGHT AURICLE ASCENDING AORTA RIGHT VENTRICLE

PECTORALIS MAJOR M. 4TH RIB

ANT. INTERVENTRICULAR A.

SUP. VENA CAVA INTERVENTRICULAR SEPTUM

LIPOMA OF UPPER LOBE OF LUNG
RIGHT ATRIUM

5TH RIB

LEFT ATRIUM

PARIETAL PERICARDIUM
& PLEURA

UPPER LOBE OF LUNG

LEFT VENTRICLE

EXT. & INT. 6TH RIB
INTERCOSTAL M.

OBLIQUE FISSURE OBLIQUE FISSURE

PLEURAL CAVITY LEFT CUSP OF
AORTIC VALVE

SERRATUS ANT. M. 7TH RIB

THORACODORSAL
VESSELS POST. INTERCOSTAL
V. & A.

ATISSIMUS DORSI M. CIRCUMFLEX A.

OWER LOBE OF LUNG LOWER LOBE OF LUNG

8TH RIB

PULMONARY V. SACROSPINALIS M. TRANSVERSOSPINAL M. BODY OF T8 DESCENDING AORTA CORONARY SINUS

AZYGOS V. TRAPEZIUS M. SPINAL CORD ESOPHAGUS PULMONARY V.

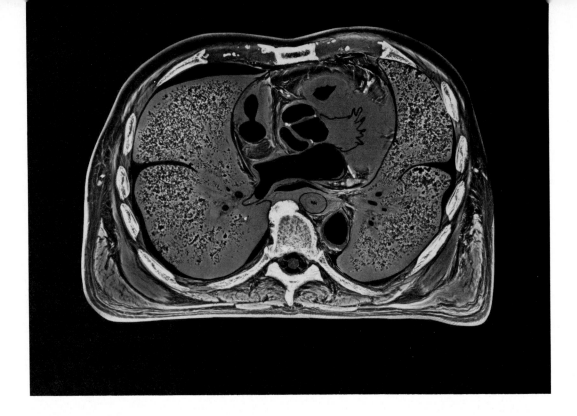

those of the pulmonary trunk. The valvules of the pulmonary trunk are called anterior, right, and left; those of the aorta are called posterior, right, and left.

Clinical Considerations

At this level, the right atrium, the right ventricle, and the left atrium are seen as sizable chambers. The left ventricle with its various trabeculae is just barely in evidence.

The student at this point must be alerted once again to the close proximity of the esophagus to the left atrium and the somewhat greater distance between the esophagus and the descending thoracic aorta. The pulmonary veins are posteriorly situated, emptying into the left atrium.

The right coronary artery is occluded in this specimen.

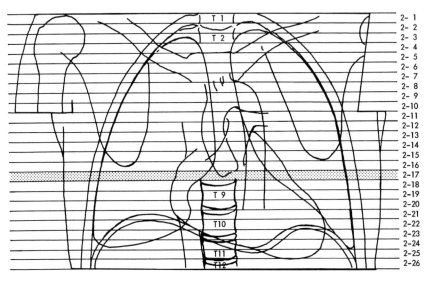

SECTION 2–17

Through the intervertebral disc between T8 and T9

Anatomic Considerations

The orifices of the aortic and pulmonary trunks are guarded by semilunar valves, which can be seen in this illustration and in Sections 2–15 and 2–16. Each orifice has three semilunar valves, which are formed by a duplication of the endocardial lining. Each consists of a free margin with a thickening at the center (the nodule) and the free margins on each side of the nodule (the lunules). Between the valves and the wall of the vessels are the sinuses.

The valves associated with the aorta are larger, thicker, and stronger than

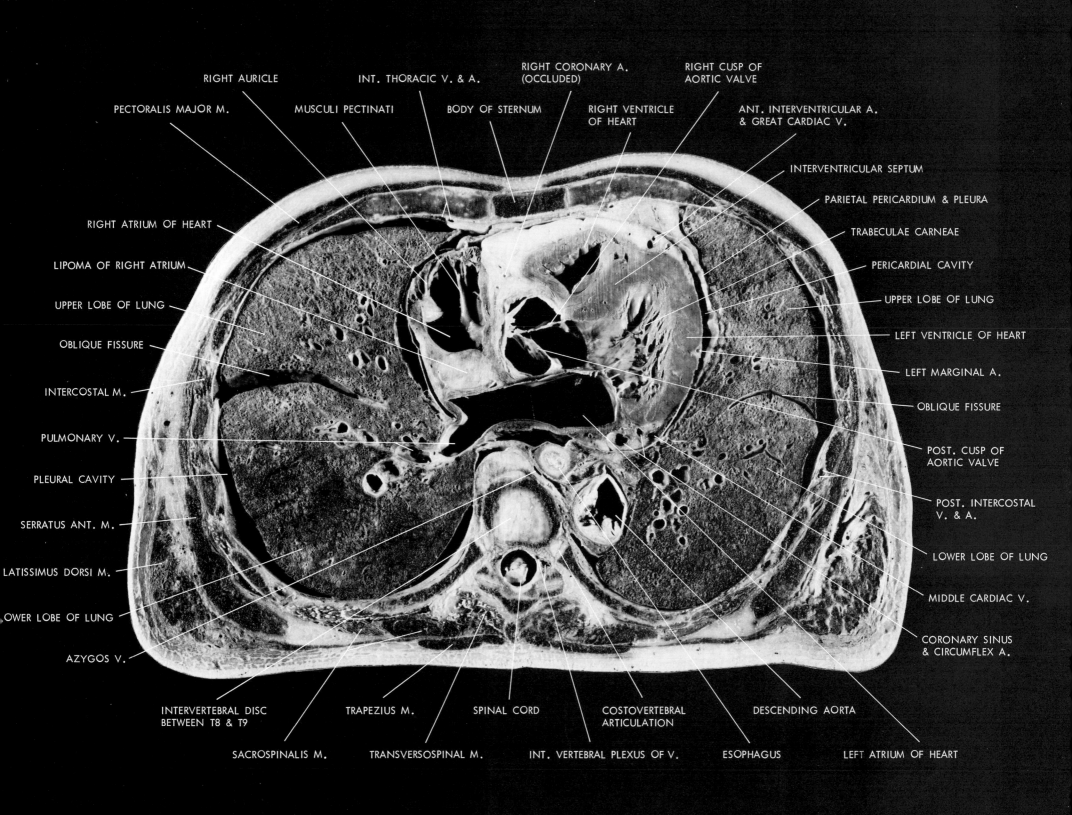

RIGHT AURICLE

INT. THORACIC V. & A.

RIGHT CORONARY A.
(OCCLUDED)

RIGHT CUSP OF
AORTIC VALVE

PECTORALIS MAJOR M.

MUSCULI PECTINATI

BODY OF STERNUM

RIGHT VENTRICLE
OF HEART

ANT. INTERVENTRICULAR A.
& GREAT CARDIAC V.

INTERVENTRICULAR SEPTUM

PARIETAL PERICARDIUM & PLEURA

TRABECULAE CARNEAE

RIGHT ATRIUM OF HEART

LIPOMA OF RIGHT ATRIUM

PERICARDIAL CAVITY

UPPER LOBE OF LUNG

UPPER LOBE OF LUNG

LEFT VENTRICLE OF HEART

OBLIQUE FISSURE

LEFT MARGINAL A.

OBLIQUE FISSURE

INTERCOSTAL M.

PULMONARY V.

POST. CUSP OF
AORTIC VALVE

PLEURAL CAVITY

POST. INTERCOSTAL
V. & A.

SERRATUS ANT. M.

LOWER LOBE OF LUNG

LATISSIMUS DORSI M.

MIDDLE CARDIAC V.

OWER LOBE OF LUNG

CORONARY SINUS
& CIRCUMFLEX A.

AZYGOS V.

INTERVERTEBRAL DISC
BETWEEN T8 & T9

TRAPEZIUS M.

SPINAL CORD

COSTOVERTEBRAL
ARTICULATION

DESCENDING AORTA

SACROSPINALIS M.

TRANSVERSOSPINAL M.

INT. VERTEBRAL PLEXUS OF V.

ESOPHAGUS

LEFT ATRIUM OF HEART

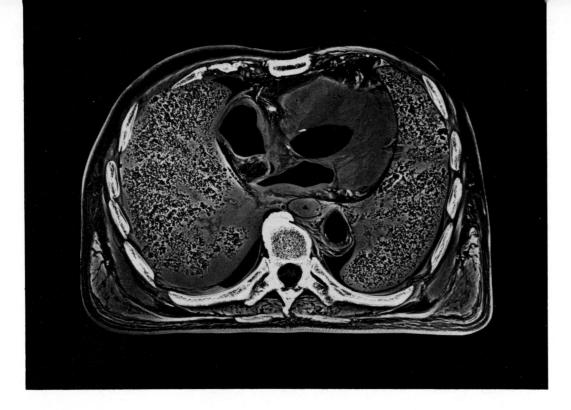

The left ventricle is approximately three times as thick as the right, and the wall is thickest around the widest portion of the cavity.

Clinical Considerations

In this section the wall of the right atrium seems quite thickly separated from the other chambers of the heart. The interventricular septum can also be differentiated, and even on 2-second computed tomography these separations may be manifested despite the pulsations of the heart.

On the other hand, the differentiation of the left ventricle and left atrium is much more difficult and the minimal blurring of a 2-second exposure could readily obscure this barrier.

Note the sigmoidal shape of the fissures in both lungs.

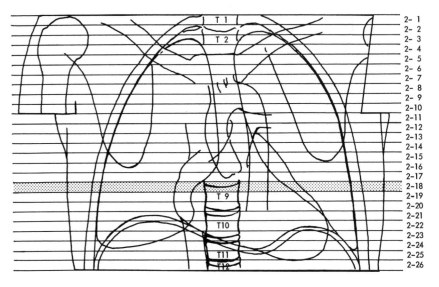

SECTION
2–18

Through the upper portion of the body of T9

Anatomic Considerations

In this section the four chambers of the heart are well defined. The atrial portion of the heart is divided into two chambers by the interatrial septum. This septum passes obliquely from the anterior wall backwards, so the right atrium lies anterior and to the right and the left atrium posterior and to the left. The ventricular portion of the heart is also divided into two chambers by the interventricular septum. It passes obliquely so the right ventricle lies anterior and the left ventricle posterior and to the left.

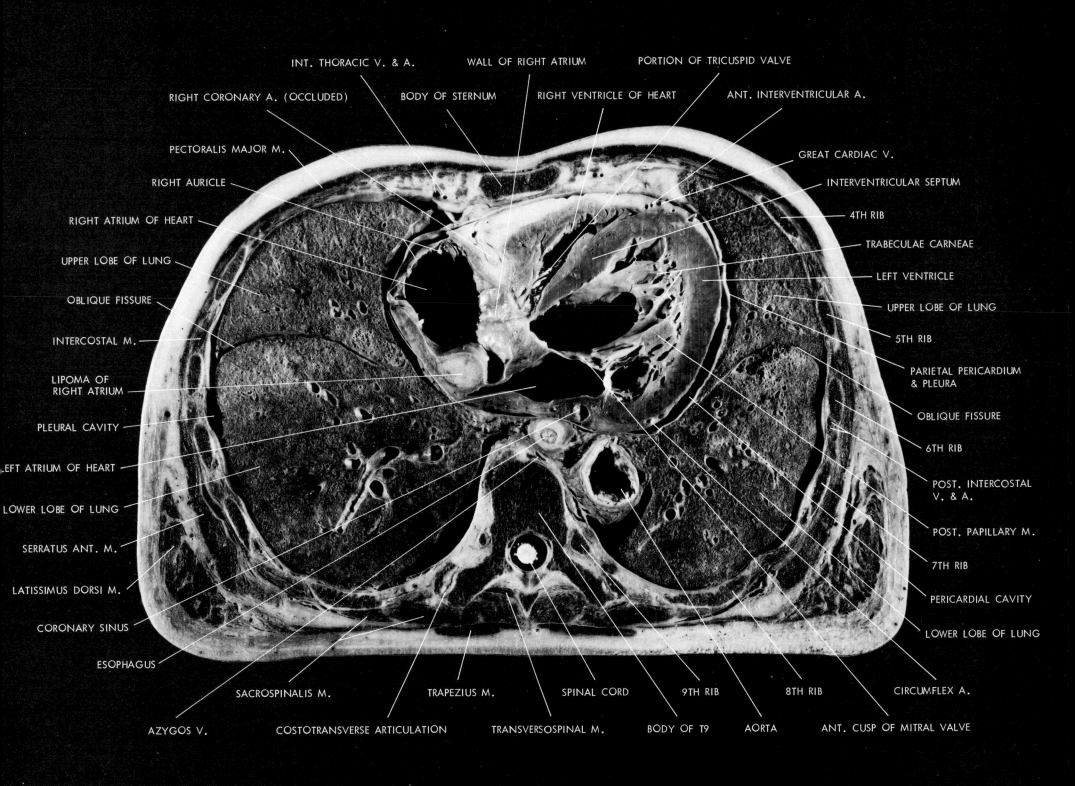

INT. THORACIC V. & A.
WALL OF RIGHT ATRIUM
PORTION OF TRICUSPID VALVE
RIGHT CORONARY A. (OCCLUDED)
BODY OF STERNUM
RIGHT VENTRICLE OF HEART
ANT. INTERVENTRICULAR A.
PECTORALIS MAJOR M.
GREAT CARDIAC V.
RIGHT AURICLE
INTERVENTRICULAR SEPTUM
RIGHT ATRIUM OF HEART
4TH RIB
UPPER LOBE OF LUNG
TRABECULAE CARNEAE
OBLIQUE FISSURE
LEFT VENTRICLE
INTERCOSTAL M.
UPPER LOBE OF LUNG
LIPOMA OF
RIGHT ATRIUM
5TH RIB
PLEURAL CAVITY
PARIETAL PERICARDIUM
& PLEURA
LEFT ATRIUM OF HEART
OBLIQUE FISSURE
LOWER LOBE OF LUNG
6TH RIB
SERRATUS ANT. M.
POST. INTERCOSTAL
V. & A.
LATISSIMUS DORSI M.
POST. PAPILLARY M.
CORONARY SINUS
7TH RIB
ESOPHAGUS
PERICARDIAL CAVITY
LOWER LOBE OF LUNG
AZYGOS V.
SACROSPINALIS M.
TRAPEZIUS M.
SPINAL CORD
9TH RIB
8TH RIB
CIRCUMFLEX A.
COSTOTRANSVERSE ARTICULATION
TRANSVERSOSPINAL M.
BODY OF T9
AORTA
ANT. CUSP OF MITRAL VALVE

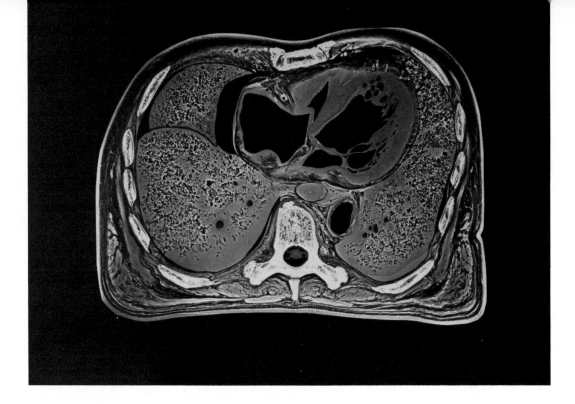

SECTION
2–19

*Through the
lower portion of
the body of T9*

Anatomic Considerations

The mitral (bicuspid) valve of the heart, which is found at the left atrioventricular opening, can be clearly seen in this illustration. It is located at the left lateral margin of the sternum at the level of the fifth intercostal space. As can be noted in the section, the two cusps are of unequal size, with the anterior cusp being larger than the posterior. The chordae tendinae, which are fibrous cords extending between the cusps and the papillary muscles, can also be clearly seen. Although the mitral valve is anatomically located at the left sternal border of the fifth intercostal space, the sound of this valve is best heard at the apex of the heart in the same interspace.

Clinical Considerations

Note the thickness of the interventricular septum, which separates the right and left ventricles. Even on 2-second CT scans this may not be obliterated by the motion of the heart. On the other hand, the other septae are readily obliterated by this motion. Note also the relative size of the cavity of the right ventricle as opposed to that of the left. The left atrium at this point has become a rather small chamber.

Although separated by an air space, the pericardial fat pad can be identified (here called "extrapericardial fat"). Whereas the pad is detached in this section, in the living it is usually closely applied to the pericardium of the heart. It may be readily differentiated by its lower absorption coefficient and fatty consistency.

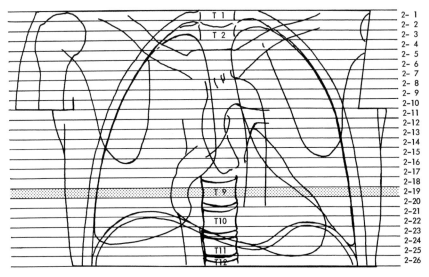

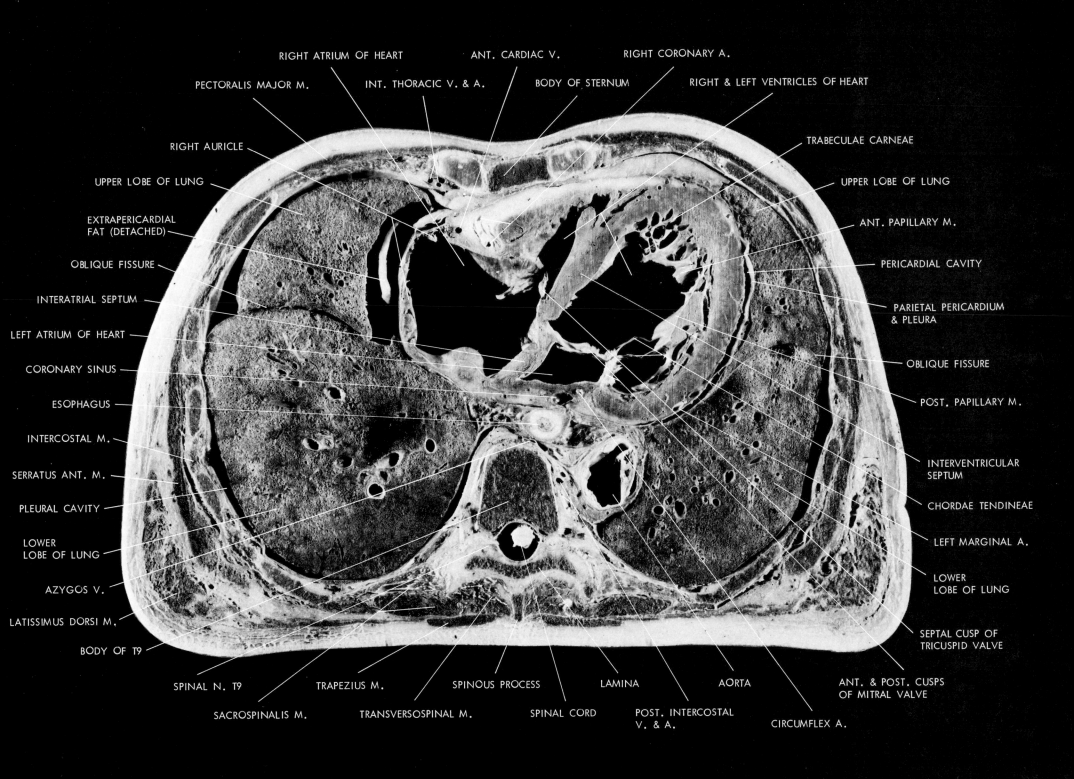

RIGHT ATRIUM OF HEART
ANT. CARDIAC V.
RIGHT CORONARY A.
PECTORALIS MAJOR M.
INT. THORACIC V. & A.
BODY OF STERNUM
RIGHT & LEFT VENTRICLES OF HEART
RIGHT AURICLE
TRABECULAE CARNEAE
UPPER LOBE OF LUNG
UPPER LOBE OF LUNG
EXTRAPERICARDIAL
FAT (DETACHED)
ANT. PAPILLARY M.
OBLIQUE FISSURE
PERICARDIAL CAVITY
INTERATRIAL SEPTUM
PARIETAL PERICARDIUM
& PLEURA
LEFT ATRIUM OF HEART
OBLIQUE FISSURE
CORONARY SINUS
ESOPHAGUS
POST. PAPILLARY M.
INTERCOSTAL M.
INTERVENTRICULAR
SEPTUM
SERRATUS ANT. M.
CHORDAE TENDINEAE
PLEURAL CAVITY
LEFT MARGINAL A.
LOWER
LOBE OF LUNG
LOWER
LOBE OF LUNG
AZYGOS V.
SEPTAL CUSP OF
TRICUSPID VALVE
LATISSIMUS DORSI M.
BODY OF T9
ANT. & POST. CUSPS
OF MITRAL VALVE
SPINAL N. T9
TRAPEZIUS M.
SPINOUS PROCESS
LAMINA
AORTA
SACROSPINALIS M.
TRANSVERSOSPINAL M.
SPINAL CORD
POST. INTERCOSTAL
V. & A.
CIRCUMFLEX A.

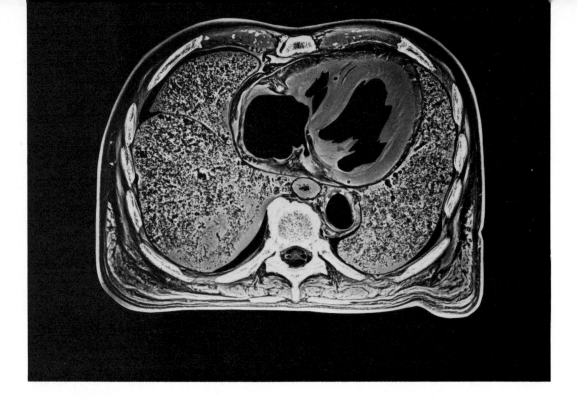

sternum. The relationship of the tricuspid valve to the mitral valve can be seen by comparing this illustration with Section 2–19. The tricuspid valve is located anterior, inferior, and to the right of the mitral valve.

Clinical Considerations

In this section the maximal chambers of the heart are the right atrium and left ventricle, with only a small portion of the right ventricle manifest anteriorly. The thick septum between the right atrium and left ventricle is readily differentiated. The close relationship of the azygos vein to the posterior wall of the esophagus is indicated.

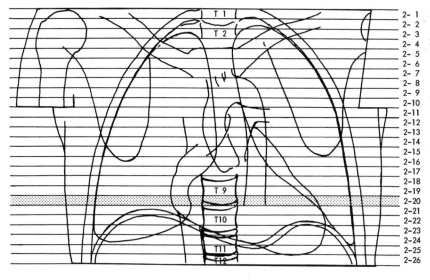

SECTION
2-20

Through the intervertebral disc between T9 and T10

Anatomic Considerations

The tricuspid valve can be seen in this section. This valve is found at the opening between the right atrium and ventricle. The anterior (infundibular) cusp is attached to the anterior wall of the right ventricle, the posterior (marginal) cusp is attached along the acute margin of the heart, and the septal cusp is attached to the interventricular septum. As can be seen in the illustration, the tricuspid valve is located near the midline, posterior to the

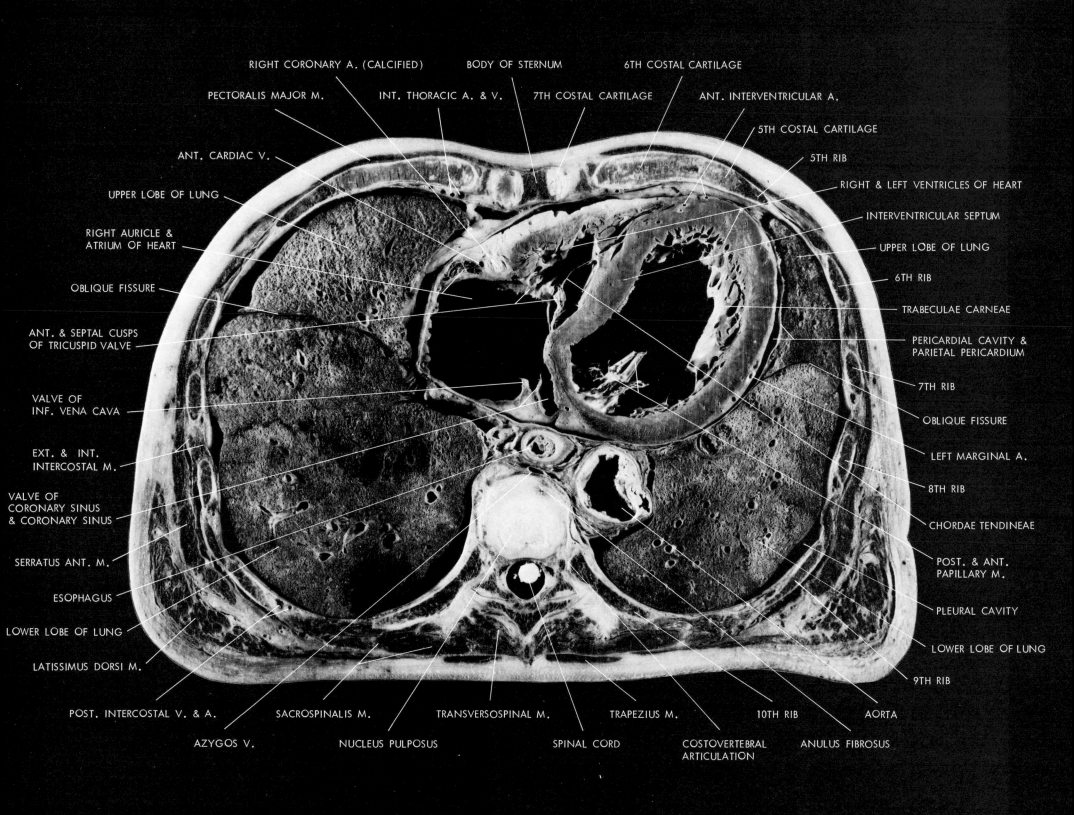

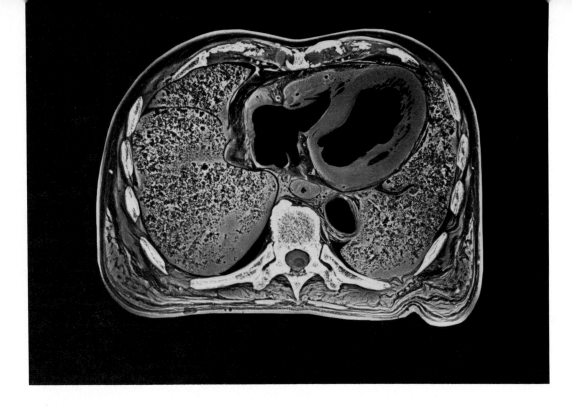

into the atrium. Some venous return from the heart flows directly into the chambers by small veins (Thebesian veins).

Clinical Considerations

In this section the diaphragm and liver are coming into view. This will vary from patient to patient, depending upon the degree of respiration. At times a small portion of the left lobe of the liver may also be visualized, depending upon its relationship to the right.

The right atrium and the left ventricle are still the two major cardiac chambers in view, with an oblique septum between these two structures that is often visualized even on the 2-second computed tomogram despite cardiac pulsations. The esophagus, if outlined by a small amount of barium intermixed with honey, lies on the posterior aspect of this septum. The azygos vein is in a more posterior relationship than it had been previously, but it is always very close in contiguity to the vertebral body.

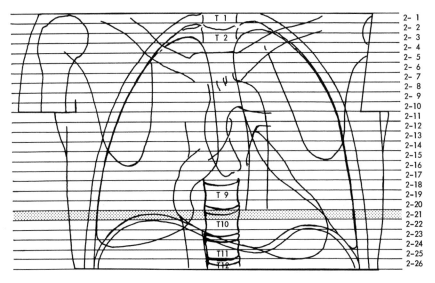

SECTION
2–21

Through the upper portion of the body of T10

Anatomic Considerations

The majority of the veins of the heart drain into the right atrium by way of the coronary sinus (Sections 2–15 to 2–20). The sinus lies in the posterior atrioventricular groove and opens into the right atrium (Section 2–20). Some of its tributaries can be observed in the illustrations; these are the great cardiac vein (Sections 2–15 to 2–18), the middle cardiac vein (Sections 2–17 to 2–23), and the small cardiac vein (Section 2–22). The great cardiac vein lies in the anterior interventricular groove, the middle cardiac vein is located in the posterior interventricular groove, and the small cardiac vein lies in the anterior atrioventricular groove. The anterior cardiac vein (Sections 2–19 to 2–20) is located on the anterior surface of the right atrium and drains directly

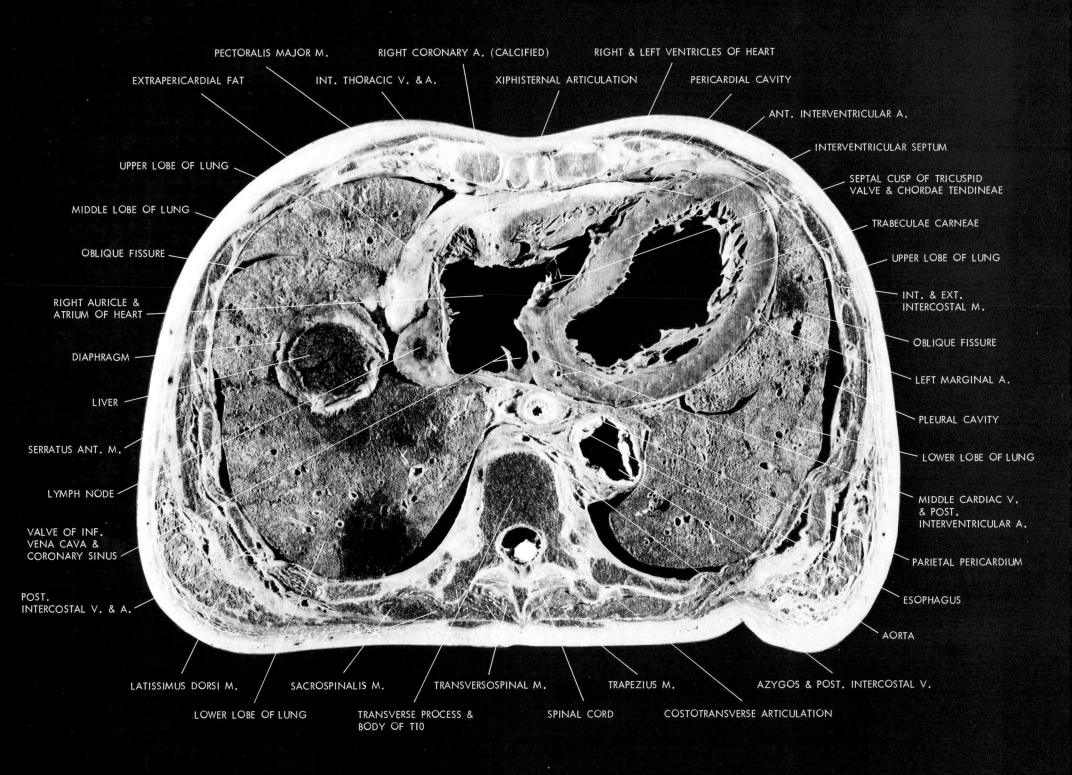

PECTORALIS MAJOR M.

RIGHT CORONARY A. (CALCIFIED)

RIGHT & LEFT VENTRICLES OF HEART

EXTRAPERICARDIAL FAT

INT. THORACIC V. & A.

XIPHISTERNAL ARTICULATION

PERICARDIAL CAVITY

ANT. INTERVENTRICULAR A.

INTERVENTRICULAR SEPTUM

UPPER LOBE OF LUNG

SEPTAL CUSP OF TRICUSPID
VALVE & CHORDAE TENDINEAE

MIDDLE LOBE OF LUNG

TRABECULAE CARNEAE

OBLIQUE FISSURE

UPPER LOBE OF LUNG

INT. & EXT.
INTERCOSTAL M.

RIGHT AURICLE &
ATRIUM OF HEART

OBLIQUE FISSURE

DIAPHRAGM

LEFT MARGINAL A.

LIVER

PLEURAL CAVITY

SERRATUS ANT. M.

LOWER LOBE OF LUNG

LYMPH NODE

MIDDLE CARDIAC V.
& POST.
INTERVENTRICULAR A.

VALVE OF INF.
VENA CAVA &
CORONARY SINUS

PARIETAL PERICARDIUM

POST.
INTERCOSTAL V. & A.

ESOPHAGUS

AORTA

LATISSIMUS DORSI M.

SACROSPINALIS M.

TRANSVERSOSPINAL M.

TRAPEZIUS M.

AZYGOS & POST. INTERCOSTAL V.

LOWER LOBE OF LUNG

TRANSVERSE PROCESS &
BODY OF T10

SPINAL CORD

COSTOTRANSVERSE ARTICULATION

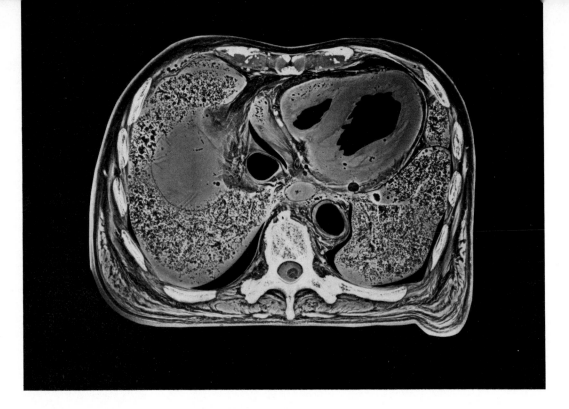

It is noteworthy that the liver may separate the middle and lower lobes of the right lung at this level.

The inferior vena cava is now in view just to the right of the right lobe of the liver. This relationship of lung, liver, inferior vena cava, esophagus, and descending thoracic aorta is important in computed tomography.

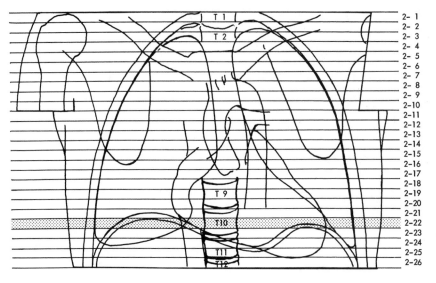

SECTION
2–22

Through the lower portion of the body of T10

Anatomic Considerations

The relationship of the dome of the liver to the right lung is shown in this illustration. Observe the diaphragm, which separates these two organs. All three lobes of the right lung are present at this level; the lower lobe of the lung is related posteriorly, laterally, and anteriorly to the liver.

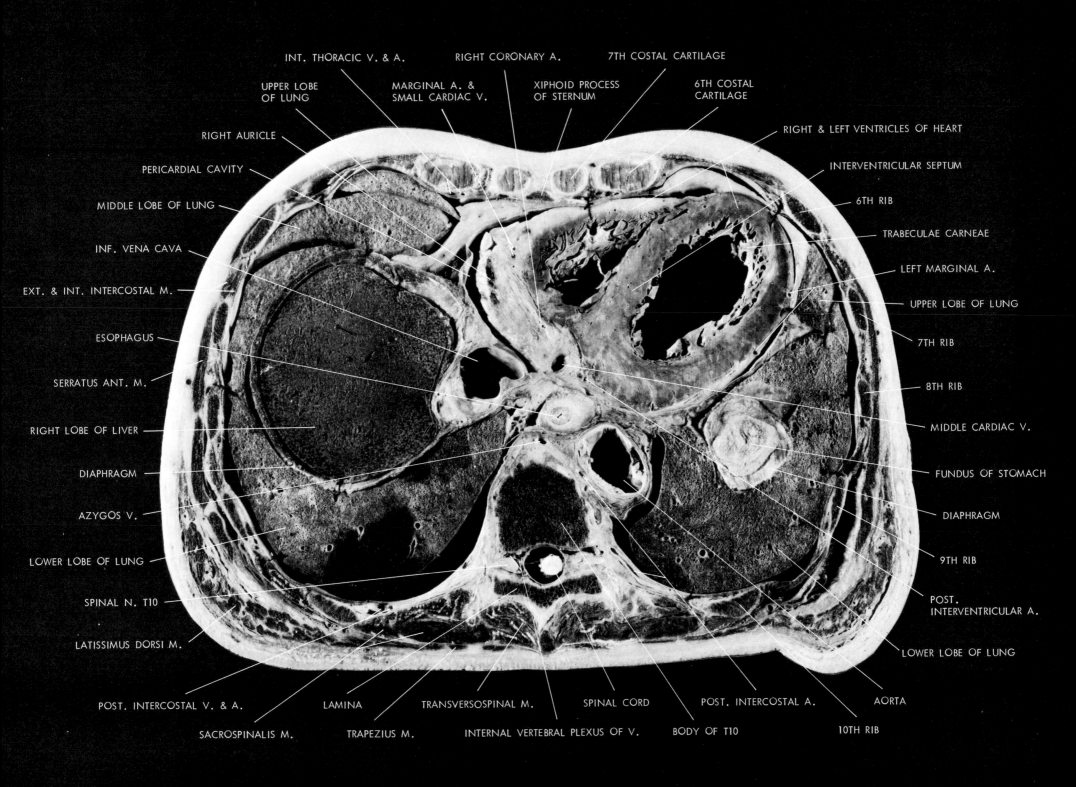

INT. THORACIC V. & A. RIGHT CORONARY A. 7TH COSTAL CARTILAGE

UPPER LOBE OF LUNG MARGINAL A. & SMALL CARDIAC V. XIPHOID PROCESS OF STERNUM 6TH COSTAL CARTILAGE

RIGHT AURICLE RIGHT & LEFT VENTRICLES OF HEART

PERICARDIAL CAVITY INTERVENTRICULAR SEPTUM

MIDDLE LOBE OF LUNG 6TH RIB

TRABECULAE CARNEAE

INF. VENA CAVA LEFT MARGINAL A.

EXT. & INT. INTERCOSTAL M. UPPER LOBE OF LUNG

7TH RIB

ESOPHAGUS 8TH RIB

SERRATUS ANT. M.

RIGHT LOBE OF LIVER MIDDLE CARDIAC V.

DIAPHRAGM FUNDUS OF STOMACH

AZYGOS V. DIAPHRAGM

LOWER LOBE OF LUNG 9TH RIB

SPINAL N. T10

LATISSIMUS DORSI M. POST. INTERVENTRICULAR A.

LOWER LOBE OF LUNG

POST. INTERCOSTAL V. & A. LAMINA TRANSVERSOSPINAL M. SPINAL CORD POST. INTERCOSTAL A. AORTA

SACROSPINALIS M. TRAPEZIUS M. INTERNAL VERTEBRAL PLEXUS OF V. BODY OF T10 10TH RIB

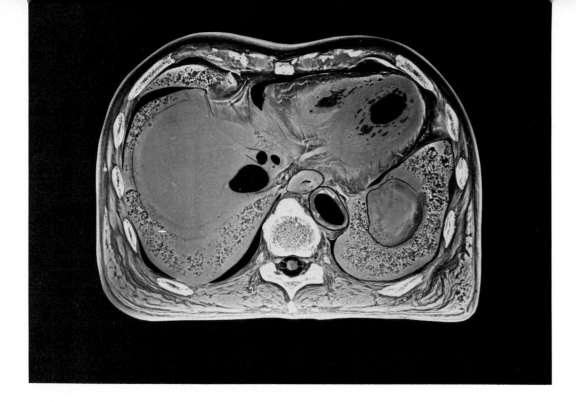

Clinical Considerations

In this section the inferior vena cava can be identified clearly, particularly when it is contrast enhanced. Immediately anterior to the inferior vena cava lies the hepatic vein of the liver. Small, semilunate portions of the lung may still be seen posteriorly in view of the dome shape of the diaphragm.

By contrast with Section 2–22, the esophagus is now in closer proximity with the fundus of the stomach and is in very close proximity with the descending thoracic aorta as it passes through the diaphragm.

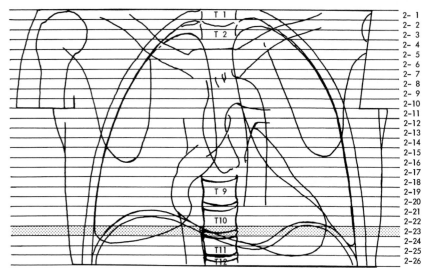

SECTION
2–23

Through the intervertebral disc between T10 and T11

Anatomic Considerations

The fundus of the stomach can be seen in this section. The diaphragm is interposed between the stomach and the left lung and heart. The left ventricle lies anterior to the fundus of the stomach; the lower lobe of the left lung lies superior, lateral, and posterior to the fundus.

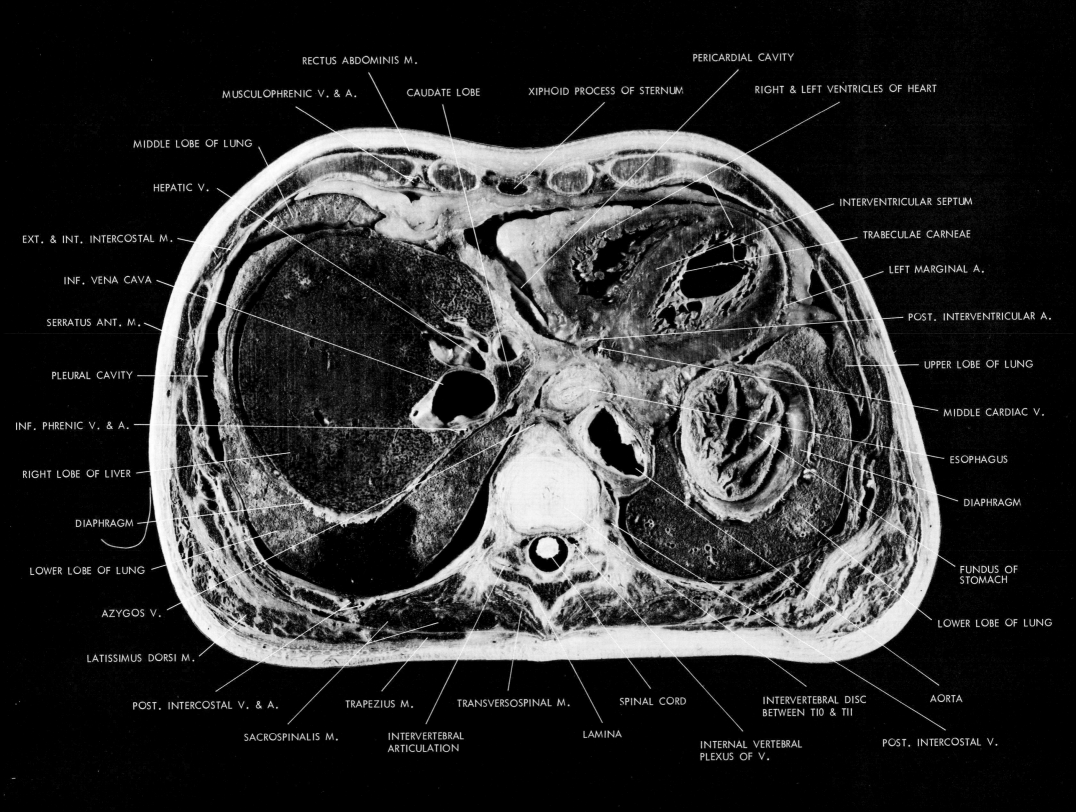

RECTUS ABDOMINIS M.

MUSCULOPHRENIC V. & A.

CAUDATE LOBE

PERICARDIAL CAVITY

XIPHOID PROCESS OF STERNUM

RIGHT & LEFT VENTRICLES OF HEART

MIDDLE LOBE OF LUNG

HEPATIC V.

INTERVENTRICULAR SEPTUM

TRABECULAE CARNEAE

EXT. & INT. INTERCOSTAL M.

LEFT MARGINAL A.

INF. VENA CAVA

POST. INTERVENTRICULAR A.

SERRATUS ANT. M.

UPPER LOBE OF LUNG

PLEURAL CAVITY

MIDDLE CARDIAC V.

INF. PHRENIC V. & A.

ESOPHAGUS

RIGHT LOBE OF LIVER

DIAPHRAGM

DIAPHRAGM

FUNDUS OF STOMACH

LOWER LOBE OF LUNG

AZYGOS V.

LOWER LOBE OF LUNG

LATISSIMUS DORSI M.

POST. INTERCOSTAL V. & A.

TRAPEZIUS M.

TRANSVERSOSPINAL M.

SPINAL CORD

INTERVERTEBRAL DISC BETWEEN T10 & T11

AORTA

SACROSPINALIS M.

INTERVERTEBRAL ARTICULATION

LAMINA

INTERNAL VERTEBRAL PLEXUS OF V.

POST. INTERCOSTAL V.

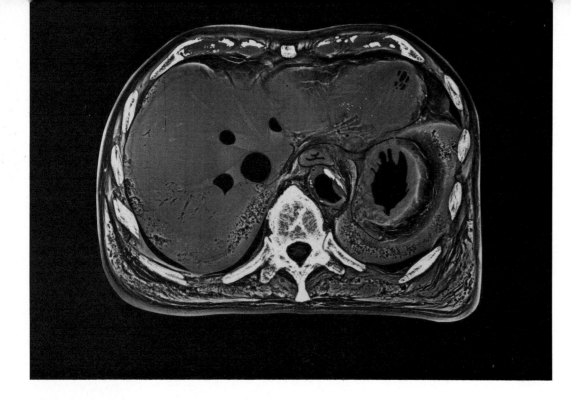

Clinical Considerations

In this section, only small "slivers" of lung, semilunate in shape, are visualized. There are three medial openings shown in the liver: two are related to the hepatic vein, the third, or medial one, being the inferior vena cava, which is buried within the substance of the liver but intensified by contrast enhancement when so desired. Anterior to the inferior vena cava is a tonguelike structure, the caudate lobe of the liver. The left lobe of the liver lies anterior to the caudate lobe. These relationships of hepatic vein, inferior vena cava, and caudate lobe of the liver are important to recall in the interpretation of CT sections at the level of T11 vertebral body.

At this level the esophagus is communicating with the fundus of the stomach just below the level of the diaphragm. This, in some of the older literature, has been referred to as the ventricle of the esophagus.

The esophagus may be contrast enhanced with barium intermixed with honey in small quantities, whereas the stomach is contrast enhanced with about 5 per cent Gastrografin, a special diatrozoate contrast substance utilized in radiography.

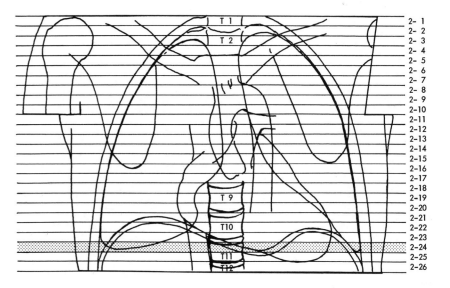

SECTION
2-24

Through the upper portion of the body of T11

Anatomic Considerations

In Sections 2–22 to 2–25 the lower lobes of the lungs and the pleura are seen between the diaphragm and the body wall. This is due to the high extension of some of the abdominal organs. The base of each lung is concave and rests upon the diaphragm, which separates the right lung from the liver and the left lung from the liver, stomach, and spleen.

The thoracic duct, which is seen in this illustration and in Section 2–25, is difficult to observe in every section because it tends to collapse. An extension of the cisterna chyli, it passes through the aortic hiatus of the diaphragm and ascends through the posterior mediastinum between the aorta and azygos vein. In the superior mediastinum it passes to the left of the esophagus and enters the root of the neck. It terminates at the junction of the internal jugular and left subclavian veins. All the lymphatic vessels of the body terminate in the thoracic duct except those of the right side of the head, neck, thorax, and right upper extremity.

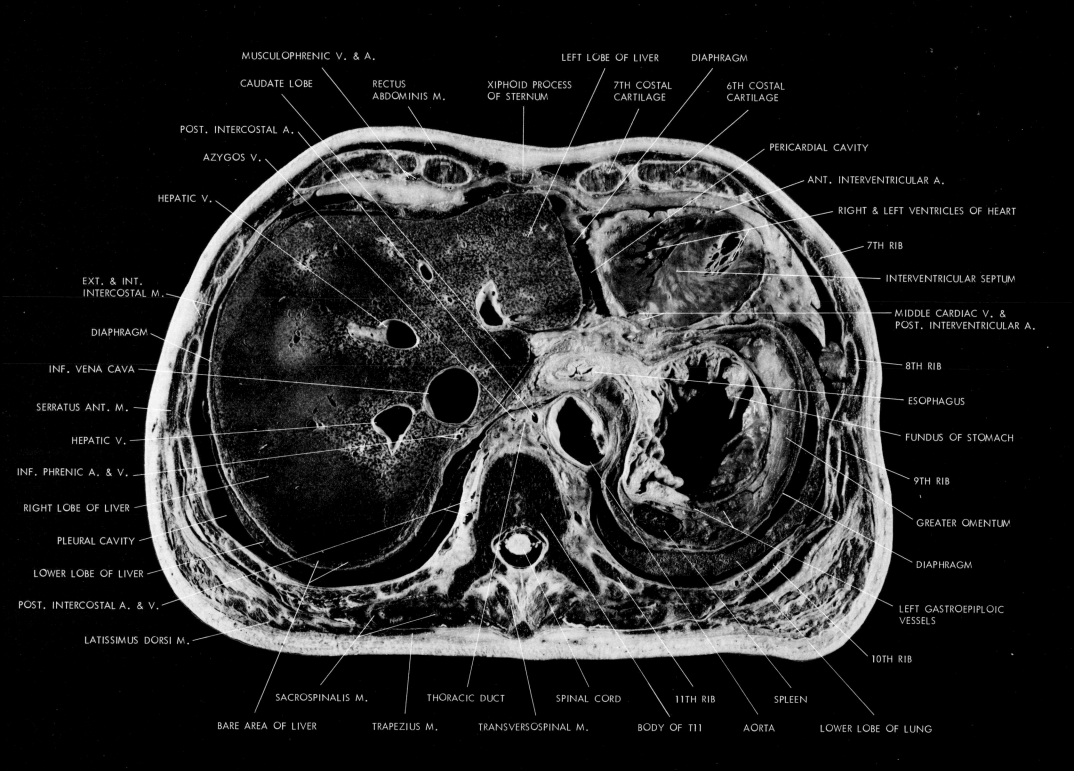

MUSCULOPHRENIC V. & A.
CAUDATE LOBE
RECTUS ABDOMINIS M.
LEFT LOBE OF LIVER
XIPHOID PROCESS OF STERNUM
DIAPHRAGM
7TH COSTAL CARTILAGE
6TH COSTAL CARTILAGE
POST. INTERCOSTAL A.
AZYGOS V.
PERICARDIAL CAVITY
ANT. INTERVENTRICULAR A.
HEPATIC V.
RIGHT & LEFT VENTRICLES OF HEART
7TH RIB
EXT. & INT. INTERCOSTAL M.
INTERVENTRICULAR SEPTUM
MIDDLE CARDIAC V. & POST. INTERVENTRICULAR A.
DIAPHRAGM
INF. VENA CAVA
8TH RIB
ESOPHAGUS
SERRATUS ANT. M.
HEPATIC V.
FUNDUS OF STOMACH
INF. PHRENIC A. & V.
9TH RIB
RIGHT LOBE OF LIVER
PLEURAL CAVITY
GREATER OMENTUM
LOWER LOBE OF LIVER
DIAPHRAGM
POST. INTERCOSTAL A. & V.
LEFT GASTROEPIPLOIC VESSELS
LATISSIMUS DORSI M.
10TH RIB
SACROSPINALIS M.
THORACIC DUCT
SPINAL CORD
11TH RIB
SPLEEN
BARE AREA OF LIVER
TRAPEZIUS M.
TRANSVERSOSPINAL M.
BODY OF T11
AORTA
LOWER LOBE OF LUNG

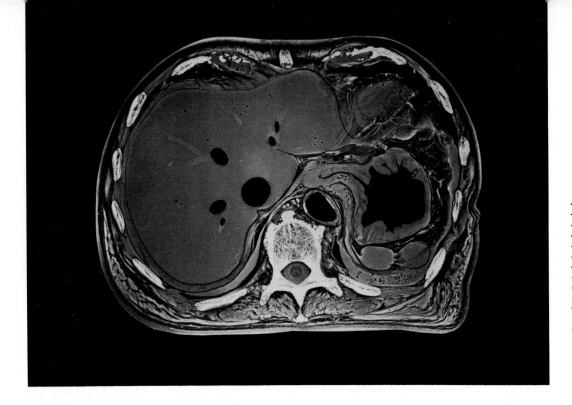

Anatomic Considerations

The apex of the heart, a portion of the left ventricle, can be seen in this section. It points inferiorly, anteriorly, and to the left. In this specimen the apex of the heart lies just below the sixth costal cartilage. The apex is usually related to the fifth intercostal space, about 8 or 9 cm to the left of the midsternal line.

Clinical Considerations

The continued relationships of the hepatic veins persist, forming a triangle with the inferior vena cava and the caudate lobe of the liver just medial to it. The left lobe of the liver is now more readily in evidence. The ductules and vascular structures within the liver may also be seen and can be differentiated on computed tomograms at this level. The falciform ligament can usually be differentiated just anterior to the left lobe of the liver and to the right of the midline.

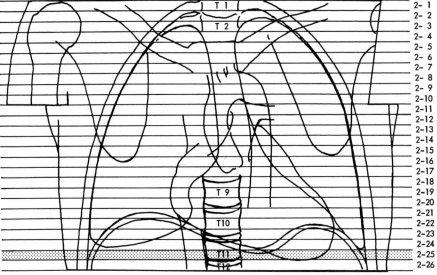

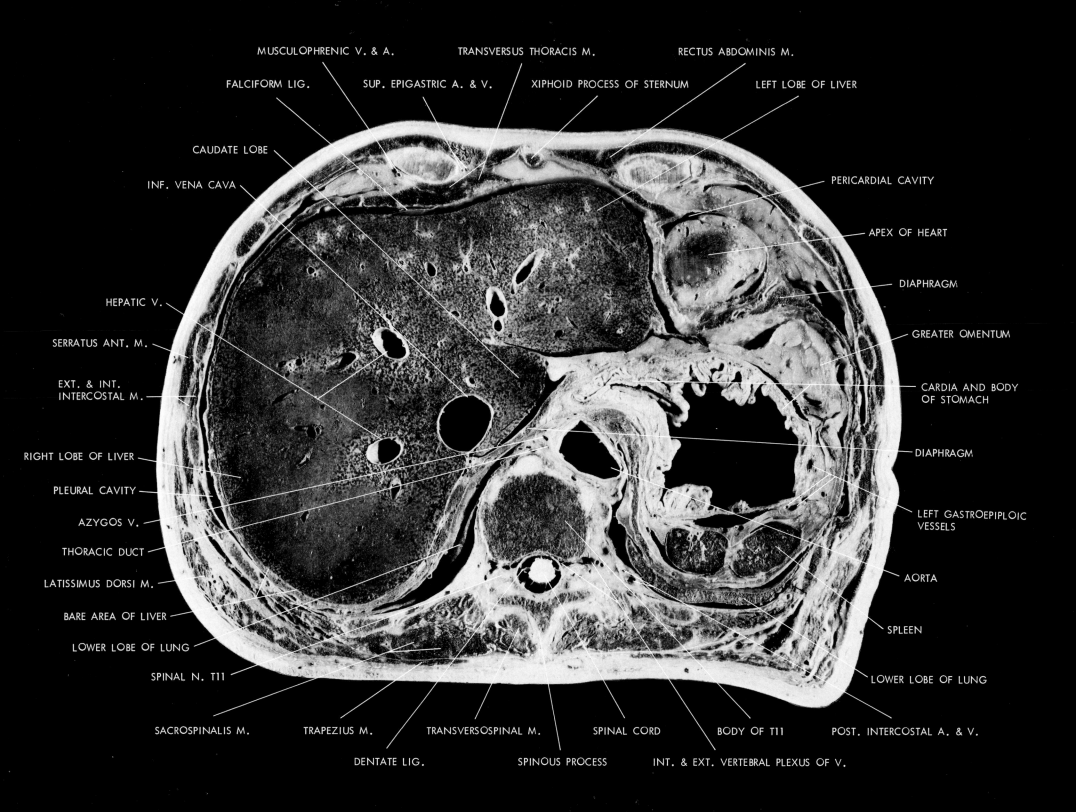

MUSCULOPHRENIC V. & A.

TRANSVERSUS THORACIS M.

RECTUS ABDOMINIS M.

FALCIFORM LIG.

SUP. EPIGASTRIC A. & V.

XIPHOID PROCESS OF STERNUM

LEFT LOBE OF LIVER

CAUDATE LOBE

PERICARDIAL CAVITY

INF. VENA CAVA

APEX OF HEART

DIAPHRAGM

HEPATIC V.

GREATER OMENTUM

SERRATUS ANT. M.

CARDIA AND BODY
OF STOMACH

EXT. & INT.
INTERCOSTAL M.

DIAPHRAGM

RIGHT LOBE OF LIVER

PLEURAL CAVITY

LEFT GASTROEPIPLOIC
VESSELS

AZYGOS V.

THORACIC DUCT

AORTA

LATISSIMUS DORSI M.

BARE AREA OF LIVER

SPLEEN

LOWER LOBE OF LUNG

LOWER LOBE OF LUNG

SPINAL N. T11

SACROSPINALIS M.

TRAPEZIUS M.

TRANSVERSOSPINAL M.

SPINAL CORD

BODY OF T11

POST. INTERCOSTAL A. & V.

DENTATE LIG.

SPINOUS PROCESS

INT. & EXT. VERTEBRAL PLEXUS OF V.

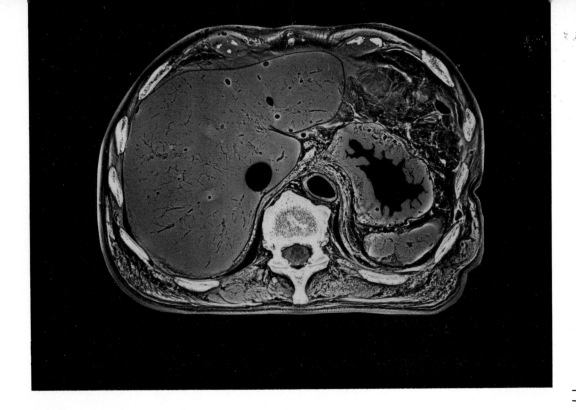

tendinous portion at the level of the eighth thoracic vertebra. The motor innervation of the diaphragm is by the phrenic nerve.

Clinical Considerations

This section shows the ligamentum venosum separating the left lobe of the liver from the caudate lobe of the liver. Just inferior to the caudate lobe of the liver is the inferior vena cava, once again readily in evidence. On the medial aspect of the ligamentum venosum are the branches of the left hepatic artery. These relationships are important to remember as one studies tomography through this area.

With contrast enhancement of appropriate types, the body of the stomach and all of the vascular structures depicted herein come readily into view and are differentiated. The fatty nature of the greater omentum allows it to be readily differentiated from the stomach proper. At times, however, the transverse colon may lie high in the abdomen at this level, but is readily differentiated if contrast media enhances its presence in this location. In most instances it can be differentiated by the absorption coefficient of its content, which is air.

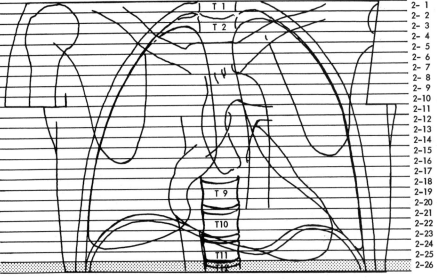

SECTION
2–26

*Through the
body of T12*

Anatomic Considerations

The relation of the diaphragm to the structures of the thorax and abdomen can be seen in Sections 2–21 to 2–26. The diaphragm is the convex musculofascial partition between the thorax and the abdomen. The peripheral portion of the diaphragm consists of muscle fibers, and the central portion is tendinous and forms the central tendon. The muscle fibers can be grouped according to their origins — sternal, costal, and lumbar. The lumbar part consists of lumbar arches and two crura. The medial lumbocostal arch surrounds the psoas major muscle and the lateral lumbocostal arch surrounds the quadratus lumborum muscle. The two crura are tendinous; the right crus extends approximately to the third lumbar vertebra, and the left extends approximately to the second.

There are three large openings in the diaphragm — the aortic, the esophageal, and the vena caval. The aortic hiatus is at the level of the 12th thoracic vertebra. It is not strictly an aperture in the diaphragm, because the aorta passes posterior to the diaphragm and is surrounded by the crura. The esophageal hiatus is located in the muscular portion of the diaphragm at the level of the tenth thoracic vertebra. The vena caval opening is situated in the

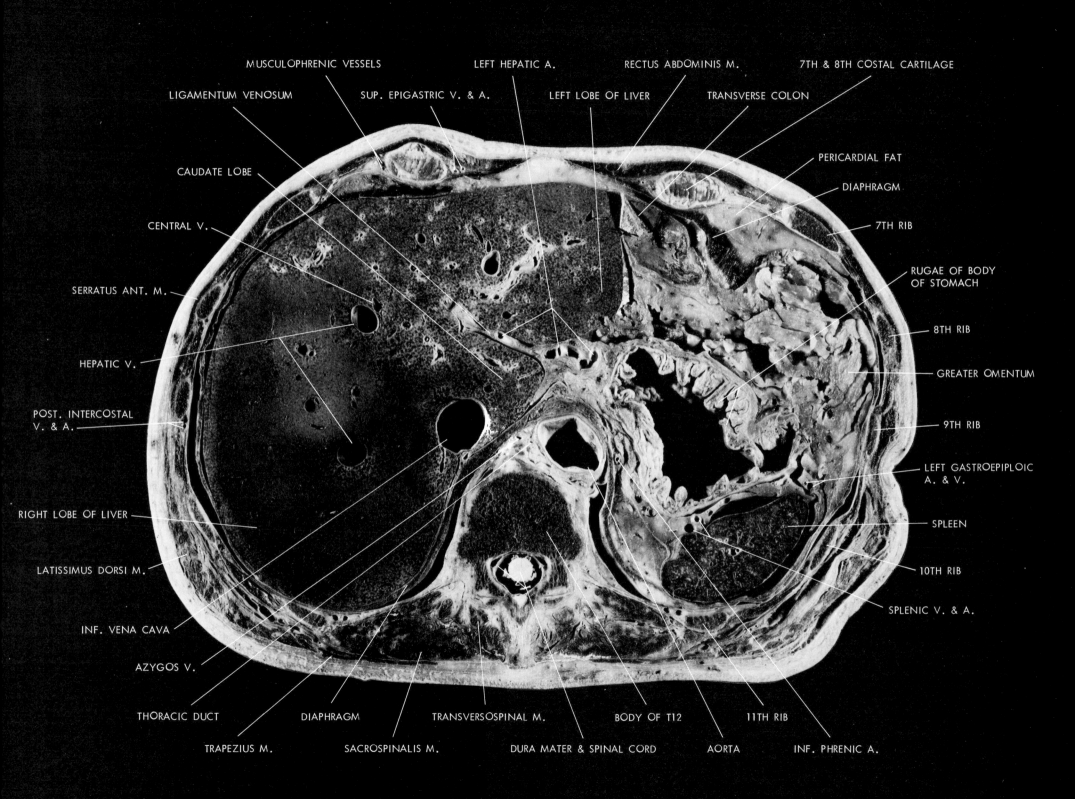

MUSCULOPHRENIC VESSELS

LEFT HEPATIC A.

RECTUS ABDOMINIS M.

7TH & 8TH COSTAL CARTILAGE

LIGAMENTUM VENOSUM

SUP. EPIGASTRIC V. & A.

LEFT LOBE OF LIVER

TRANSVERSE COLON

CAUDATE LOBE

PERICARDIAL FAT

DIAPHRAGM

CENTRAL V.

7TH RIB

RUGAE OF BODY
OF STOMACH

SERRATUS ANT. M.

8TH RIB

HEPATIC V.

GREATER OMENTUM

POST. INTERCOSTAL
V. & A.

9TH RIB

LEFT GASTROEPIPLOIC
A. & V.

RIGHT LOBE OF LIVER

SPLEEN

LATISSIMUS DORSI M.

10TH RIB

INF. VENA CAVA

SPLENIC V. & A.

AZYGOS V.

THORACIC DUCT

DIAPHRAGM

TRANSVERSOSPINAL M.

BODY OF T12

11TH RIB

TRAPEZIUS M.

SACROSPINALIS M.

DURA MATER & SPINAL CORD

AORTA

INF. PHRENIC A.

3

Abdomen

INTRODUCTION

The accompanying sketch shows that the sections extend from the intervertebral disc between T11 and T12 to the vertebral body of L5. These sections are from the same specimen used in Chapter 4, "Male Pelvis and Perineum," but from a specimen different from that used in Chapter 2, "Thorax"; therefore, a few of the sections are duplicated.

Sonographic Imaging of the Abdomen

In discussing the clinical relevance of cross-sectional anatomy, we have largely confined ourselves to the application of computed tomography. Ultrasound studies have contributed significantly to imaging of the abdominal areas, however.

LIVER. The following clinical applications can be enumerated:
1. Occasionally it is possible to differentiate second-order branches of the hepatic arterial system.
2. The caudate and quadrate segments of the left lobe of the liver can be clearly identified.
3. Jaundice due to diffuse parenchymal disease of the liver or due to hemolysis can be differentiated.

GALL BLADDER. Normal bile is readily traversed by the acoustic beam; hence the gall bladder is often visualized by ultrasound. Gallstones are readily detected by ultrasound.

PANCREAS. Although the pancreas is very clearly delineated by computed tomography and its morphology shown more accurately than with ultrasonography, one cannot dispute the importance of ultrasonography in visualization of the pancreas, particularly when reliable boundary landmarks are utilized for proper identification (Berger et al., 1977; Ghorashi and Rector, 1977; Sample et al., 1975; Sample, 1977; Weil et al., 1977).

KIDNEYS. Usually ultrasonographic techniques require various positions of the patient for a complete approach to the examination of the kidneys. Considerable anatomic detail may be gained. Computed tomography, however, is employed when greater morphologic detail is required.

ABDOMINAL VASCULATURE. Variable portions of the inferior vena cava and abdominal aorta and its branches can be delineated in most patients with considerable accuracy by sonography. A great advantage of ultrasound is the facility with which the abdominal aorta can be examined in its sagittal relationship. The sagittal relationship of the aorta is most revealing of disease processes such as abdominal aortic aneurysms.

Computed Tomographic Imaging of the Abdomen

Abdominal slices may be obtained either at 2-cm or 1-cm increments, depending upon the organ specificity desired. Usually an initial set of scans without any contrast enhancement is obtained. Thereafter, contrast enhancement of the gastrointestinal tract with 5 per cent Gastrografin is often employed, and intravenous infusion of a diatrizoate, using 12 ml of Renografin in 390 ml of water, is employed for contrast enhancement of the vascular system. The scanning is performed in the supine position primarily, but the patient may be placed in a lateral position for verification or enhancement of morphology. Occasionally, contrast enemas of 400 to 800 ml of 5 per cent Gastrografin may be administered, particularly if pelvic abnormalities are suspected. Urinary bladder opacification is accomplished sufficiently by the intravenous administration of 25 ml of the 60 per cent diatrizoate mixture. One may use either the single bolus injection technique or a drip-type intravenous infusion. Of course, cardiac and renal functions, as well as sensitivity to the contrast agents, are taken into account prior to their introduction.

In planning radiation therapy, the patients are scanned in the positions in which therapy is to be administered.

Manipulation of window width and level is essential for complete and appropriate evaluation. This is particularly true when one is seeking liver metastases and bone destruction.

At times it is highly desirable to magnify certain areas, such as the adrenal, and many of the commercially available instruments are capable of such magnification.

LIVER. Appearance of the normal liver varies considerably in CT imaging; hence, variations of normal must be thoroughly understood. The transmission coefficient of the normal liver is possibly greater than that of any other soft tissue organ. In this respect it is very helpful to measure absorption coefficients, since fatty infiltration (liver too lucent) and hemochromatosis (liver too dense) can thereby readily be recognized.

Analysis of the porta hepatis is very important. The common bile duct, the portal vein, and the hepatic artery may be differentiated by contrast enhancement if not readily detected otherwise.

The inferior vena cava ordinarily lies just caudad and medial to the caudate lobe of the liver and sometimes appears to be encased by liver substance unless it is contrast enhanced. The ligamentum teres can almost always be differentiated. At times the left lobe of the liver is so small that one must differentiate it from a neoplasm by other modes, such as radioisotopic scans or ultrasonography. The quadrate lobe of the liver can usually be differentiated just caudal to and to the right of the ligamentum teres.

With contrast enhancement, particularly of the bolus type, the hepatic artery can readily be differentiated. The splenic artery can usually be differentiated as almost corresponding to the hepatic artery, but with a somewhat greater curvature and curving toward the left. Usually the left gastric artery is the first branch of the celiac axis, and it runs ventrocranially and to the left to enter the body of the stomach. It is often visualized with the aid of 5 per cent Gastrografin.

Unfortunately, the axis of the portal vein is quite variable, ranging from horizontal to practically vertical. The portal vein lies dorsal and medial to the main bile duct and dorsal in relation to the hepatic artery at the porta hepatis. Branches of the portal vein may be identified coming from the caudate and also the left lobe of the liver. Because of the considerable variability of all of these structures, contrast enhancement involving intravenous cholangiography as well as angiography of blood vessels plays an important part.

Without contrast enhancement, dilated bile ducts, having a distribution somewhat similar to portal veins, offer some difficulty in differentiation.

Since most mass lesions (not all) involving the liver are of a lesser attenuation coefficient than the liver itself, they can be detected readily if the operator carefully studies window width and levels employed. Metastases are the most common tumors identified, but primary neoplasms, such as hepatomas, have also been discovered in this fashion, as have abscesses. Contrast enhancement produces a more pronounced appearance in avascular lesions, such as abscess cavities, and those solid mass lesions that are diminished in vascularity.

As in the case with ultrasonography, computed tomography is helpful in differentiating obstructive jaundice from hemolytic jaundice. The site of obstruction can usually be ascertained with considerable accuracy.

Since the contents of the gall bladder usually have an attenuation coefficient lower than that of normal liver, the gall bladder when it is distended is almost routinely seen. On the other hand, gallstones, which are of biliary consistency, may not be differentiated. In this respect sonography is superior to computed tomography. Calcification and thickening of the gall bladder wall, however, are readily demonstrated by computed tomography.

PANCREAS. The pancreas generally has a very specific morphologic relationship to several vascular landmarks: The body and tail of the pancreas are ventral to the splenic vein and superior mesenteric artery. The head of the pancreas is caudal to the portal vein. The uncinate process is commonly observed as a projection of the head of the pancreas, which passes dorsal to the superior mesenteric vein from right to left. The superior mesenteric artery points to the head of the pancreas.

The axis of the pancreas is ordinarily visualized on two or three contiguous 1-cm sections in most patients. It does, however, have considerable variation in its shape and may appear either as an inverted "U" or as an "S." The fat plane between the splenic vein and pancreas must not be mistaken for a dilated pancreatic duct (Seidelmann et al., 1977).

Various criteria for a normal-sized pancreas have been published (Haaga et al., 1976; Kreel et al., 1977). The pancreas is smaller in older patients than in middle-aged groups, and its appearance may vary from smooth to lobulated. It has a feathery pattern, especially in obese patients in whom fatty infiltration is also present. This is shown especially in the xeroradiographic sections. Measurements of the pancreas are somewhat variable; they lie in the range of 2.5 to 3.5 cm for the head, 1.5 to 3 cm for the body, and 2.8 to 3.5 cm for the tail (Haber et al., 1976; Lutz et al., 1976; MacCarty et al., 1977).

The splenic vein originates from five or six tributaries coming off the splenic hilum and forms a single vein, passing from left to right, close to the superior and dorsal part of the pancreas. A space that is often identifiable between these two structures should not be misinterpreted as the pancreatic duct. The splenic vein is a good reference point for identification of the pancreas. Haaga and Reich (1978) have pointed out that lesions of the adrenal gland displace the splenic vein anteriorly, whereas lesions of the pancreas displace this same vein posteriorly, which they have referred to as the "splenic vein sign."

When it is desired to delineate the gastrointestinal tract contiguous with the pancreas, a diluted water-soluble contrast agent is given orally 15 to 24 minutes before the examination (40 cc of Gastrografin in 1000 cc of water). This may be followed by 1 mg of glucagon, injected intramuscularly or intravenously, to decrease the peristaltic action of the gastrointestinal tract.

Unfortunately, diagnosis of pancreatic carcinoma is based upon the demonstration of alterations in size and shape of the gland and is most accurately demonstrated radiologically by the coordinated use of endoscopic retrograde cholangiographic pancreatography (ERCP), which involves intuba-

tion of the patient; cannulation of the pancreatic duct (and common bile duct as desired); and injection of contrast agent.

SPLEEN. The spleen is usually readily detected with computed tomography even though it varies considerably in its size and shape. The splenic parenchyma appears homogeneous without a contrast bolus. Occasionally an accessory spleen is demonstrated. The splenic artery ranges from 8 to 32 cm, is very often tortuous and partially calcified, and is retrogastric (contrast enhancement of the stomach is helpful).

RETROPERITONEAL LYMPHADENOPATHY (Zelch and Haaga, 1979). Generally, the retroperitoneal lymph nodes completely surround the aorta and inferior vena cava, and it is particularly when these structures are enlarged posteriorly that they can be most readily detected. With computed tomography, however, enlargement of lymph nodes in the retroperitoneum is variable in appearance. Once enlargement progresses, the fat angles between the aorta and vena cava are obliterated and the margins of these important vessels can no longer be differentiated. The aorta may actually be displaced anteriorly.

KIDNEYS (Love et al., 1979). The utilization of computed tomography for visualization of the kidneys has taken on great significance. Kidneys are generally scanned before and after contrast enhancement with diatrizoate. One or both renal arteries and renal veins can then be visualized, and cortical areas can even be distinguished from the collecting systems. The various fascial planes, including the anterior renal fascia, the posterior renal fascia, and the so-called lateroconal fascia, are readily identified, as are the pararenal, perirenal, and posterior pararenal spaces, as defined by Myers (1976).

The following are some of the pathologic entities that may be identified quite accurately with the aid of computed tomography: renal masses due to cysts or neoplasms; extrarenal masses that deflect the kidneys; hydronephrosis of undetermined origin; nonfunctioning kidneys; complications of renal transplantation and renal surgery; and equivocal findings on excretory urography. Computed tomography is also helpful when planning for surgery and radiation therapy.

Renal trauma, with associated retroperitoneal hemorrhage, and subscapular or intracapsular hematoma can be defined accurately by computed tomography.

ADRENAL GLANDS (Reynes et al., 1979). Generally, once the position of the adrenal glands is ascertained by surveying the position of the kidneys, no more than ten sections are necessary at 0.5- to 1-cm increments.

Both adrenal glands are situated within the confines of Gerota's fascia and are usually surrounded by abundant perirenal fat. Computed tomography for normal adrenal gland visualization has been described in much greater detail by Brownlie and Kreel (1978) and also Montagne et al. (1978), and the student may refer to these for further study.

GASTROINTESTINAL TRACT. Since the more conventional techniques for investigation of the gastrointestinal tract, employing full column barium and double contrast techniques, are highly accurate and display the gastrointestinal tract *in vivo* in almost its entirety, the cross-sectional approach is of lesser value in this organ system, except to denote relationships. When treatment is being planned and the surgeon wants to know the full extent of the lesion in its cross-sectional relationship, demonstration in cross-section becomes particularly valuable. Usually this is accomplished with the aid of contrast enhancement by the oral administration of 5 per cent Gastrografin or by Gastrografin enema.

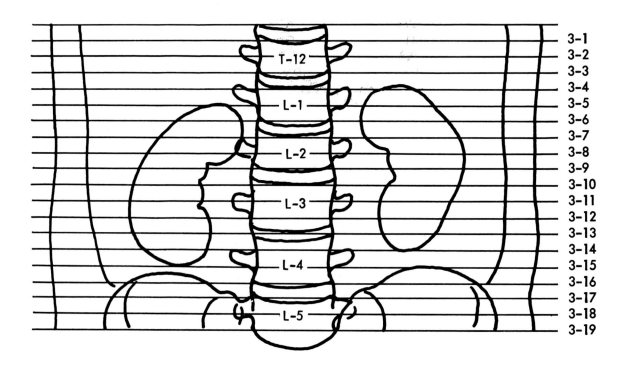

Berger M, Smith EH, Bartrum RJ Jr, Holm HH, and Mascatello V: False/positive diagnoses of pancreatic tail lesions caused by colon. JCU 5:343–345, 1977.

Brownlie K and Kreel L: Computer assisted tomography of normal adrenal glands. J Compututer Assisted Tomography 2:1–10, 1978.

Ghorashi B and Rector WR: Gray scale sonographic anatomy of the pancreas. JCU 5:25–29, 1977.

Haaga J, Alfidi RJ, Zelch MG, Meany TF, Boller M, Gonzalez L, and Jelden GL: Computed tomography of the pancreas. Radiology 120:589–595, 1976.

Haaga J and Reich NE: Computed Tomography of Abdominal Abnormalities. C. V. Mosby Co., St. Louis, Missouri, 1978.

Haber K, Feimanis AK, and Asher WM: Demonstration and dimensional analysis of the normal pancreas with gray scale echography. AJR 126:624–628, 1976.

Kreel L, Haertel M, and Katz D: Computed tomography of the normal pancreas. J Computer Assisted Tomography 1:290–299, 1977.

Love L, Reynes CJ, Churchill R, and Moncada R: Third generation C/T scanning in renal disease. Radiol Clin North Am 16:77–90, 1979.

Lutz H, Petzold TR, and Fuchs HF: Ultrasonic diagnosis of chronic pancreatitis. Acta Gastroenterol Belg 39:458–464, 1976.

MacCarty RL, Wahner HW, Stephens DH, Sheedy PF, and Hattery RR: Retrospective comparison of radionuclide scans and computed tomography of the liver and pancreas. AJR 129:23–28, 1977.

Meyers MA: Dynamic Radiology of the Abdomen. Springer-Verlag, Berlin, 1976, pp 113–194.

Montagne JP, Kressel HY, Korbkin M and Moss AA: Computed tomography of the normal adrenal glands. AJR 130:963–966, 1978.

Reynes CJ, Churchill R, Moncada R, and Love L: Computed tomography of adrenal glands. Radiol Clin North Am 17:91–104, 1979.

Sample WF: Techniques for the improved delineation of normal anatomy of the upper abdomen and high retroperitoneum with gray scale ultrasound. Radiology 124:197–202, 1977.

Sample WF, Po JB, Gray RK, and Cahill PJ: Gray scale ultrasonography. Techniques in pancreatic scanning. Applied Radiol 4:63–67; 90–91, 1975.

Seidelmann FF, Cohen WN, Bryan TJ, and Brown J: C/T demonstration of the splenic vein-pancreatic relationship: The pseudodilated pancreatic duct. AJR 129:17–21, 1977.

Weil F, Eisencher A, and Zeltner F: Ultrasonography of the normal pancreas. Radiology 123:417–423, 1977.

Zelch MG and Haaga JR: Clinical comparison of computed tomography and lymphangiography for detection of retroperitoneal lymphadenopathy. Radiol Clin North Am 17:157–168, 1979.

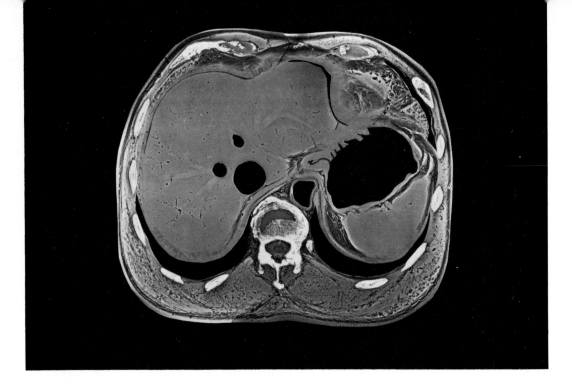

Clinical Considerations

Computed axial tomography of the liver and biliary tract is significantly accurate in diagnosing disorders of these structures (Levitt et al., 1977). Such disease entities as liver metastases, primary liver neoplasms, and benign hepatic cysts may be detected with a high degree of accuracy. Even abscesses of the liver may likewise be defined. Of particular help to diagnosis is the demonstration of subcapsular or intrahepatic hematomas.

Since obstructive jaundice is very often associated with dilatation of the intrahepatic biliary tree, this may be identified not only by computed axial tomography but also with the aid of cross-sectional ultrasound. In general, obstructive and nonobstructive jaundice can be distinguished with a high degree of accuracy.

Computed axial tomography is also helpful in guiding biopsy techniques, especially with thin-walled small caliber needles (the so-called Chiba or its equivalent). Fluoroscopic and ultrasonic guidance is also used, however (Haaga et al., 1977).

The position of the caudate lobe in this section with respect to the liver and stomach should also be noted. In conventional radiography, the caudate lobe of the liver, if enlarged from a pathologic process, may displace the stomach anteriorly or to the left. On the other hand, the other lobes of the liver usually displace the stomach posteriorly and to the left, and thus there is a significant difference. Also, note the position of the inferior vena cava in respect to the caudate lobe and the aorta to the left of the midline. When the inferior vena cava is outlined with contrast media, it must not be confused with the gall bladder.

Levitt RG, Sagel SS, Stanley RJ, and Jost RG: Accuracy of computed tomography of the liver and biliary tract. Radiology 124:123–128, 1977.

Haaga JR, Reich NE, Havrilla TR, Alfidi RJ, and Meaney TF: CT guided biopsy. Cleve Clin Q. 44:27–33, 1977.

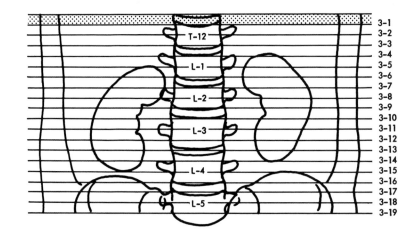

SECTION 3–1

Through the intervertebral disc between T11 and T12

Anatomic Considerations

The liver occupies almost the whole right hypochondrium and a great part of the epigastrium and may extend to the left hypochondrium. It rests under the diaphragm, which separates it from the pleurae, lungs, pericardium, and heart.

By following the liver in the various sections it can be observed that the visceral surface is related to the stomach, duodenum, hepatic flexure of the colon, right kidney, right suprarenal gland, and gall bladder. The liver is enclosed by peritoneum except for a small portion, the bare area, where the peritoneum is reflected from the diaphragm onto the posterior portion of the liver, which can be seen in this section.

Based on the external configuration, the liver is divided into four lobes. The large right lobe is separated from the small left lobe by the falciform ligament on the anterior surface and by the ligamentum teres and ligamentum venosum on the visceral surface. The caudate lobe is located between the fossa of the inferior vena cava and the ligamentum venosum, and the quadrate lobe is found between the fossa of the gall bladder and the ligamentum teres. The two lobes are separated from each other by the porta hepatis.

The hepatic triad, which can be seen in this section, consists of the hepatic duct, portal vein, and hepatic artery. The hepatic veins, which are formed by the union of central veins, drain into the inferior vena cava. There are usually three large hepatic veins and a variable number of small hepatic veins. The ligamentum venosum is a remnant of the ductus venosus, which conveyed blood in the fetus from the left branch of the portal vein to the left hepatic vein.

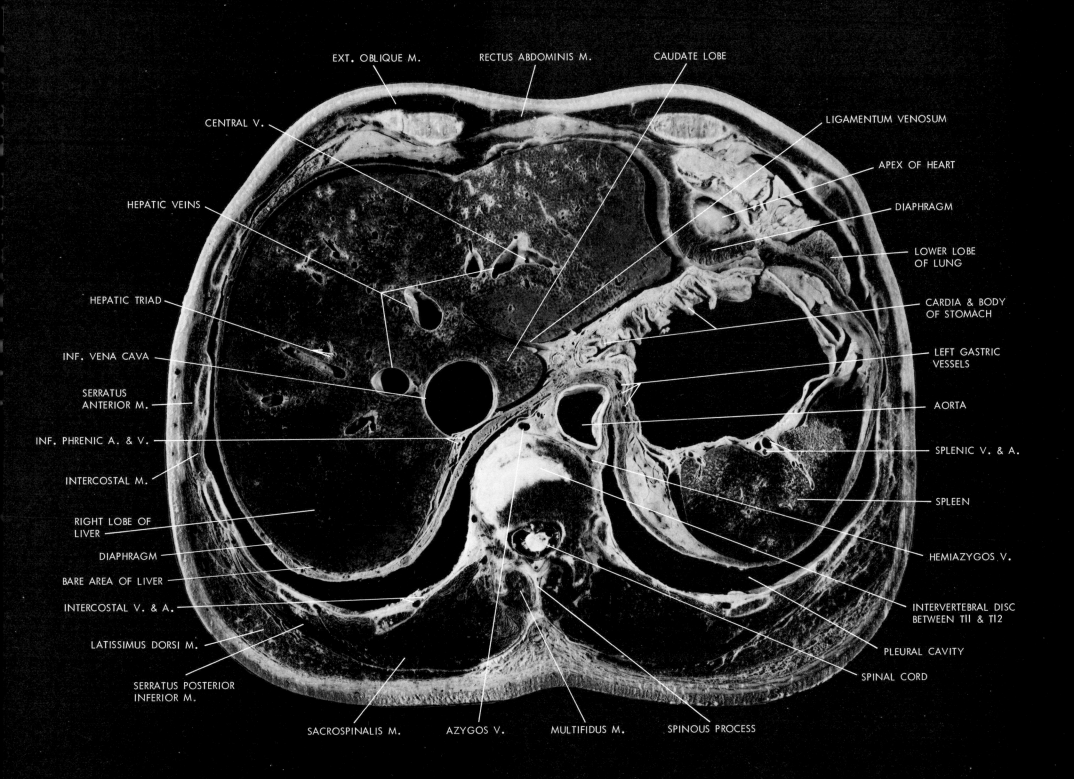

EXT. OBLIQUE M.

RECTUS ABDOMINIS M.

CAUDATE LOBE

CENTRAL V.

LIGAMENTUM VENOSUM

APEX OF HEART

HEPATIC VEINS

DIAPHRAGM

LOWER LOBE
OF LUNG

HEPATIC TRIAD

CARDIA & BODY
OF STOMACH

INF. VENA CAVA

LEFT GASTRIC
VESSELS

SERRATUS
ANTERIOR M.

AORTA

INF. PHRENIC A. & V.

SPLENIC V. & A.

INTERCOSTAL M.

RIGHT LOBE OF
LIVER

SPLEEN

DIAPHRAGM

HEMIAZYGOS V.

BARE AREA OF LIVER

INTERCOSTAL V. & A.

INTERVERTEBRAL DISC
BETWEEN TII & TI2

LATISSIMUS DORSI M.

PLEURAL CAVITY

SERRATUS POSTERIOR
INFERIOR M.

SPINAL CORD

SACROSPINALIS M.

AZYGOS V.

MULTIFIDUS M.

SPINOUS PROCESS

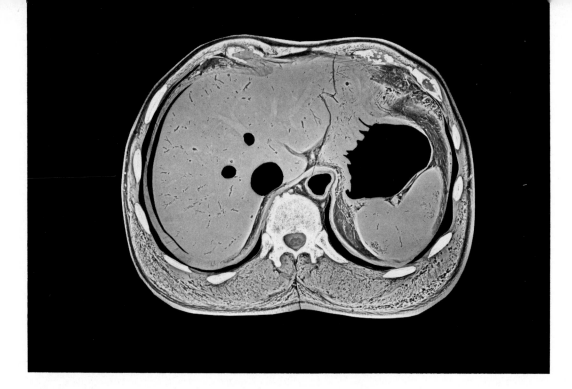

The arterial supply to the spleen is from the splenic artery, which is one of the branches of the celiac axis.

Clinical Considerations

In this section it is important to note the relationship of the crura of the diaphragm in respect to the aorta and the inferior vena cava. At times this posterior attachment of the diaphragm can appear somewhat nodular and be readily mistaken for an enlarged pathologic process.

The complete peritonealization of the liver, except for the bare area posteriorly, can be readily identified. It is this complete peritonealization of the liver that allows the egress of free air released from a ruptured hollow viscus to surround the liver, and when the patient is in the erect position, it lies between the diaphragm and the liver giving a typical semilunate appearance.

The relationship of the spleen to the stomach in this section, as in Sections 3-1 and 3-3, is important. The splenic artery and vein are readily identified in the hilus of the spleen, and in computed axial tomography, at times, the entire branch from the aorta or to the inferior vena cava is readily seen. It forms an important structure for identification and separation from the contiguous structures.

Enlargement of the spleen will occasionally cause an edema and thickening of the rugae of the stomach in the immediate vicinity of the spleen. In the intracapsular hematoma of the spleen, there is a displacement of the stomach with an occasional thickening of the rugae that is quite significant in the diagnosis of this condition.

SECTION

3-2

Through the body of T12

Anatomic Considerations

The stomach, the first abdominal subdivision of the gastrointestinal tract, has two surfaces (anterior and posterior) and two borders (greater and lesser curvatures). The size, configuration, and position of this organ depend upon the physiological state of the stomach and general body build. The stomach is divided into the cardiac portion, which is continuous with the esophagus; the fundus, which is the part superior to the esophageal junction; the body or main part of the stomach; and the pyloric region. The mucous lining of the stomach is thrown into longitudinal ridges called rugae.

The blood supply to the lesser curvature is by the left and right gastric arteries. The arterial supply to the greater curvature is from the left and right gastroepiploic arteries and the short gastric arteries. The veins accompany the corresponding arteries and terminate in the portal vein.

The spleen, located in the left hypochondriac region, has a diaphragmatic and visceral surface. As can be observed in this and in subsequent sections, the diaphragmatic surface is related to the 9th, 10th, and 11th ribs, and the visceral surface is related to the stomach, large intestine, tail of the pancreas, left suprarenal gland, and kidney.

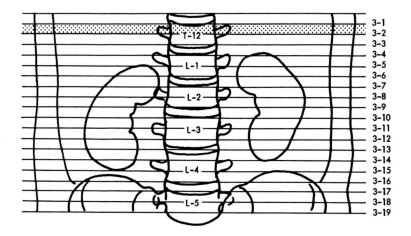

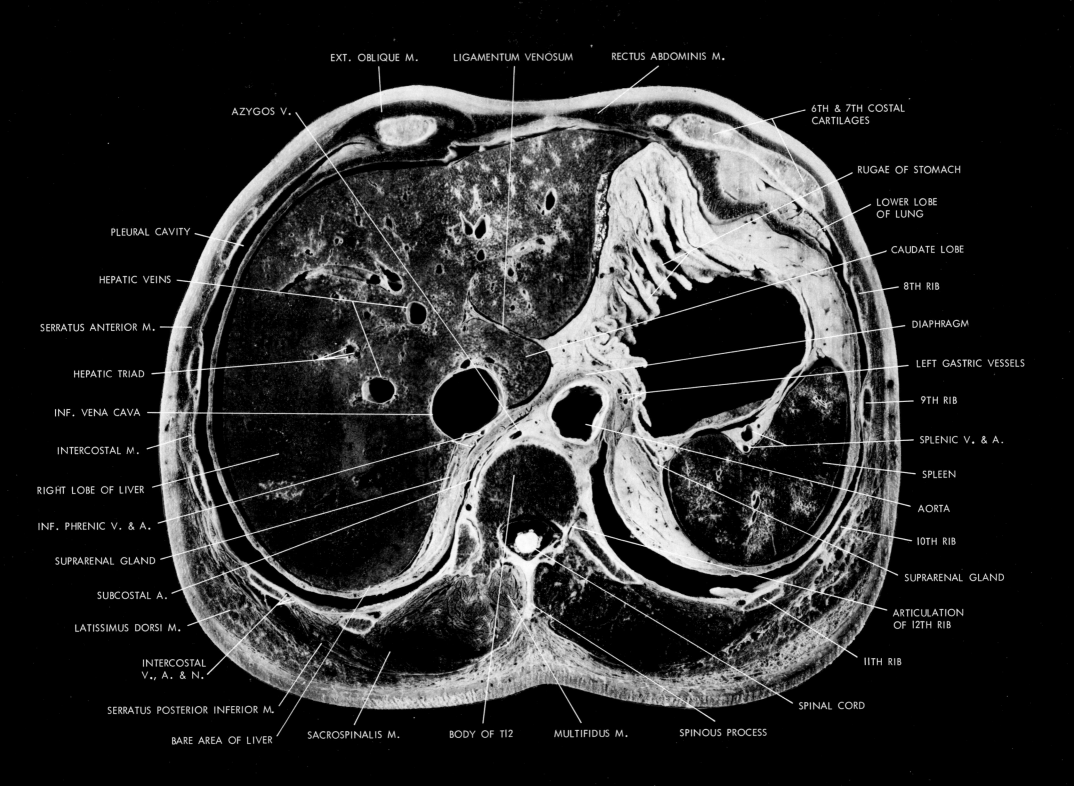

EXT. OBLIQUE M.

LIGAMENTUM VENOSUM

RECTUS ABDOMINIS M.

AZYGOS V.

6TH & 7TH COSTAL CARTILAGES

RUGAE OF STOMACH

LOWER LOBE OF LUNG

PLEURAL CAVITY

CAUDATE LOBE

HEPATIC VEINS

8TH RIB

SERRATUS ANTERIOR M.

DIAPHRAGM

LEFT GASTRIC VESSELS

HEPATIC TRIAD

9TH RIB

INF. VENA CAVA

SPLENIC V. & A.

INTERCOSTAL M.

SPLEEN

RIGHT LOBE OF LIVER

AORTA

INF. PHRENIC V. & A.

10TH RIB

SUPRARENAL GLAND

SUPRARENAL GLAND

SUBCOSTAL A.

ARTICULATION OF 12TH RIB

LATISSIMUS DORSI M.

INTERCOSTAL V., A. & N.

11TH RIB

SERRATUS POSTERIOR INFERIOR M.

SPINAL CORD

BARE AREA OF LIVER

SACROSPINALIS M.

BODY OF T12

MULTIFIDUS M.

SPINOUS PROCESS

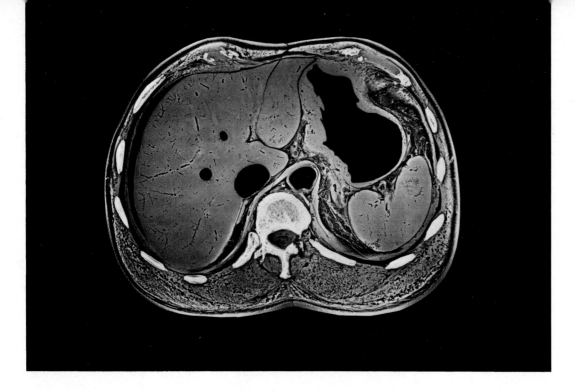

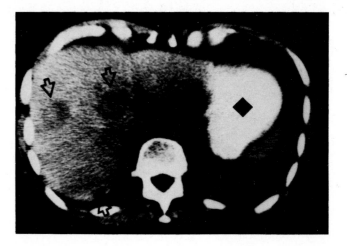

SECTION 3–3

Through the intervertebral disc between T12 and L1

Anatomic Considerations

The paired suprarenal glands first make their appearance in the previous section and continue until Section 3–6. The right suprarenal gland is closely related to the visceral surface of the liver, inferior vena cava, and right crus of the diaphragm; the left suprarenal gland is related to the stomach, spleen, aorta, and left crus of the diaphragm. In this specimen, the glands are separated from the kidneys by a large amount of perirenal fat.

The suprarenals receive their blood supply from the inferior phrenic arteries, the aorta, and the renal arteries. On the left side the suprarenal vein drains into the renal vein and on the right into the inferior vena cava.

Clinical Considerations

This CT scan through the liver demonstrates several metastatic tumors with absorption coefficients less than that of the surrounding liver substance (open arrows). The stomach (closed diamond) is contrast enhanced with 5 per cent Gastrografin. The remainder of the scan is similar to the cadaveric slice corresponding to this section. (Courtesy of Dr. Neil Wolfman.)

In the cadaveric section the slitlike appearance of the suprarenal gland is identified. In computed axial tomography this appearance can be identified in the normal and the abnormal situations. When abnormal, the suprarenal gland becomes enlarged and changed in its contour from that depicted here, so that this section is of importance in these conditions.

In this section also, the slitlike appearance of the splenic artery is becoming evident and should be followed in subsequent sections because of its importance in identification and separation, particularly from shadows related to the pancreas, in computed axial tomography and in ultrasound.

The blood supply and venous drainage of the suprarenals are of considerable importance angiographically.

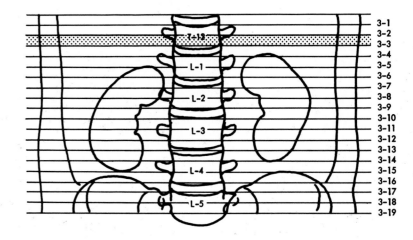

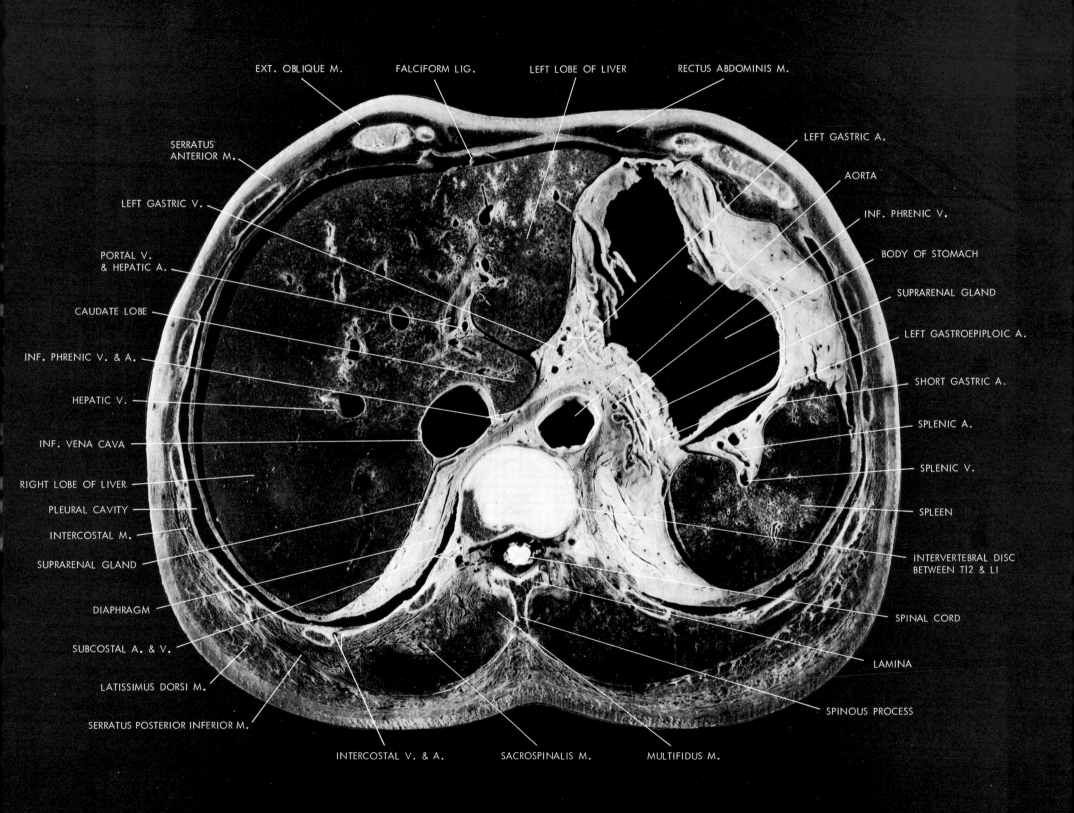

EXT. OBLIQUE M.   FALCIFORM LIG.   LEFT LOBE OF LIVER   RECTUS ABDOMINIS M.

SERRATUS ANTERIOR M.

LEFT GASTRIC V.

PORTAL V. & HEPATIC A.

CAUDATE LOBE

INF. PHRENIC V. & A.

HEPATIC V.

INF. VENA CAVA

RIGHT LOBE OF LIVER

PLEURAL CAVITY

INTERCOSTAL M.

SUPRARENAL GLAND

DIAPHRAGM

SUBCOSTAL A. & V.

LATISSIMUS DORSI M.

SERRATUS POSTERIOR INFERIOR M.

LEFT GASTRIC A.

AORTA

INF. PHRENIC V.

BODY OF STOMACH

SUPRARENAL GLAND

LEFT GASTROEPIPLOIC A.

SHORT GASTRIC A.

SPLENIC A.

SPLENIC V.

SPLEEN

INTERVERTEBRAL DISC BETWEEN T12 & L1

SPINAL CORD

LAMINA

SPINOUS PROCESS

INTERCOSTAL V. & A.   SACROSPINALIS M.   MULTIFIDUS M.

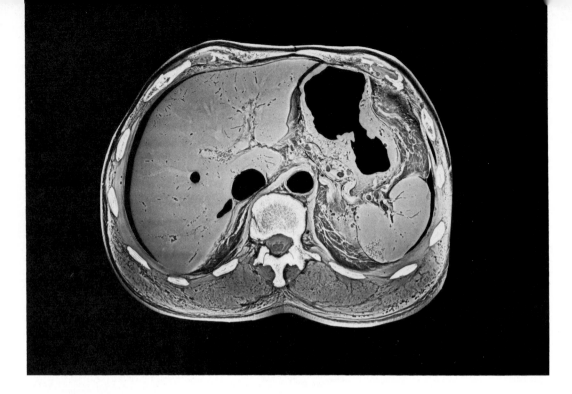

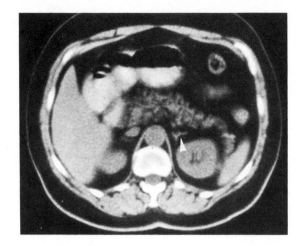

SECTION

3–4

*Through the
upper portion of
the body of L1*

Anatomic Considerations

As can be seen in Sections 2–24 to 3–7, the posterior relations of the stomach (stomach bed) consist of the spleen, splenic vessels, pancreas, transverse mesocolon, diaphragm, left suprarenal gland, and left kidney.

This illustration shows the celiac axis, which is the first unpaired branch of the abdominal aorta. The celiac axis divides to form the left gastric, common hepatic, and splenic arteries, which supply the caudal portions of the foregut and its derivatives.

The superior pole of the left kidney is present in this section. The left kidney usually lies at a higher level than the right. In this specimen, the superior pole of the right kidney lies 2 cm below the superior pole of the left kidney.

Clinical Considerations

This CT scan of the abdomen beautifully demonstrates the left adrenal gland (arrow). A portion of the right adrenal gland can be seen just posterior to the inferior vena cava. There is Gastrografin in the gastrointestinal tract for contrast enhancement. (Courtesy of Dr. George Flouty and Dr. Sadek Hilal.)

In the cadaveric section the suprarenal gland appears as a slightly larger structure but still very small normally. It is helpful to combine the information obtained from this section with that in the preceding section and in subsequent sections to obtain a complete view of this very important anatomic structure. Note that the left suprarenal gland is more anteriorly situated than the right suprarenal gland, which can be identified normally immediately ventral to the inferior vena cava and the hepatic vein. These last two structures can be intensified or enhanced with contrast substance.

In this section a small portion of the pancreas is identified, impressing itself upon the stomach and tending to approach the hilus of the spleen. When it becomes enlarged, the pancreas can be identified under these circumstances, particularly if it is surrounded by sufficient fat.

The portal vein is a large structure that usually can be identified in good ultrasound depictions of this section; it lies just to the right and slightly anterior to the caudate lobe of the liver.

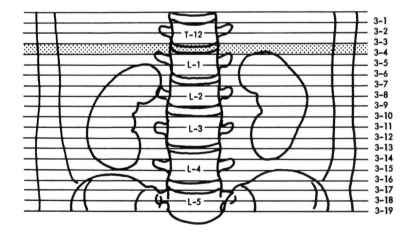

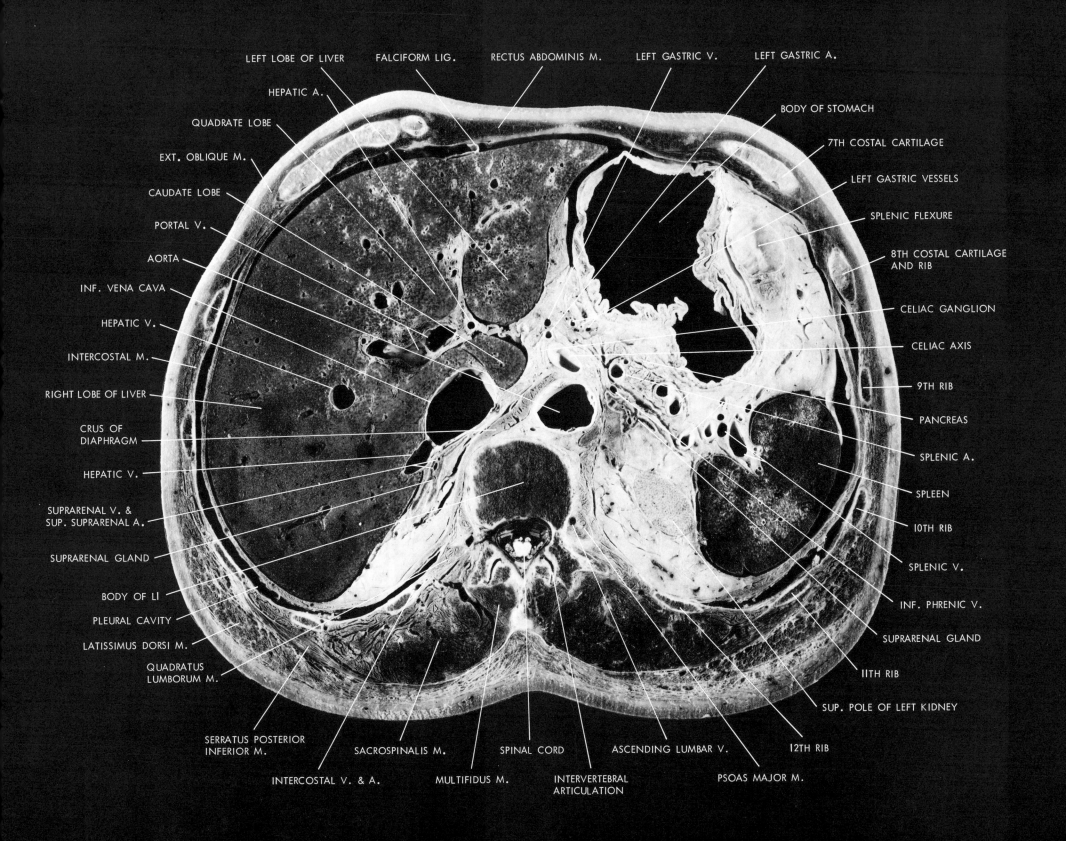

LEFT LOBE OF LIVER FALCIFORM LIG. RECTUS ABDOMINIS M. LEFT GASTRIC V. LEFT GASTRIC A.

HEPATIC A.

QUADRATE LOBE

EXT. OBLIQUE M.

CAUDATE LOBE

PORTAL V.

AORTA

INF. VENA CAVA

HEPATIC V.

INTERCOSTAL M.

RIGHT LOBE OF LIVER

CRUS OF DIAPHRAGM

HEPATIC V.

SUPRARENAL V. & SUP. SUPRARENAL A.

SUPRARENAL GLAND

BODY OF LI

PLEURAL CAVITY

LATISSIMUS DORSI M.

QUADRATUS LUMBORUM M.

BODY OF STOMACH

7TH COSTAL CARTILAGE

LEFT GASTRIC VESSELS

SPLENIC FLEXURE

8TH COSTAL CARTILAGE AND RIB

CELIAC GANGLION

CELIAC AXIS

9TH RIB

PANCREAS

SPLENIC A.

SPLEEN

10TH RIB

SPLENIC V.

INF. PHRENIC V.

SUPRARENAL GLAND

11TH RIB

SUP. POLE OF LEFT KIDNEY

SERRATUS POSTERIOR INFERIOR M. SACROSPINALIS M. SPINAL CORD ASCENDING LUMBAR V. 12TH RIB

INTERCOSTAL V. & A. MULTIFIDUS M. INTERVERTEBRAL ARTICULATION PSOAS MAJOR M.

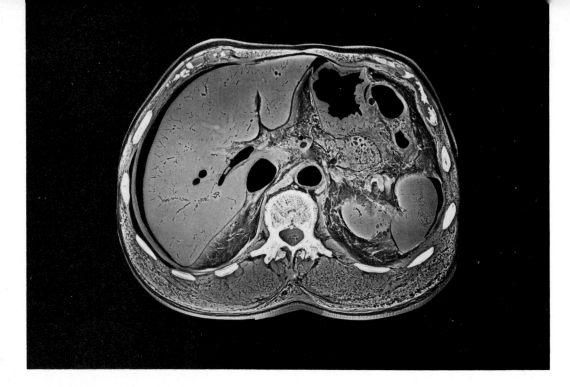

anterior to the splenic artery. It also lies anterior to the left suprarenal gland on the left. The right aspect of the pancreas as visualized here becomes contiguous with the common hepatic artery. This, too, is a very important relationship. Visualization of the pancreas by computed axial tomography is becoming increasingly important, since this method allows us to evaluate the pancreas most accurately by noninvasive techniques.

Note the position of the falciform ligament. In pneumoperitoneum of the newborn, the falciform ligament can be readily identified, since all of the structures contiguous to it become separated from the abdominal wall by the air in the peritoneal space. This identification of the falciform ligament has given rise to the so-called "football sign," since the entire distended peritoneal space, with the falciform ligament appearing in the cephalad part of the abdomen, gives the appearance of the "lacework" on a football.

Note also in this section the appearance of the transverse colon and descending colon. Very often the transverse colon as it appears on this section is misconstrued as representing the splenic flexure, because in a straight anteroposterior supine projection of the abdomen it is projected near the hilus of the spleen.

In this section the cortex of the kidney becomes evident. The kidney can be readily identified by its architecture, both in computed axial tomography and in ultrasound; in this and succeeding sections, the clear identification of the kidney in its full architectural pattern is an extremely important landmark.

SECTION 3–5

Through the lower portion of the body of L1

Anatomic Considerations

In this section and in the following section the structures of the porta hepatis can be observed. The porta hepatis is approximately 5 cm long and through it pass the hepatic duct, hepatic artery, portal vein, sympathetic fibers from the celiac ganglion, parasympathetic fibers of the anterior branch of the vagus nerve, and lymphatics. It separates the caudate lobe of the liver from the quadrate lobe, and its margins serve as attachment for the lesser omentum. The above structures are found in the free margin of the lesser omentum, which forms the anterior boundary of the epiploic foramen. The foramen is bounded dorsally by the peritoneum covering the inferior vena cava, superiorly by the peritoneum on the caudate lobe of the liver, and inferiorly by the peritoneum covering the beginning of the duodenum.

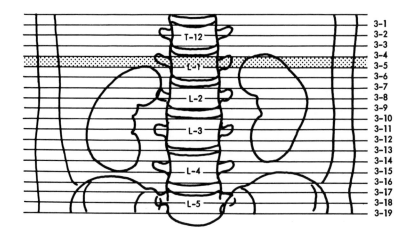

Clinical Considerations

Note that the pancreas has become a significantly larger structure in this section and is situated just posterior to the body of the stomach, somewhat

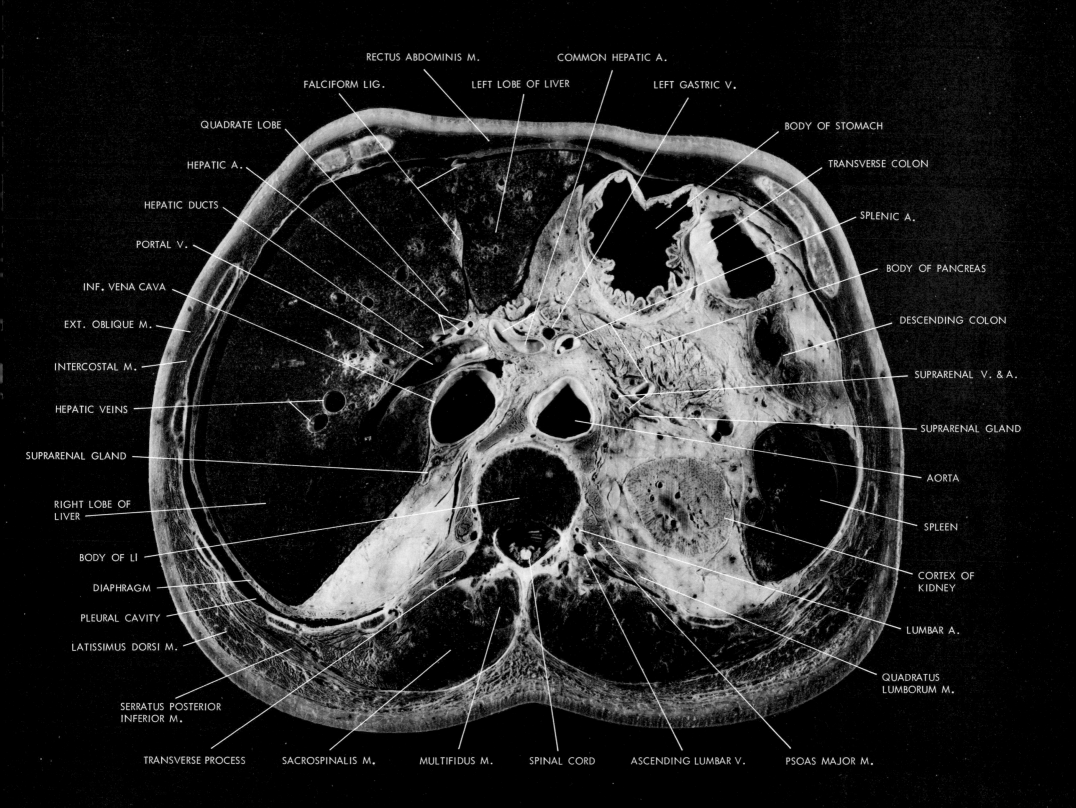

RECTUS ABDOMINIS M.

COMMON HEPATIC A.

FALCIFORM LIG.

LEFT LOBE OF LIVER

LEFT GASTRIC V.

QUADRATE LOBE

BODY OF STOMACH

HEPATIC A.

TRANSVERSE COLON

HEPATIC DUCTS

SPLENIC A.

PORTAL V.

BODY OF PANCREAS

INF. VENA CAVA

DESCENDING COLON

EXT. OBLIQUE M.

INTERCOSTAL M.

SUPRARENAL V. & A.

HEPATIC VEINS

SUPRARENAL GLAND

SUPRARENAL GLAND

AORTA

RIGHT LOBE OF LIVER

SPLEEN

BODY OF LI

CORTEX OF KIDNEY

DIAPHRAGM

PLEURAL CAVITY

LUMBAR A.

LATISSIMUS DORSI M.

QUADRATUS LUMBORUM M.

SERRATUS POSTERIOR INFERIOR M.

TRANSVERSE PROCESS

SACROSPINALIS M.

MULTIFIDUS M.

SPINAL CORD

ASCENDING LUMBAR V.

PSOAS MAJOR M.

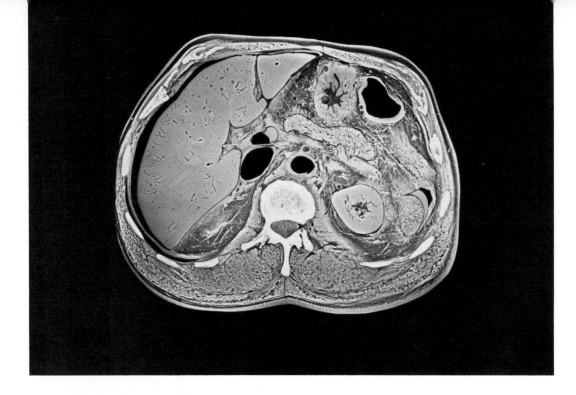

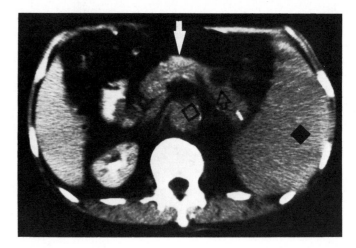

Clinical Considerations

This CT scan through the pancreas (white solid arrow) demonstrates a cyst near the tail of the pancreas (open arrow). The superior mesenteric artery (open diamond) is clearly shown branching from the aorta. Although the pancreas appears here almost in its entirety, the superior mesenteric artery is a very important landmark in respect to pointing toward the pancreas. The pancreas contains calcification (white spots). The spleen (closed diamond) is also very large in this patient, who was an alcoholic. (Courtesy of Dr. Neil Wolfman.)

In the cadaveric section the pyloric region of the stomach and transverse colon are adjacent to one another. When enhanced with contrast media, these structures can be readily identified as being anterior to the pancreas. The close relationship of the descending colon to the caudal end of the spleen must likewise be clearly identified, since occasionally the descending colon can also be intensified or enhanced with contrast agent.

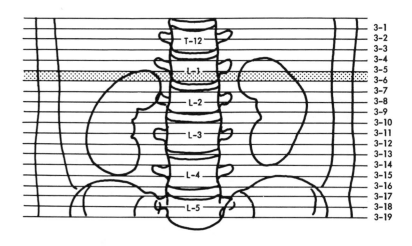

SECTION
3–6

Through the intervertebral disc between L1 and L2

Anatomic Considerations

The pancreas, which can be seen in Sections 3–4 to 3–12, is both an endocrine and an exocrine gland. The pancreas is subdivided into a head, neck, body, and tail. The head is located within the concavity of the duodenum and is related posteriorly to the aorta and inferior vena cava and anteriorly to the transverse colon. The uncinate process is an extension of the head of the pancreas, which lies posterior to the superior mesenteric vessels and anterior to the aorta. The neck of the pancreas connects the head and body and lies anterior to the portal vein. The body of the pancreas is related posteriorly to the left crus of the diaphragm, left suprarenal gland, left kidney, left renal vein, and splenic vein. The transverse mesocolon is attached along the anterior aspect of the body of the pancreas. The tail of the pancreas extends to the hilus of the spleen.

The arterial blood supply to the pancreas is derived from the splenic, common hepatic, gastroduodenal, and superior mesenteric arteries. Most of the veins draining the pancreas terminate in the splenic vein; some end in the superior mesenteric or portal veins.

The superior mesenteric artery is the second unpaired branch of the abdominal aorta. In this specimen the artery arose at the inferior border of L1. In addition to the pancreas, the superior mesenteric artery supplies the intestinal tract from the duodenum to the splenic flexure of the large intestine.

The relationships of the superior mesenteric artery to the aorta and to the pancreas are important landmarks for identification. The superior mesenteric artery, particularly if identified as arising from the aorta, points to the body of the pancreas. The left aspect of the pancreas, on the other hand, tends to point toward the spleen and the kidney.

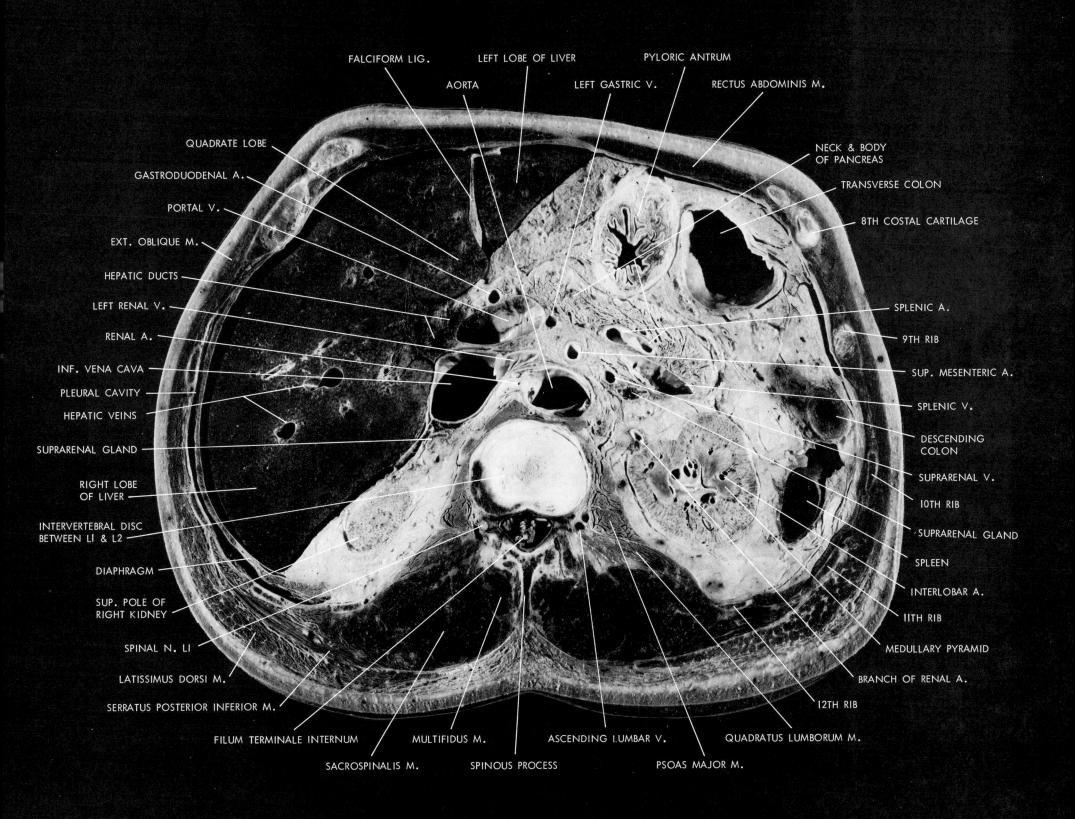

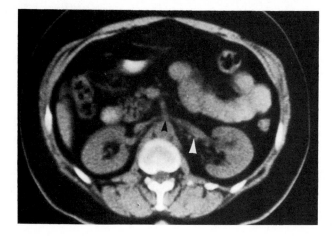

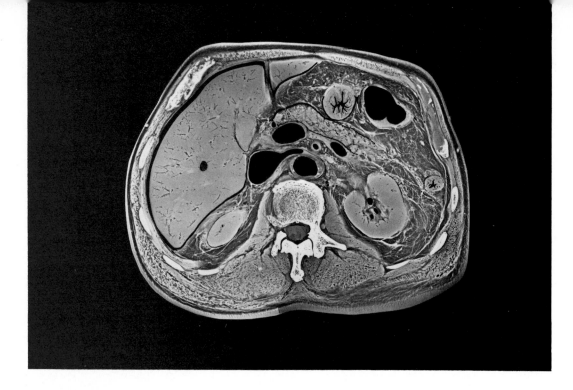

SECTION 3–7

Through the upper portion of the body of L2

Anatomic Considerations

The portal vein is formed posterior to the neck of the pancreas by the union of the splenic and superior mesenteric veins. In this section the left gastric vein is shown entering the portal vein. The portal vein passes obliquely to the right into the porta hepatis.

The left renal vein passes anterior to the aorta and terminates in the inferior vena cava. Observe the proximity of the superior mesenteric artery to the left renal vein.

The gall bladder is first seen in this section and continues inferiorly to Section 3–12. As can be observed, the gall bladder is closely related to the anterior abdominal wall inferiorly. The gall bladder lies in a small fossa on the visceral surface of the liver and is divided into a neck, body, and fundus. The fundus projects beyond the inferior margin of the liver. The anterior surface of the body is closely related to the liver and the posterior surface is related to the transverse colon and the second portion of the duodenum. The neck is continuous with the cystic duct, which passes into the hepatoduodenal ligament and joins the hepatic duct to form the common bile duct.

Clinical Considerations

In this CT scan of the abdomen, the superior mesenteric artery (black arrow) is well visualized pointing toward a portion of the pancreas. The left renal vein (white arrow) can be seen crossing the abdomen and entering the inferior vena cava. (Courtesy of Dr. George Flouty and Dr. Sadek Hilal.)

In the cadaveric section the gall bladder is clearly seen lying anterior to the inferior vena cava and to the right of the portal vein. Visualization of the gall bladder by cross-sectional anatomy, using ultrasonic techniques as well as computed axial tomography, has become extremely important. In the latter technique the detection of very small stones within the gall bladder has become feasible. This is especially important when contrast enhancement of the gall bladder is impossible by noninvasive techniques because of poor function of the gall bladder.

Note the large, fatty envelope that surrounds both kidneys. This fatty envelope is responsible for the clear definition of the kidneys on both planar type tomographic studies of the kidney and CT studies.

The quadratus lumborum muscle on either side of the vertebral body has the appearance of a symmetrical mass. The relationship of this muscle mass in respect to each kidney is important for identification, since these muscle masses must not be misinterpreted as representing abnormalities.

It will be noticed that the left aspect of the pancreas lies immediately anterior to the splenic vein. Contrast enhancement of the splenic vein is very helpful in measurements of this portion of the pancreas.

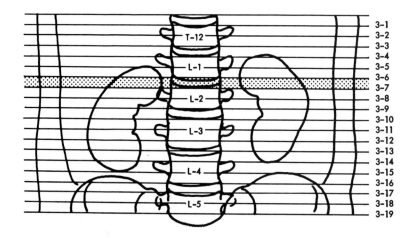

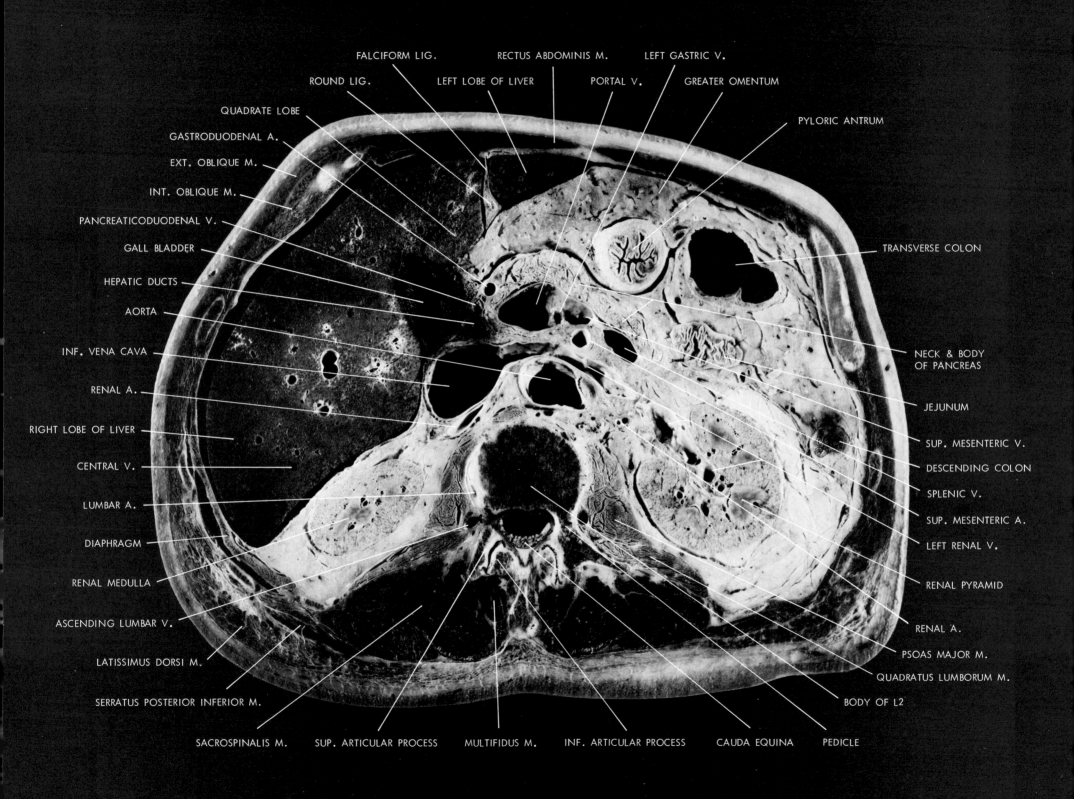

FALCIFORM LIG.

RECTUS ABDOMINIS M.

LEFT GASTRIC V.

ROUND LIG.

LEFT LOBE OF LIVER

PORTAL V.

GREATER OMENTUM

QUADRATE LOBE

PYLORIC ANTRUM

GASTRODUODENAL A.

EXT. OBLIQUE M.

INT. OBLIQUE M.

PANCREATICODUODENAL V.

GALL BLADDER

TRANSVERSE COLON

HEPATIC DUCTS

AORTA

INF. VENA CAVA

NECK & BODY
OF PANCREAS

RENAL A.

JEJUNUM

RIGHT LOBE OF LIVER

SUP. MESENTERIC V.

CENTRAL V.

DESCENDING COLON

LUMBAR A.

SPLENIC V.

DIAPHRAGM

SUP. MESENTERIC A.

LEFT RENAL V.

RENAL MEDULLA

RENAL PYRAMID

ASCENDING LUMBAR V.

RENAL A.

LATISSIMUS DORSI M.

PSOAS MAJOR M.

QUADRATUS LUMBORUM M.

SERRATUS POSTERIOR INFERIOR M.

BODY OF L2

SACROSPINALIS M.

SUP. ARTICULAR PROCESS

MULTIFIDUS M.

INF. ARTICULAR PROCESS

CAUDA EQUINA

PEDICLE

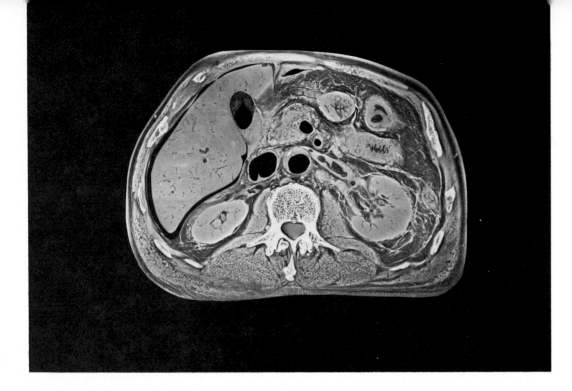

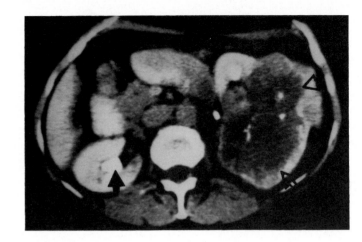

contains contrast agent in the collecting system (closed arrow). (Courtesy of Dr. Neil Wolfman.)

In the cadaveric section the gall bladder is in clear view and it should be noted how anteriorly situated the gall bladder usually is found. It lies anterior to the inferior vena cava and forms an ovoid filling defect in the adjoining portion of the anterior aspect of the liver.

Note the relationship between the left renal vein and artery, with the left renal vein lying anterior to the artery. Likewise, the right renal artery and vein are similarly related, with the exception that the right renal artery may impress itself upon the inferior vena cava, producing a small nodular appearance therein; this must not be misinterpreted as being abnormal.

By separate or consecutive enhancement of the blood vessels against the gastrointestinal tract, one can readily separate these two systems in this type of cross section. Diatrozoates are used in both instances, a methyl or sodium diatrozoate for the blood vessels and Gastrografin in dilute solution for the gastrointestinal structures. (Gastrografin is meglumine diatrozoate in a specially formed solution.)

SECTION
3–8

Through the lower portion of the body of L2

Anatomic Considerations

The duodenum is the first part of the small intestine and extends from the pylorus to the duodenojejunal flexure. The duodenum can be seen in this section and those that follow, through Section 3–15. The duodenum is somewhat C-shaped, with the concavity enclosing the head of the pancreas. The superior portion of the duodenum (duodenal bulb) extends from the pylorus to the neck of the gall bladder and is the most movable part of the duodenum, since it is almost entirely covered by peritoneum. This portion of the duodenum is related to the quadrate lobe of the liver, gall bladder, gastroduodenal artery, portal vein, and common bile duct. The second or descending portion of the duodenum is the longest one, usually extending to the fourth lumbar vertebra (Section 3–15); it receives the common bile duct and pancreatic duct. As can be seen in the illustrations, the major relations of the descending portion of the duodenum are the gall bladder, liver, pancreas, inferior vena cava, right kidney, and ascending and transverse colon. The horizontal portion of the duodenum passes to the left between the aorta and superior mesenteric artery. The ascending or fourth part of the duodenum ascends along the left side of the aorta for approximately 3 cm, where it turns ventralward to become continuous with the jejunum.

The blood supply to the duodenum is from the common hepatic, gastroduodenal, and superior mesenteric arteries. The venous drainage is to the portal system.

Clinical Considerations

This CT scan at the level of the kidneys demonstrates a large left clear cell carcinoma (open arrows). The slice through the opposite normal kidney

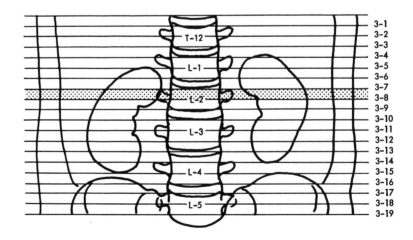

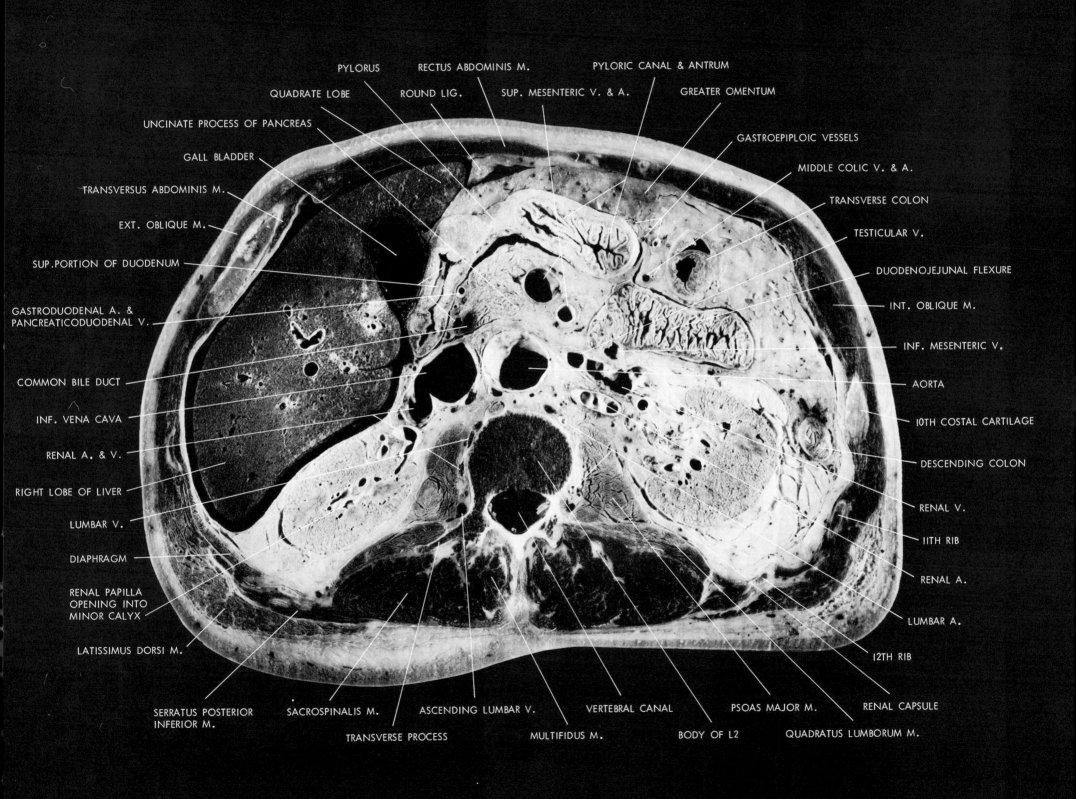

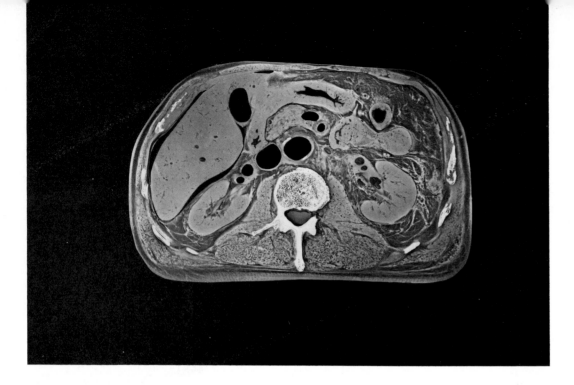

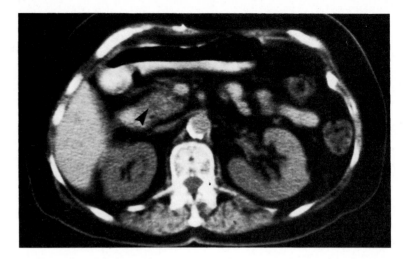

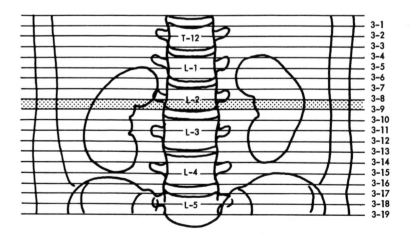

SECTION 3–9

Through the upper portion of the intervertebral disc between L2 and L3

Anatomic Considerations

As can be seen in this illustration, the kidneys are paired retroperitoneal organs that lie lateral to the vertebral column. The right kidney usually lies at a lower level than the left one. In this specimen, the right kidney extends from the intervertebral disc between L1 and L2 (Section 3–6) to the lower aspect of the fourth lumbar vertebra (Section 3–15). The left kidney extends from the upper end of L1 (Section 3–4) to the upper part of L4 (Section 3–14). In this specimen, the left kidney is slightly longer (approximately 11 cm) than the right (10 cm).

The anterior surface of the right kidney is related to the duodenum, liver, ascending colon, and suprarenal gland, while the left kidney is related to the spleen, stomach, jejunum, descending colon, and suprarenal gland. The posterior surface of each kidney has similar relations to four muscles: the quadratus lumborum and psoas major are related to the kidney throughout its entire extent; the diaphragm is related to the kidney at its superior end; and the transverse abdominis is at the inferior end.

Perirenal fat is the adipose tissue that lies adjacent to and completely invests the kidney. In this specimen (Sections 3–2 to 3–6), the suprarenal glands are separated from the kidney by several centimeters owing to the abundance of this perirenal fat.

Clinical Considerations

The CT scan through the head of the pancreas (arrow) shows it to be at the upper limits of normal as to size. This patient had been operated upon one year ago and a very hard pancreas had been demonstrated at the time of cholecystectomy. It was not biopsied. The long-term survival of this patient would suggest that this hard pancreas is due to a chronic pancreatitis. It is difficult to determine the difference between a carcinoma involving the pancreas and pancreatitis. There are small flakes of calcium in the head of the pancreas, suggesting pancreatitis. (Courtesy of Dr. Neil Wolfman.)

Computed axial tomography has become especially valuable in the diagnosis of renal mass lesions such as abscesses, cysts, and tumors. Ultrasound is an alternative method for demonstration of the kidneys and their mass lesions.

In this section the anterior relationship of the gall bladder to the descending part of the duodenum should also be noted. The descending part of the duodenum may be contrast-enhanced with Gastrografin. The semilunate appearance of the right renal vein, posterior to the shadow of the inferior vena cava, with both of these structures being posterior to the descending part of the duodenum, takes on clinical significance in that these three structures must be clearly defined and differentiated for accurate diagnosis.

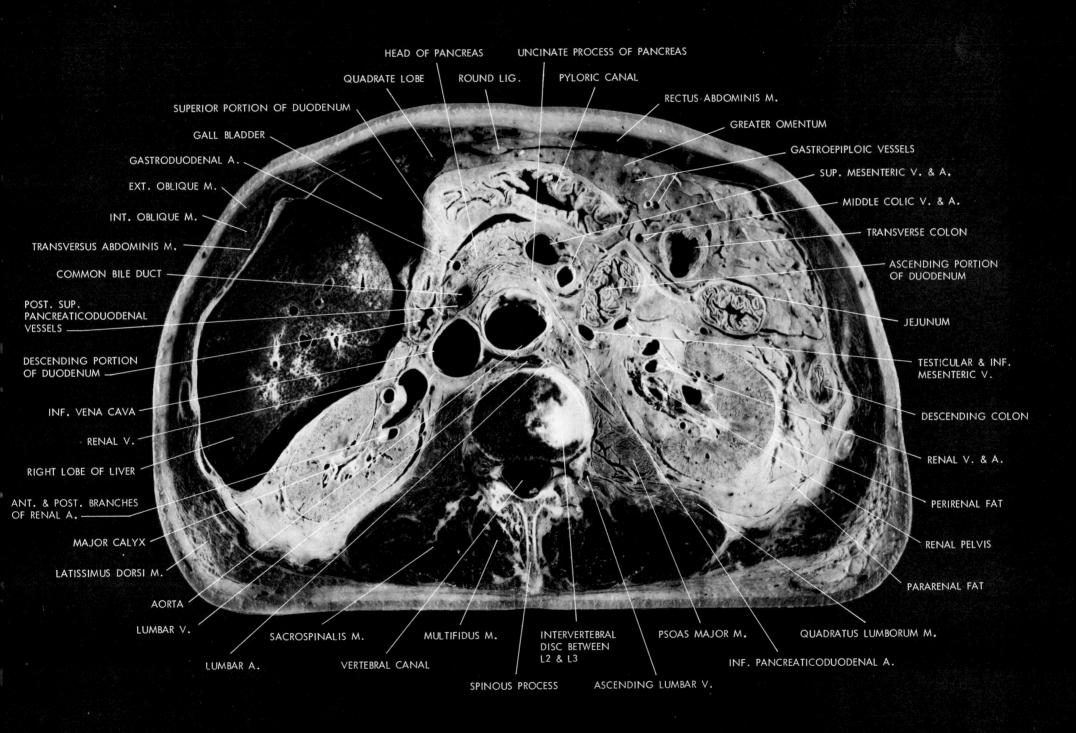

HEAD OF PANCREAS UNCINATE PROCESS OF PANCREAS

QUADRATE LOBE ROUND LIG. PYLORIC CANAL

RECTUS ABDOMINIS M.

SUPERIOR PORTION OF DUODENUM

GREATER OMENTUM

GALL BLADDER

GASTROEPIPLOIC VESSELS

GASTRODUODENAL A.

SUP. MESENTERIC V. & A.

EXT. OBLIQUE M.

MIDDLE COLIC V. & A.

INT. OBLIQUE M.

TRANSVERSE COLON

TRANSVERSUS ABDOMINIS M.

ASCENDING PORTION OF DUODENUM

COMMON BILE DUCT

POST. SUP. PANCREATICODUODENAL VESSELS

JEJUNUM

DESCENDING PORTION OF DUODENUM

TESTICULAR & INF. MESENTERIC V.

INF. VENA CAVA

DESCENDING COLON

RENAL V.

RENAL V. & A.

RIGHT LOBE OF LIVER

ANT. & POST. BRANCHES OF RENAL A.

PERIRENAL FAT

MAJOR CALYX

RENAL PELVIS

LATISSIMUS DORSI M.

PARARENAL FAT

AORTA

LUMBAR V.

SACROSPINALIS M. MULTIFIDUS M. INTERVERTEBRAL DISC BETWEEN L2 & L3 PSOAS MAJOR M. QUADRATUS LUMBORUM M.

LUMBAR A. VERTEBRAL CANAL INF. PANCREATICODUODENAL A.

SPINOUS PROCESS ASCENDING LUMBAR V.

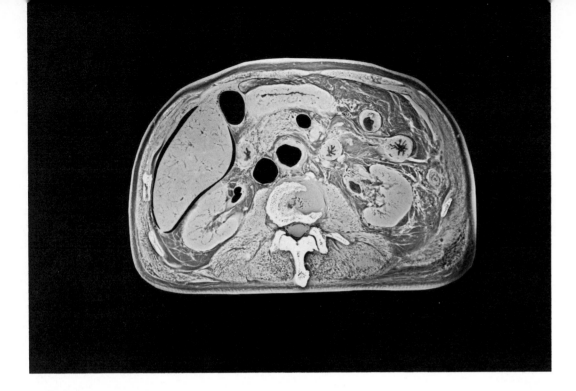

The gall bladder may still be seen just beneath the anterior abdominal wall, as was apparent in Section 3–9. This marked anterior relationship of the gall bladder is not always obtained but is so frequently found in this relationship that it is best to examine a patient for gall bladder disease in the prone position (in conventional radiography, in which the film is beneath the patient).

The transverse mesocolon is identified in this section. It may act as a conduit of fluid, inflammatory substance, or neoplasm from the pancreas toward the transverse colon, even involving the latter structure on occasion. At times, exudative processes may pass ventrally through this structure from the transverse colon to the pancreas. It holds a special place as a conduit and important space marker in the abdomen.

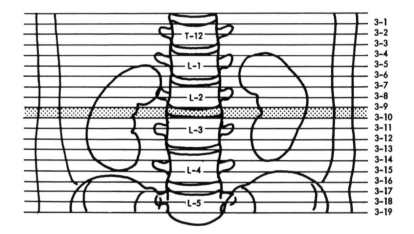

SECTION
3–10

Through the intervertebral disc between L2 and L3

Anatomic Considerations

Various aspects of the internal morphology of the kidney can be seen in this section and in the adjacent illustrations. The renal cortex lies deep to the capsule of the kidney, overlies the bases of the renal pyramids, and extends as renal columns between adjacent pyramids. A major feature of the renal medulla, or central portion of the kidney, is a series of pyramids that contain the collecting tubules. The renal papillae are located at the apices of the pyramids. The minor calyxes surround one or several papillae, and several of these minor calyxes unite to form a major calyx. The major calyxes (usually numbering from three to five) empty into the renal pelvis, which is the dilated cranial portion of the ureter.

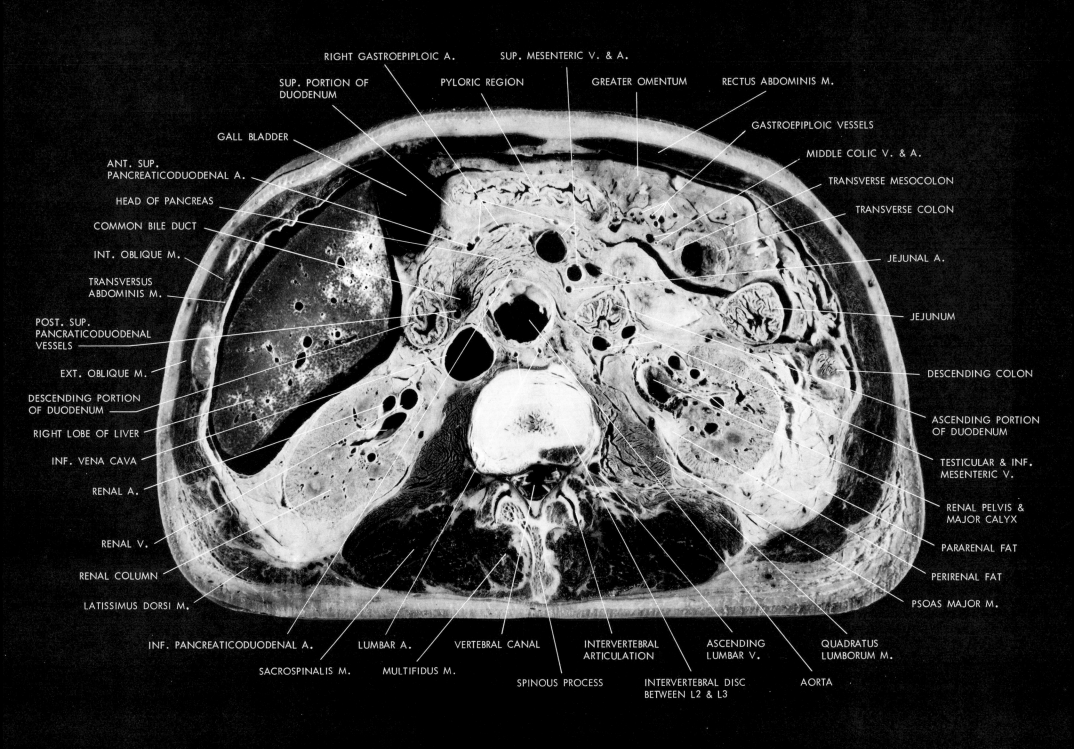

RIGHT GASTROEPIPLOIC A.

SUP. MESENTERIC V. & A.

SUP. PORTION OF
DUODENUM

PYLORIC REGION

GREATER OMENTUM

RECTUS ABDOMINIS M.

GALL BLADDER

GASTROEPIPLOIC VESSELS

ANT. SUP.
PANCREATICODUODENAL A.

MIDDLE COLIC V. & A.

TRANSVERSE MESOCOLON

HEAD OF PANCREAS

TRANSVERSE COLON

COMMON BILE DUCT

INT. OBLIQUE M.

JEJUNAL A.

TRANSVERSUS
ABDOMINIS M.

JEJUNUM

POST. SUP.
PANCREATICODUODENAL
VESSELS

EXT. OBLIQUE M.

DESCENDING COLON

DESCENDING PORTION
OF DUODENUM

ASCENDING PORTION
OF DUODENUM

RIGHT LOBE OF LIVER

INF. VENA CAVA

TESTICULAR & INF.
MESENTERIC V.

RENAL A.

RENAL PELVIS &
MAJOR CALYX

RENAL V.

PARARENAL FAT

RENAL COLUMN

PERIRENAL FAT

LATISSIMUS DORSI M.

PSOAS MAJOR M.

INF. PANCREATICODUODENAL A.

LUMBAR A.

VERTEBRAL CANAL

INTERVERTEBRAL
ARTICULATION

ASCENDING
LUMBAR V.

QUADRATUS
LUMBORUM M.

SACROSPINALIS M.

MULTIFIDUS M.

SPINOUS PROCESS

INTERVERTEBRAL DISC
BETWEEN L2 & L3

AORTA

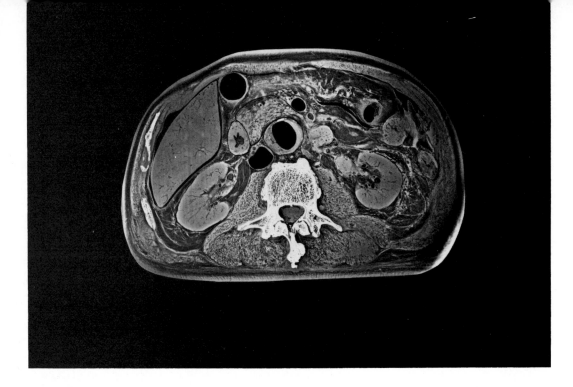

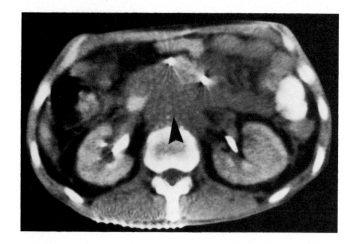

widened and aneurysmal or its wall shows evidence of dissection, there is cause for concern. A measurement of the aorta of more than 5 cm or dissection is a grave prognostic feature, suggesting impending rupture or further dissection.

In relation to the skeleton, the ureters lie along the tips of the transverse processes (L2 to L5), cross just medial to the sacroiliac joint, pass laterally to the tip of the spine of the ischium, and then pass medially to the urinary bladder. This relationship is important when searching for a ureteric stone on plain radiography of the abdomen.

The ureter is relatively narrow at three sites: at the junction of the renal pelvis with the abdominal portion, as it passes over the brim of the pelvis, and at the entrance into the urinary bladder. A ureteric calculus is likely to lodge at one of these three levels.

The relationships of the following structures should be carefully studied in this section because of their importance: (a) the descending portion of the duodenum, which may be enhanced with Gastrografin; (b) the gall bladder, which may be enhanced with iopanoic acid (Telepaque) by its administration orally 4 to 14 hours previously or by intravenous administration of an appropriate contrast agent; (c) the pancreas; (d) the aorta; and (e) the inferior vena cava.

SECTION
3–11

Through the upper portion of the body of L3

Anatomic Considerations

The ureter extends from the kidney to the urinary bladder. It begins as a funneled expansion, the renal pelvis, which is partly inside and partly outside the kidney. The portion of the renal pelvis outside the kidney tapers to become the ureter proper near the lower end of the organ. The ureter is approximately 25 cm long and is divided into abdominal and pelvic portions. The abdominal portion passes from lateral to medial on the surface of the psoas major muscle and enters the pelvis at the bifurcation of the common iliac artery.

Both ureters are crossed anteriorly by the gonadal vessels. The right ureter is covered by the duodenum at its origin, passes lateral to the inferior vena cava, and is crossed by the right colic and ileocolic vessels and the root of the mesentery. The left ureter is crossed by the left colic vessels and root of the sigmoid mesocolon.

Clinical Considerations

This CT scan demonstrates the abdomen of a patient with malignant lymphoma (arrow) producing a large retroperitoneal mass that extends cephalad and completely obscures the normal retroperitoneal anatomy, which ordinarily would be identifiable in this location. The artifacts are metal clips producing stellate secondary radiations, which extend somewhat into the lymphomatous mass. Gastrografin was administered to this patient for intensification of the gastrointestinal tract and Renografin was administered for contrast enhancement of the collecting system of both kidneys. (Courtesy Dr. Neil Wolfman.)

In the cadaveric section the aorta has an intimal plaque, which often contains calcification, seen not only by CT but also in conventional radiography. In some individuals, the aorta is elongated and tortuous. When it is

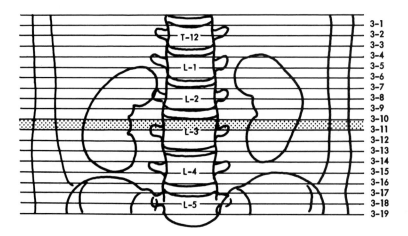

3–1
3–2
3–3
3–4
3–5
3–6
3–7
3–8
3–9
3–10
3–11
3–12
3–13
3–14
3–15
3–16
3–17
3–18
3–19

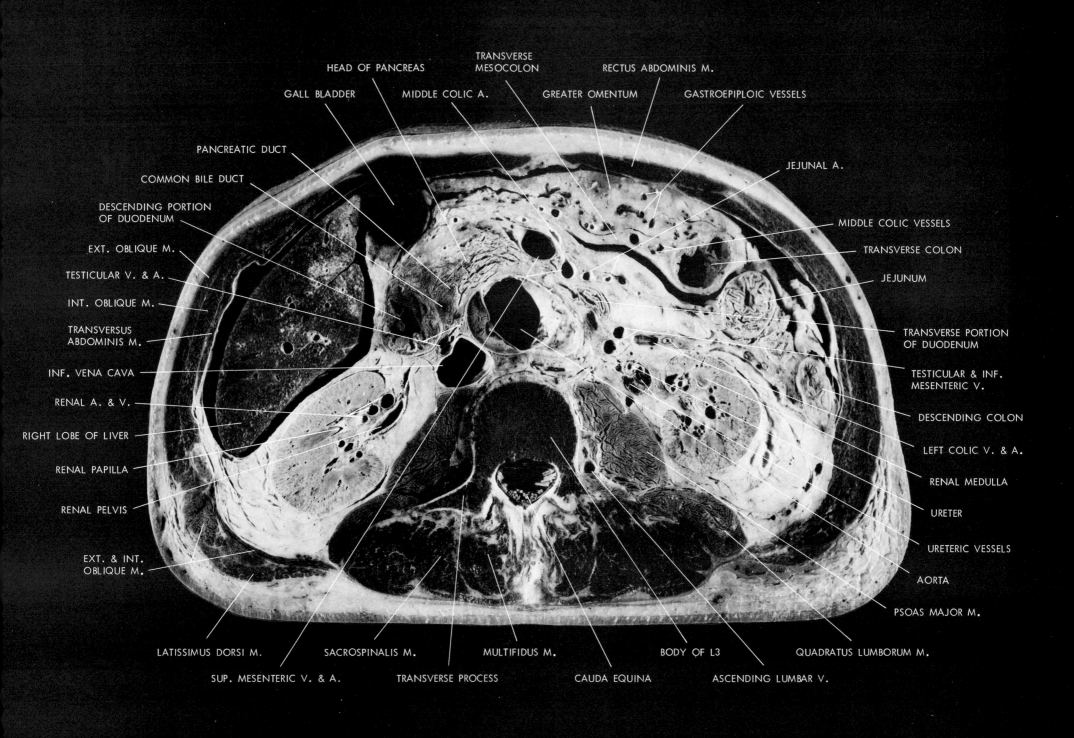

HEAD OF PANCREAS

TRANSVERSE
MESOCOLON

RECTUS ABDOMINIS M.

GALL BLADDER

MIDDLE COLIC A.

GREATER OMENTUM

GASTROEPIPLOIC VESSELS

PANCREATIC DUCT

JEJUNAL A.

COMMON BILE DUCT

DESCENDING PORTION
OF DUODENUM

MIDDLE COLIC VESSELS

EXT. OBLIQUE M.

TRANSVERSE COLON

TESTICULAR V. & A.

JEJUNUM

INT. OBLIQUE M.

TRANSVERSUS
ABDOMINIS M.

TRANSVERSE PORTION
OF DUODENUM

INF. VENA CAVA

TESTICULAR & INF.
MESENTERIC V.

RENAL A. & V.

DESCENDING COLON

RIGHT LOBE OF LIVER

LEFT COLIC V. & A.

RENAL PAPILLA

RENAL MEDULLA

RENAL PELVIS

URETER

EXT. & INT.
OBLIQUE M.

URETERIC VESSELS

AORTA

PSOAS MAJOR M.

LATISSIMUS DORSI M.

SACROSPINALIS M.

MULTIFIDUS M.

BODY OF L3

QUADRATUS LUMBORUM M.

SUP. MESENTERIC V. & A.

TRANSVERSE PROCESS

CAUDA EQUINA

ASCENDING LUMBAR V.

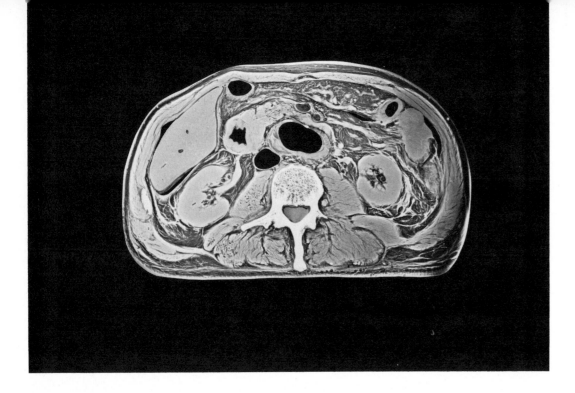

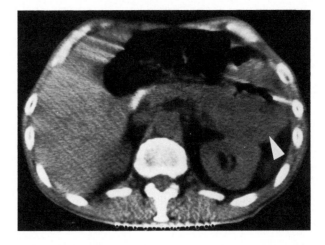

There has been considerable discussion of the importance of clear definition of the pancreatic duct, which at times may be dilated in lesions that obstruct at the level of the major duodenal papilla or in the more proximal portions of the head of the pancreas. Although a good roentgenographic sign of abnormality, it must be interpreted with caution, since its definition is variable, depending upon the amount of adjoining fat.

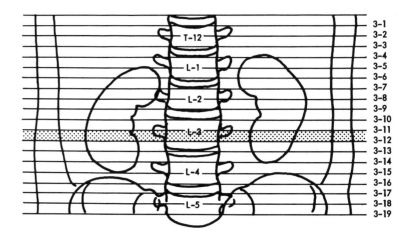

SECTION

3–12

Through the lower portion of the body of L3

Anatomic Considerations

This section demonstrates the termination of the biliary duct system on the summit of the major duodenal papilla. The right and left hepatic ducts unite in the porta hepatis to form the common hepatic duct, which joins the cystic duct to form the bile duct. There is a great range of variation in the morphology of this area with regard to the manner in which the cystic duct joins the common hepatic duct and its relations to the neighboring arteries.

The bile duct begins near the porta hepatis, descends in the free margin of the lesser omentum, passes posterior to the first part of the duodenum, descends in a groove on the posterior portion of the head of the pancreas, and enters the second portion of the duodenum a little below its middle on the posteromedial surface.

The bile duct penetrates the duodenal wall obliquely and expands to form the ampulla of the bile duct (ampulla of Vater); the bulging of the ampulla forms the duodenal papilla. The pancreatic duct (of Wirsung) joins the bile duct before or during the passage through the duodenal wall.

Clinical Considerations

This CT scan presents a patient with a recurrent carcinoma of the colon (arrow) displacing the lumen of the descending colon anteriorly and interposed between the colon and the left kidney. (Courtesy of Dr. Neil Wolfman.)

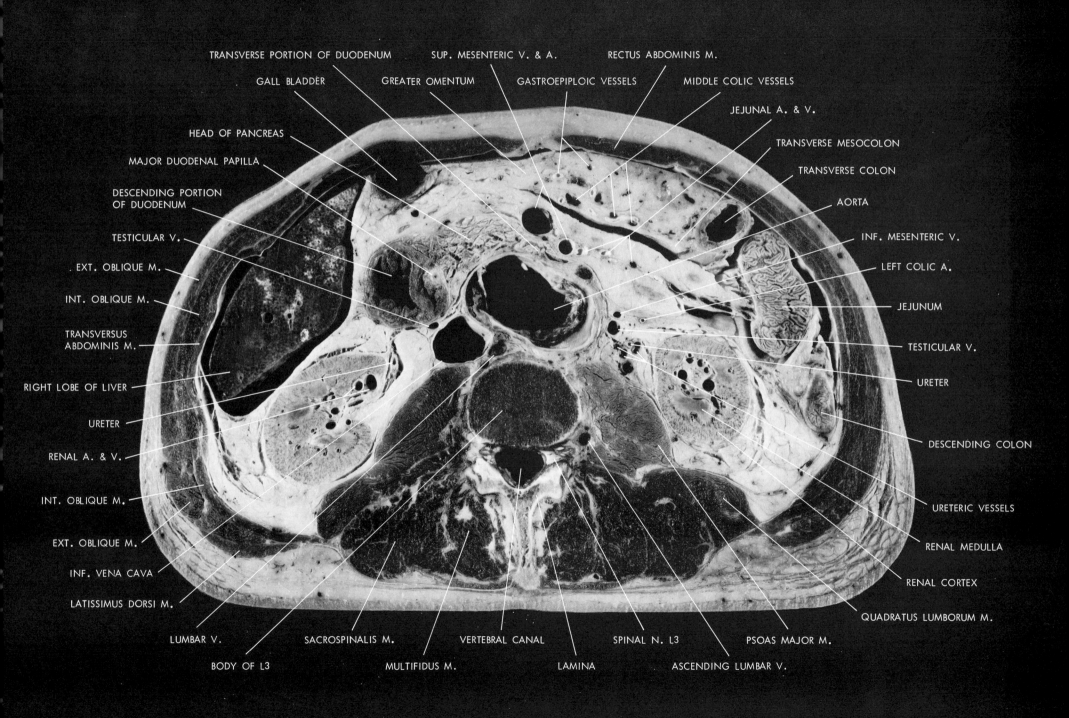

TRANSVERSE PORTION OF DUODENUM SUP. MESENTERIC V. & A. RECTUS ABDOMINIS M.

GALL BLADDER GREATER OMENTUM GASTROEPIPLOIC VESSELS MIDDLE COLIC VESSELS

JEJUNAL A. & V.

HEAD OF PANCREAS TRANSVERSE MESOCOLON

MAJOR DUODENAL PAPILLA TRANSVERSE COLON

DESCENDING PORTION OF DUODENUM AORTA

TESTICULAR V. INF. MESENTERIC V.

EXT. OBLIQUE M. LEFT COLIC A.

INT. OBLIQUE M. JEJUNUM

TRANSVERSUS ABDOMINIS M. TESTICULAR V.

RIGHT LOBE OF LIVER URETER

URETER DESCENDING COLON

RENAL A. & V.

URETERIC VESSELS

INT. OBLIQUE M. RENAL MEDULLA

EXT. OBLIQUE M. RENAL CORTEX

INF. VENA CAVA

LATISSIMUS DORSI M. QUADRATUS LUMBORUM M.

LUMBAR V. SACROSPINALIS M. VERTEBRAL CANAL SPINAL N. L3 PSOAS MAJOR M.

BODY OF L3 MULTIFIDUS M. LAMINA ASCENDING LUMBAR V.

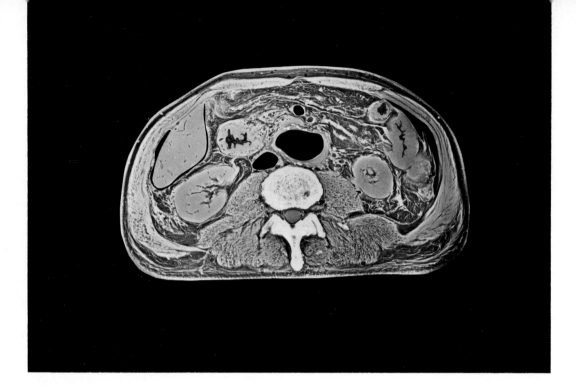

circumference; it consists of fibrocartilage and laminae of fibrous tissue. The nucleus pulposus is the soft elastic portion that is located in the center of the disc. The nucleus pulposus appears especially pronounced in the lumbar region, as is shown in this illustration.

Clinical Considerations

In this section the relationship of the hepatic flexure to the anterior portion of the right lobe of the liver is clearly indicated. It is only when the colon is distended with gas or other contrast agent that one can define the adjoining right lobe of the liver clearly, since the hepatic flexure of the colon is virtually a completely peritonealized structure and is otherwise not clearly defined.

The marked posterior relationship of the descending colon and the very minimal angle that exists in the peritoneal space between the descending colon and the parietal peritoneum of the peritoneal space are clearly indicated in this section. Although this space is minimal, it may contain exudate or neoplasm or produce a bulge of the adjoining flank or a displacement of the adjoining descending colon. If this angle is occupied by a fluid substance, there may be an overflow into the peritoneal space, causing a separation of the adjoining jejunal loops.

SECTION 3–13

Through the intervertebral disc between L3 and L4

Anatomic Considerations

In this section the inferior mesenteric artery can be observed for the first time. This artery is the last of the unpaired visceral arteries that come from the aorta; it usually arises at the level of the third lumbar vertebra or at the level of the disc below L3, as occurs in this specimen. The inferior mesenteric artery has a left colic branch, which supplies the descending colon, and numerous sigmoidal branches to the sigmoid colon; it terminates as the superior rectal artery.

The intervertebral discs are located between adjacent vertebrae and are the chief connection of the vertebrae. The discs constitute approximately 25 per cent of the length of the vertebral column. Although the size and shape of the intervertebral discs vary in different parts of the vertebral column, all possess similar morphologic structure. The anulus fibrosus is found at the

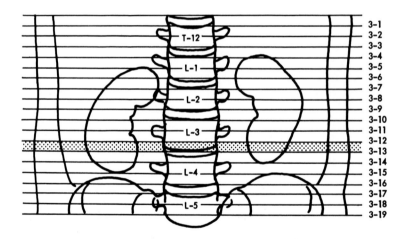

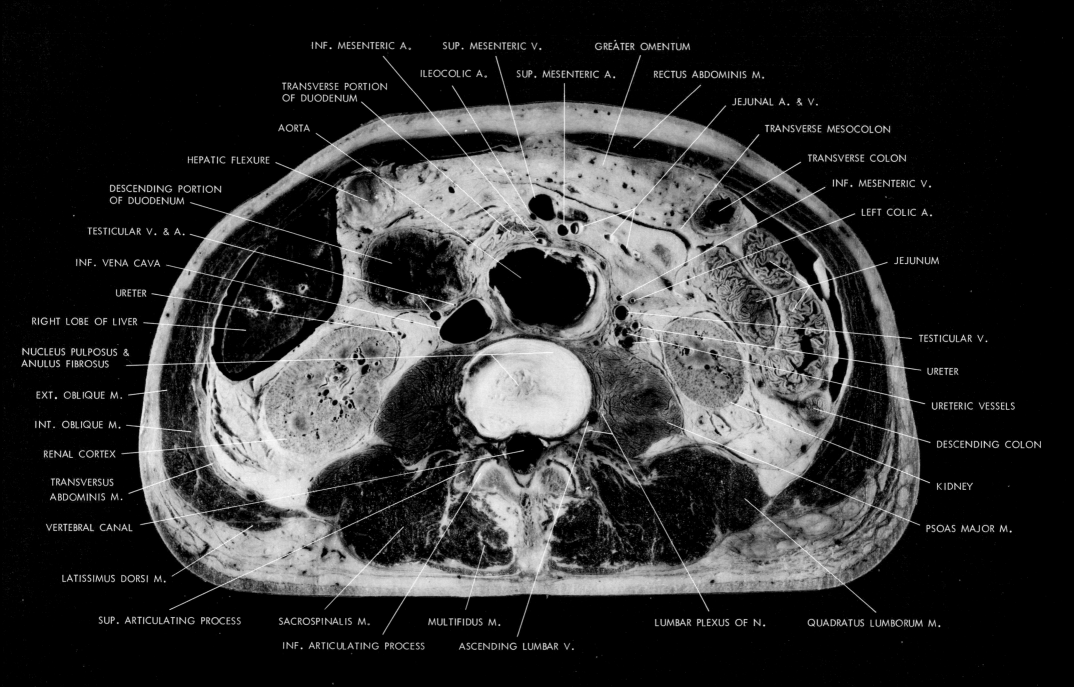

INF. MESENTERIC A.

SUP. MESENTERIC V.

GREATER OMENTUM

ILEOCOLIC A.

SUP. MESENTERIC A.

RECTUS ABDOMINIS M.

TRANSVERSE PORTION
OF DUODENUM

JEJUNAL A. & V.

AORTA

TRANSVERSE MESOCOLON

HEPATIC FLEXURE

TRANSVERSE COLON

INF. MESENTERIC V.

DESCENDING PORTION
OF DUODENUM

LEFT COLIC A.

TESTICULAR V. & A.

JEJUNUM

INF. VENA CAVA

URETER

RIGHT LOBE OF LIVER

TESTICULAR V.

NUCLEUS PULPOSUS &
ANULUS FIBROSUS

URETER

EXT. OBLIQUE M.

URETERIC VESSELS

INT. OBLIQUE M.

DESCENDING COLON

RENAL CORTEX

KIDNEY

TRANSVERSUS
ABDOMINIS M.

PSOAS MAJOR M.

VERTEBRAL CANAL

LATISSIMUS DORSI M.

SUP. ARTICULATING PROCESS

SACROSPINALIS M.

MULTIFIDUS M.

LUMBAR PLEXUS OF N.

QUADRATUS LUMBORUM M.

INF. ARTICULATING PROCESS

ASCENDING LUMBAR V.

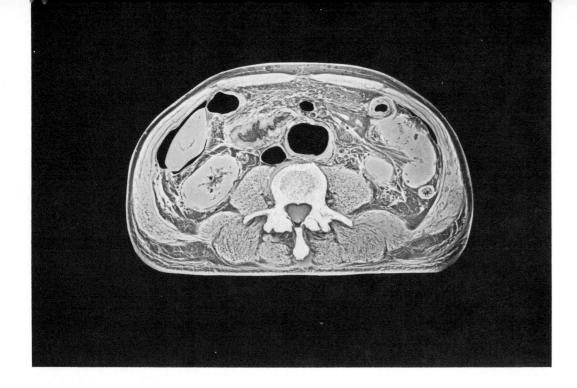

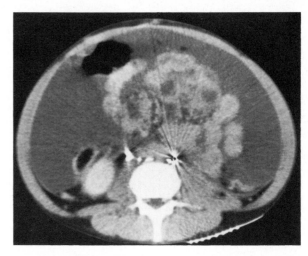

contrast enhancement of the collecting system, and the right ureter and renal pelvis are just barely in evidence. (Courtesy of Dr. Neil Wolfman.)

The psoas major muscle is enclosed in a strong fascia called the psoas sheath. Pus from diseased vertebrae can pass into the sheath (psoas abscess) and spread beneath the inguinal ligament into the femoral triangle.

In the cadaveric section the nodular appearance of the psoas major muscles on either side of the body of the fourth lumbar vertebra is even more clearly defined than has been previously indicated. This "mass suggestion" should not be interpreted as an abnormality.

SECTION
3–14

Through the upper portion of the body of L4

Anatomic Considerations

A prominent landmark of the posterior abdominal wall is the psoas major muscle. The muscle arises from the transverse processes of the lumbar vertebrae, from the intervertebral discs and the contiguous margins of the bodies of the vertebrae (T12 to L5), and from the tendinous arches that bridge over the lumbar arteries. As it passes downward and laterally, it narrows to a tendon that passes in front of the hip joint beneath the inguinal ligament and inserts with the iliacus muscle into the lesser trochanter of the femur.

Clinical Considerations

This CT scan of the abdomen demonstrates a patient with a tremendous ascites encasing all of the small intestinal loops centrally situated. There is an artifact from metallic secondary radiation overlying the left aspect of the lumbar vertebra and stellate radiation therefrom. Renografin was administered for

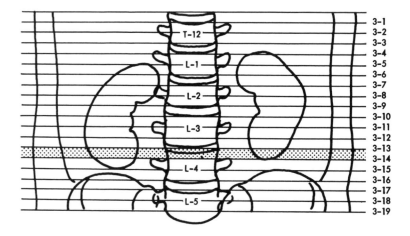

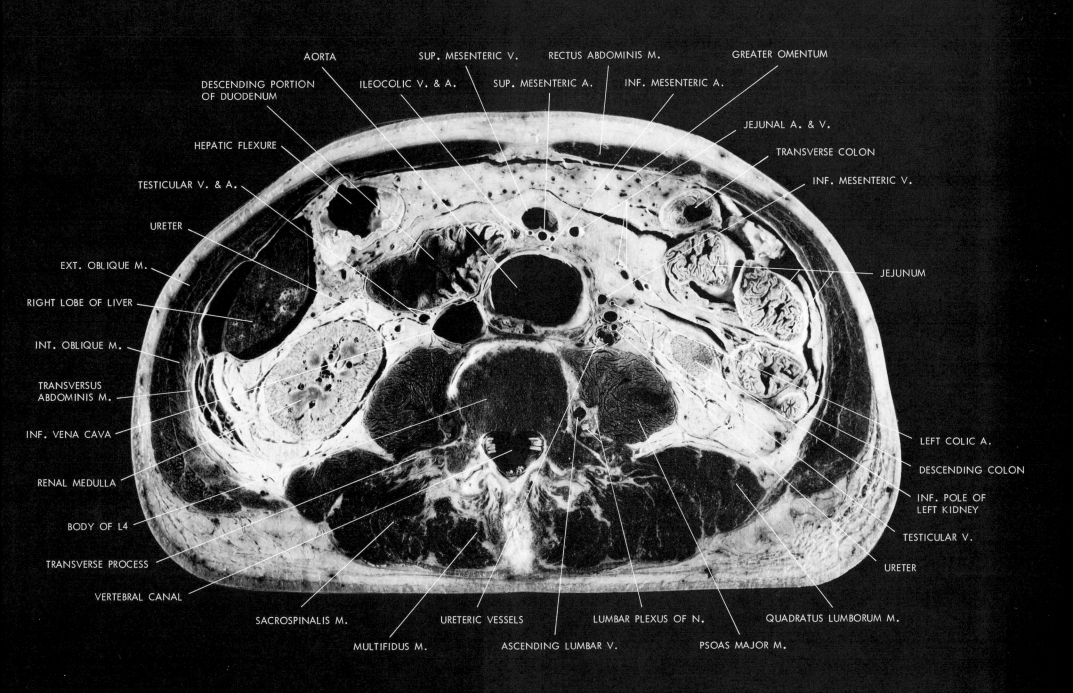

AORTA

SUP. MESENTERIC V.

RECTUS ABDOMINIS M.

GREATER OMENTUM

DESCENDING PORTION
OF DUODENUM

ILEOCOLIC V. & A.

SUP. MESENTERIC A.

INF. MESENTERIC A.

HEPATIC FLEXURE

JEJUNAL A. & V.

TRANSVERSE COLON

TESTICULAR V. & A.

INF. MESENTERIC V.

URETER

EXT. OBLIQUE M.

JEJUNUM

RIGHT LOBE OF LIVER

INT. OBLIQUE M.

TRANSVERSUS
ABDOMINIS M.

INF. VENA CAVA

LEFT COLIC A.

RENAL MEDULLA

DESCENDING COLON

INF. POLE OF
LEFT KIDNEY

BODY OF L4

TESTICULAR V.

TRANSVERSE PROCESS

URETER

VERTEBRAL CANAL

SACROSPINALIS M.

URETERIC VESSELS

LUMBAR PLEXUS OF N.

QUADRATUS LUMBORUM M.

MULTIFIDUS M.

ASCENDING LUMBAR V.

PSOAS MAJOR M.

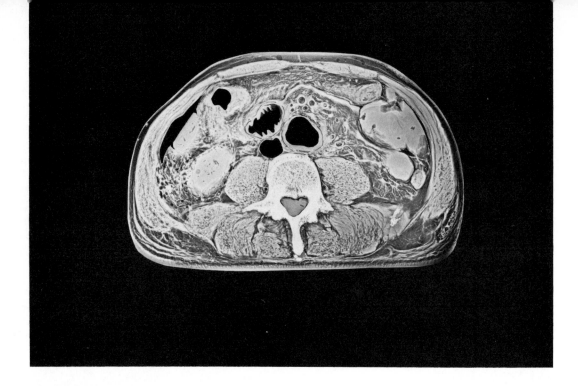

The lumbar plexus is formed in the psoas major muscle. Two of the larger nerves from this plexus are the femoral and obturator, each of which receives contributions from L2 through L4. The obturator nerve, which is formed from the anterior divisions of L2 through L4, innervates the muscles in the adductor (preaxial) chamber of the thigh. The femoral nerve, which is formed from the posterior divisions of L2 through L4, innervates the muscles in the anterior (postaxial) compartment of the thigh.

Clinical Considerations

The ascending colon, just posterior to the hepatic flexure and transverse colon, is beginning to appear. It can be enhanced by contrast agent such as Gastrografin.

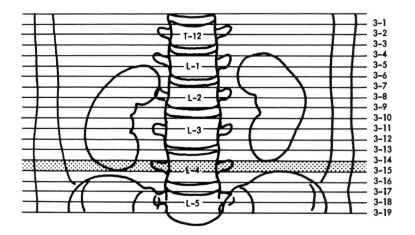

SECTION
3–15

Through the lower portion of the body of L4

Anatomic Considerations

The lumbar plexus is formed from the anterior primary rami of the first three lumbar nerves and a part of the fourth. At times the 12th thoracic (subcostal) nerve participates. The part of the fourth lumbar nerve that is not involved with the lumbar plexus joins the fifth lumbar nerve to form the lumbosacral trunk, which contributes in the formation of the sacral plexus.

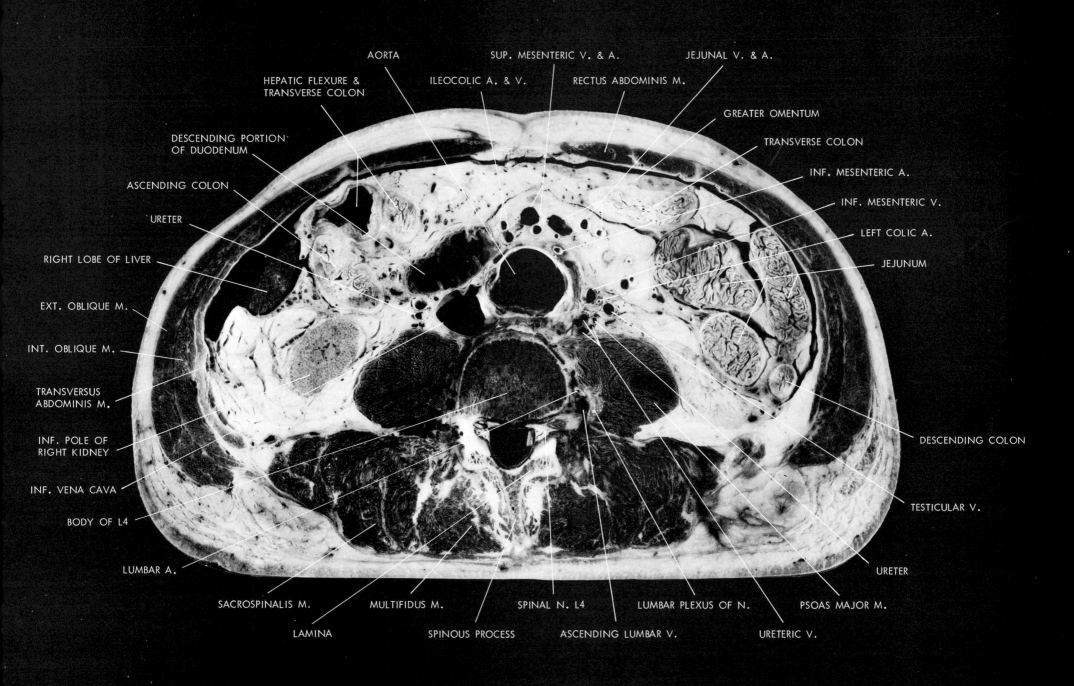

AORTA

SUP. MESENTERIC V. & A.

JEJUNAL V. & A.

HEPATIC FLEXURE &
TRANSVERSE COLON

ILEOCOLIC A. & V.

RECTUS ABDOMINIS M.

GREATER OMENTUM

DESCENDING PORTION
OF DUODENUM

TRANSVERSE COLON

INF. MESENTERIC A.

ASCENDING COLON

INF. MESENTERIC V.

URETER

LEFT COLIC A.

RIGHT LOBE OF LIVER

JEJUNUM

EXT. OBLIQUE M.

INT. OBLIQUE M.

TRANSVERSUS
ABDOMINIS M.

INF. POLE OF
RIGHT KIDNEY

DESCENDING COLON

INF. VENA CAVA

TESTICULAR V.

BODY OF L4

LUMBAR A.

URETER

SACROSPINALIS M.

MULTIFIDUS M.

SPINAL N. L4

LUMBAR PLEXUS OF N.

PSOAS MAJOR M.

LAMINA

SPINOUS PROCESS

ASCENDING LUMBAR V.

URETERIC V.

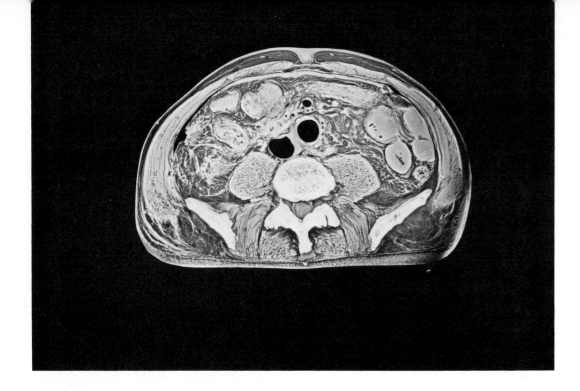

bifurcation of the aorta. The umbilicus can serve as another reference point: The segmental nerve supply overlying the skin of the anterior abdominal wall can be mapped out approximately by remembering that the area of the umbilicus is supplied by anterior primary rami of the tenth thoracic spinal nerve and the area just superior to the pubis by the first lumbar spinal nerve.

Clinical Considerations

Note the relatively large space to the right of the ascending colon as compared with that to the left of the descending colon. This becomes important when there is an accumulation of an inflammatory material or exudate in the so-called right paracolic gutter as against the left paracolic gutter, since the right gutter is so very much larger than the left.

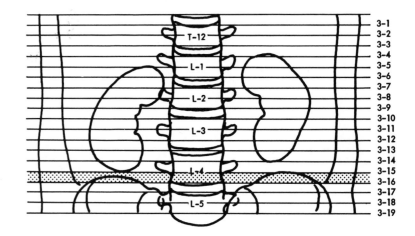

SECTION 3–16

Through the intervertebral disc between L4 and L5

Anatomic Considerations

The umbilicus can be seen in this illustration. It is located at the level of the intervertebral disc between L4 and L5 in this specimen, which is slightly lower than usual. The umbilicus is most often located at the disc between the third and fourth lumbar vertebrae or at the level of the fourth lumbar vertebra. The location of the umbilicus serves as an approximate reference point for the

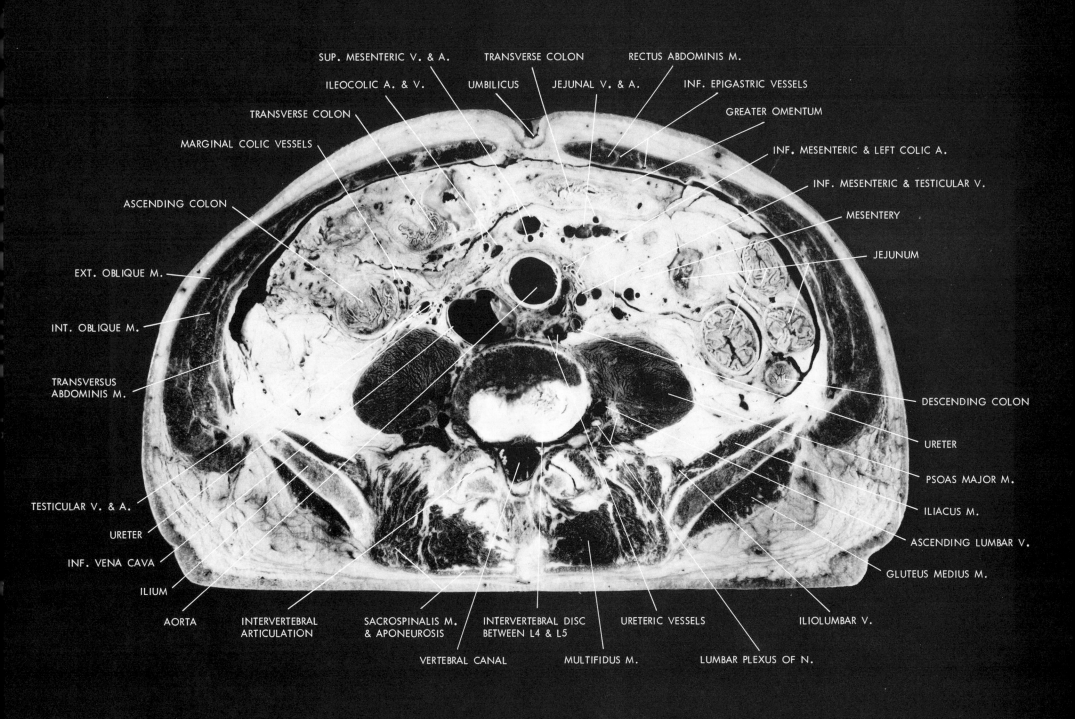

SUP. MESENTERIC V. & A. TRANSVERSE COLON RECTUS ABDOMINIS M.

ILEOCOLIC A. & V. UMBILICUS JEJUNAL V. & A. INF. EPIGASTRIC VESSELS

TRANSVERSE COLON GREATER OMENTUM

MARGINAL COLIC VESSELS INF. MESENTERIC & LEFT COLIC A.

INF. MESENTERIC & TESTICULAR V.

ASCENDING COLON MESENTERY

JEJUNUM

EXT. OBLIQUE M.

INT. OBLIQUE M.

TRANSVERSUS
ABDOMINIS M. DESCENDING COLON

URETER

PSOAS MAJOR M.

TESTICULAR V. & A. ILIACUS M.

URETER ASCENDING LUMBAR V.

INF. VENA CAVA GLUTEUS MEDIUS M.

ILIUM

AORTA INTERVERTEBRAL SACROSPINALIS M. INTERVERTEBRAL DISC URETERIC VESSELS ILIOLUMBAR V.
ARTICULATION & APONEUROSIS BETWEEN L4 & L5

VERTEBRAL CANAL MULTIFIDUS M. LUMBAR PLEXUS OF N.

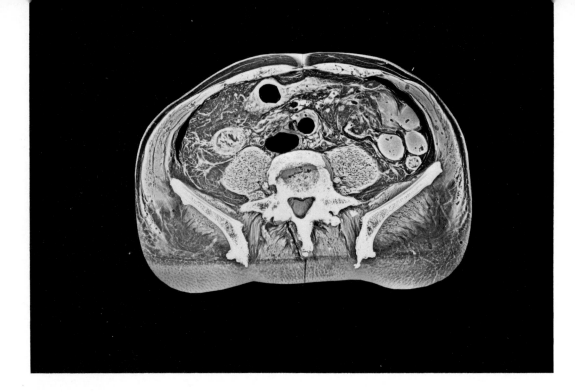

external intercostal muscles. The internal oblique muscle fibers are directed primarily upward and forward and correspond to the internal intercostal muscles. Most of the muscle fibers of the transverse abdominis are directed horizontally. The difference in direction of the muscle fibers is a source of strength of the abdominal wall.

The segmental nerve supply of the abdominal muscles is derived from anterior primary rami of spinal nerves from the seventh thoracic to the first lumbar.

Clinical Considerations

Here and in the previous section the close approximation of the iliacus muscle to the ilium is well demonstrated with the fatty space between this muscle and the psoas major muscle. In this space, exudative processes may descend from regions more cephalad in the thorax or abdomen down into the pelvis, ultimately even into the inguinal canal. Such inflammatory processes as tuberculosis are particularly apt to descend in this fascial plane.

SECTION
3–17

Through the upper portion of the body of L5

Anatomic Considerations

The anterior abdominal wall, which appears in many of the sections, consists of five pairs of muscles. Anteriorly, there are the rectus abdominis and pyramidalis muscles. The rectus abdominis is located alongside the linea alba and extends from the fifth, sixth, and seventh costal cartilages to the crest of the pubis; the pyramidalis, not always present, is located in front of the lowest part of the rectus abdominis muscle. Laterally, there are the external oblique, internal oblique, and the transversus abdominis muscles. The direction of the muscle fibers of each muscle is different. The external oblique muscle fibers pass obliquely downward and forward and correspond in direction to the

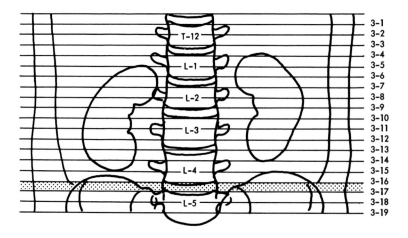

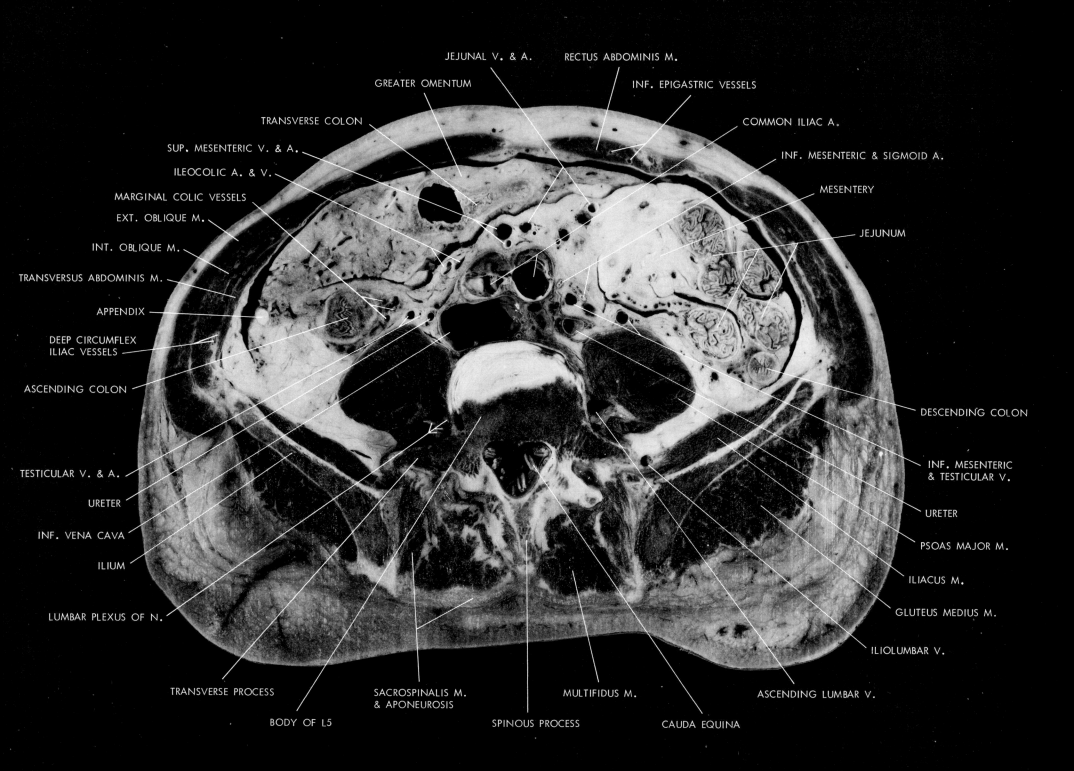

JEJUNAL V. & A.

RECTUS ABDOMINIS M.

GREATER OMENTUM

INF. EPIGASTRIC VESSELS

TRANSVERSE COLON

COMMON ILIAC A.

SUP. MESENTERIC V. & A.

INF. MESENTERIC & SIGMOID A.

ILEOCOLIC A. & V.

MESENTERY

MARGINAL COLIC VESSELS

EXT. OBLIQUE M.

JEJUNUM

INT. OBLIQUE M.

TRANSVERSUS ABDOMINIS M.

APPENDIX

DEEP CIRCUMFLEX
ILIAC VESSELS

ASCENDING COLON

DESCENDING COLON

INF. MESENTERIC
& TESTICULAR V.

TESTICULAR V. & A.

URETER

URETER

INF. VENA CAVA

PSOAS MAJOR M.

ILIUM

ILIACUS M.

LUMBAR PLEXUS OF N.

GLUTEUS MEDIUS M.

ILIOLUMBAR V.

TRANSVERSE PROCESS

SACROSPINALIS M.
& APONEUROSIS

MULTIFIDUS M.

ASCENDING LUMBAR V.

BODY OF L5

SPINOUS PROCESS

CAUDA EQUINA

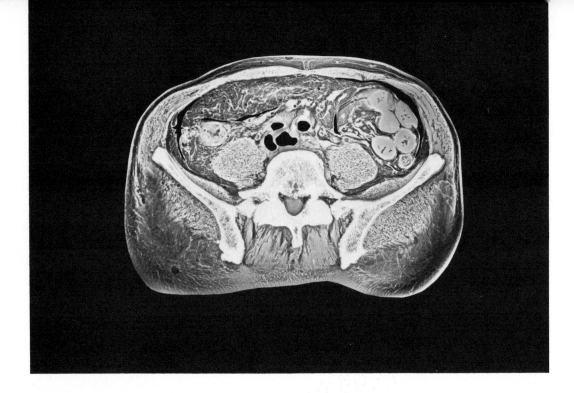

frequently it lies just below the cecum, hangs down into the pelvis, or passes in front or behind the terminal ilium. In this section the appendix is seen posterior and slightly lateral to the ascending colon.

The appendix is supplied by branches from the ileocolic artery.

Clinical Considerations

As seen in this section, the appendix lies in the loose fascial plane to the right of the ascending colon. This is highly variable, depending upon the mesenteric attachments of the cecum and the relationship of the appendix to the cecum. When the appendix is in this fascial plane, it can be readily visualized how appendicitis and its adjoining inflammation can significantly affect the "gutter" between the ascending colon and the right flank. Also, it is readily apparent how inflammatory processes of the appendix can affect the fatty planes overlying the iliacus muscle and extend to the psoas major muscle.

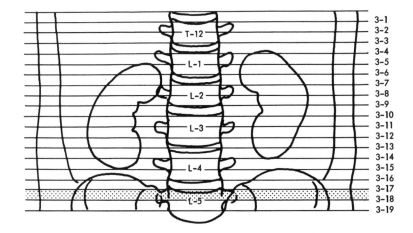

SECTION
3–18

Through the middle portion of the body of L5

Anatomic Considerations

The appendix arises from the posteromedial surface of the cecum. Its orifice is a small opening in the cecum about an inch below the ileocecal valve. It is a blind tube, and its length varies from 5 to 20 cm. The appendix has a small mesentery (mesosalpinx) connecting it to the mesentery of the small intestine.

The position of the appendix is quite variable. Most frequently it lies posterior to the cecum and may extend behind the ascending colon. Less

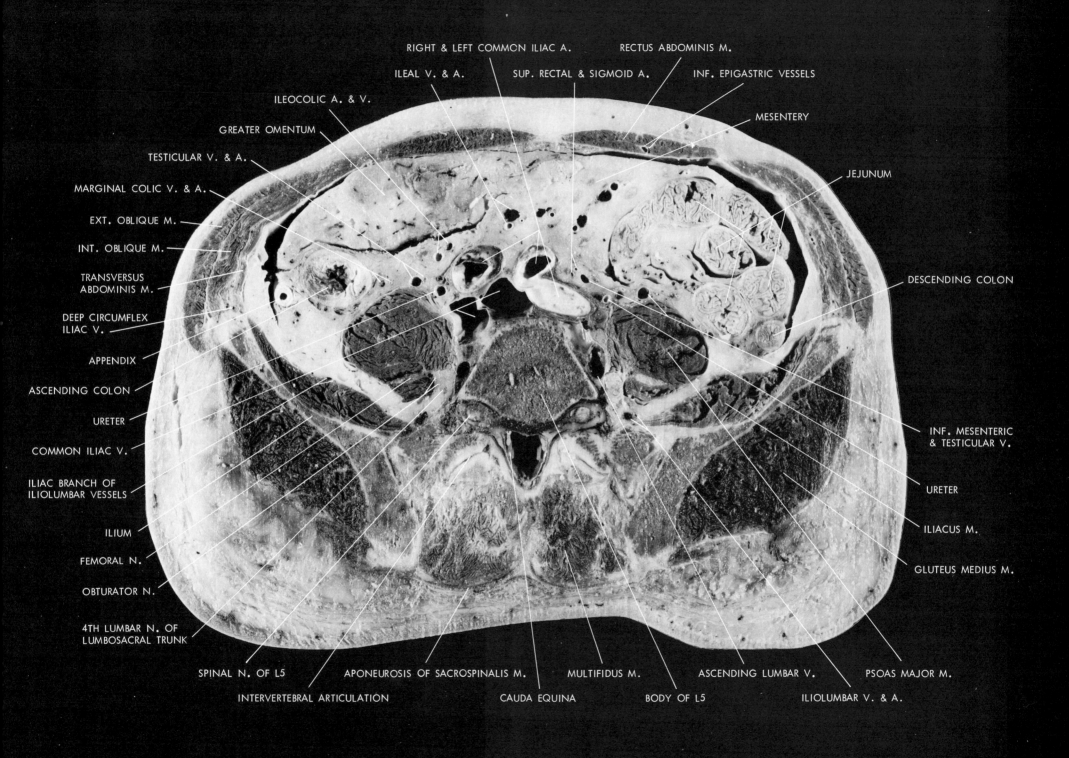

RIGHT & LEFT COMMON ILIAC A.

RECTUS ABDOMINIS M.

ILEAL V. & A.

SUP. RECTAL & SIGMOID A.

INF. EPIGASTRIC VESSELS

ILEOCOLIC A. & V.

MESENTERY

GREATER OMENTUM

JEJUNUM

TESTICULAR V. & A.

MARGINAL COLIC V. & A.

EXT. OBLIQUE M.

INT. OBLIQUE M.

DESCENDING COLON

TRANSVERSUS
ABDOMINIS M.

DEEP CIRCUMFLEX
ILIAC V.

APPENDIX

ASCENDING COLON

INF. MESENTERIC
& TESTICULAR V.

URETER

COMMON ILIAC V.

URETER

ILIAC BRANCH OF
ILIOLUMBAR VESSELS

ILIUM

ILIACUS M.

FEMORAL N.

GLUTEUS MEDIUS M.

OBTURATOR N.

4TH LUMBAR N. OF
LUMBOSACRAL TRUNK

SPINAL N. OF L5

APONEUROSIS OF SACROSPINALIS M.

MULTIFIDUS M.

ASCENDING LUMBAR V.

PSOAS MAJOR M.

INTERVERTEBRAL ARTICULATION

CAUDA EQUINA

BODY OF L5

ILIOLUMBAR V. & A.

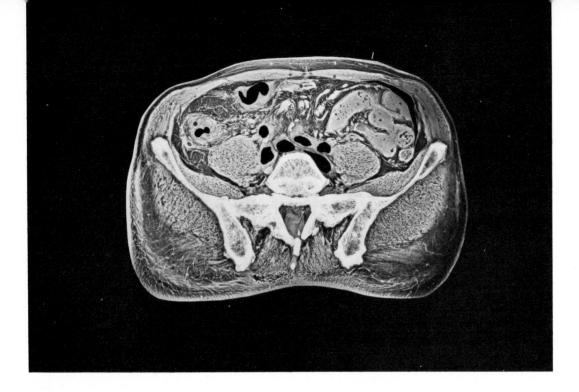

azygos, portal, and vertebral, which is of clinical importance when the inferior vena cava is obstructed.

Clinical Considerations

In this section, the ascending colon in its relationship to the right flank and the descending colon in relationship to the left flank are more closely parallel, but still the descending colon is more dorsally situated than is the ascending colon. The fatty envelope surrounding the descending colon is an important aspect of inflammatory processes that may involve the descending colon and sigmoid by extension from inflammation of diverticuli of the sigmoid colon. It can, therefore, be visualized how a so-called "left-sided appendicitis" may mimic in every respect (except for location) an appendicitis that truly has originated in the appendix on the right side of the patient.

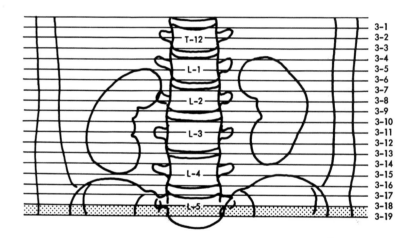

SECTION
3–19

Through the lower portion of the body of L5

Anatomic Considerations

Within the thickness of this 1-cm slice, the two iliac veins unite to form the inferior vena cava, the formation of which is usually related to the body of the fifth lumbar vertebra. The inferior vena cava, which receives venous drainage from the lower extremity, pelvis, and abdomen, can be observed in Sections 2–21 to 3–18. The tributaries of the inferior vena cava are the hepatic, renal, lumbar, right gonadal, suprarenal, and inferior phrenic veins. The anastomoses of the inferior vena cava are important in collateral circulation. The inferior vena cava communicates with three major venous systems:

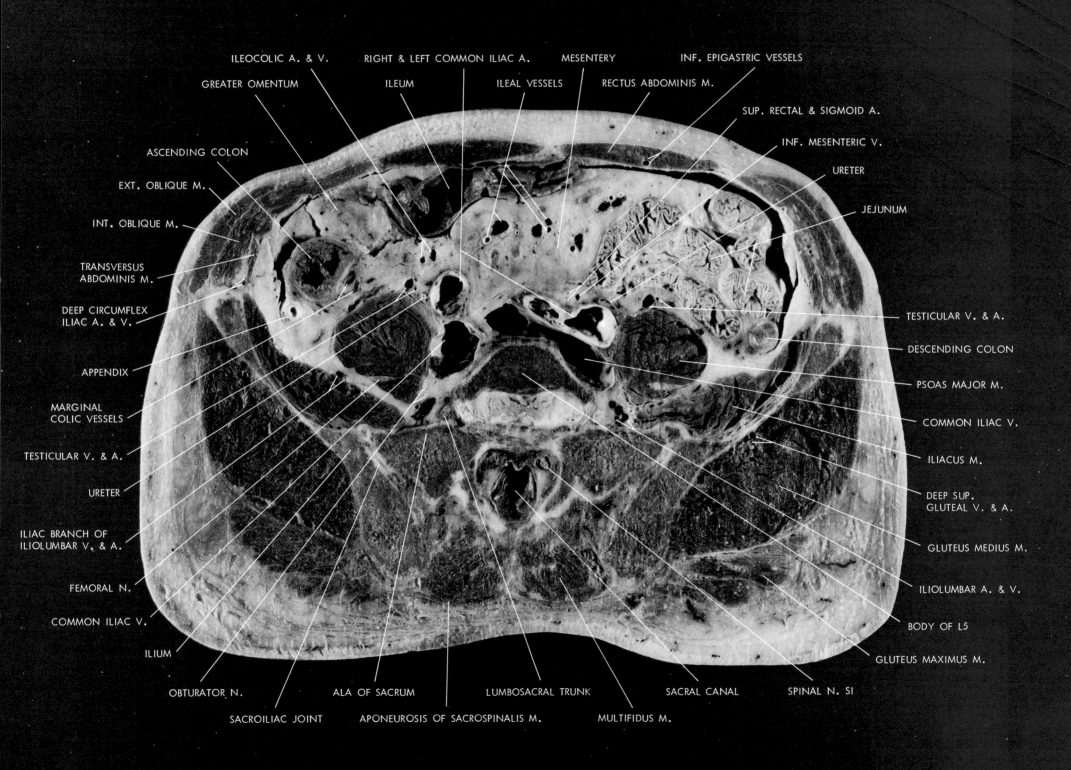

ILEOCOLIC A. & V.   RIGHT & LEFT COMMON ILIAC A.   MESENTERY   INF. EPIGASTRIC VESSELS

GREATER OMENTUM   ILEUM   ILEAL VESSELS   RECTUS ABDOMINIS M.

SUP. RECTAL & SIGMOID A.

ASCENDING COLON

INF. MESENTERIC V.

URETER

EXT. OBLIQUE M.

JEJUNUM

INT. OBLIQUE M.

TRANSVERSUS
ABDOMINIS M.

DEEP CIRCUMFLEX
ILIAC A. & V.

TESTICULAR V. & A.

DESCENDING COLON

APPENDIX

PSOAS MAJOR M.

MARGINAL
COLIC VESSELS

COMMON ILIAC V.

TESTICULAR V. & A.

ILIACUS M.

URETER

DEEP SUP.
GLUTEAL V. & A.

ILIAC BRANCH OF
ILIOLUMBAR V. & A.

GLUTEUS MEDIUS M.

FEMORAL N.

ILIOLUMBAR A. & V.

COMMON ILIAC V.

BODY OF L5

ILIUM

GLUTEUS MAXIMUS M.

OBTURATOR N.   ALA OF SACRUM   LUMBOSACRAL TRUNK   SACRAL CANAL   SPINAL N. SI

SACROILIAC JOINT   APONEUROSIS OF SACROSPINALIS M.   MULTIFIDUS M.

4

Male Pelvis and Perineum

INTRODUCTION

The accompanying sketch shows that the sections pertaining to this area extend from the lumbosacral articulation through the scrotum and therefore include sections through the upper portion of the thigh.

The 1-cm thick sections were taken from the same specimen as those of the abdomen; therefore, Section 4–1 is below Section 3–19.

The anatomic features of the male pelvis that are particularly advantageous for computed tomographic (CT) study are:

1. The urinary bladder and its associated genitourinary organs.
2. The pelvic muscle groups, which adjoin the urinary bladder and the perineum proper.
3. The peripelvic fat, which helps delineate these structures.
4. The confinement of the various soft tissue structures by the bony pelvis.
5. For the pelvic organs 2- to 18-second scans are adequate, but if one wants to paralyze completely the involved gastrointestinal organs, intramuscular administration of 0.5 to 1.0 mg of glucagon is helpful for a period of 15 to 30 minutes.

The urinary bladder may or may not be distended with contrast agent, such as 20 cc of diatrizoate, 60 per cent in approximately 200 cc of water. A Foley catheter may be inserted into the urinary bladder or the rectum, and the 5-cc balloon filled with air just prior to the CT examination to accentuate these structures (Levitt et al., 1978).

Normally, pelvic vessels, particularly when they are intensified with contrast agent, and lymph nodes, which may or may not be intensified with Ethiodol, can be identified quite readily as rather rounded soft tissue densities. Generally, pelvic lymph nodes greater than 8 mm in diameter are considered suspect in the pelvis on CT scans (Levitt et al., 1978).

PRESACRAL MASSES. Presacral masses may be of several consistencies: (1) excessive fat or (2) solid or cystic tumors, such as meningiomas. Occasionally a large pear-shaped iliopsoas muscle will produce an identical appearance and impression upon the urinary bladder identical to those of a pelvic lipomatosis (Chang, 1978).

Computed tomography is also effective in demonstrating abdominal abscesses and their relation to surrounding structures. Not only are such lesions demonstrable, but computed tomography permits an approach with a percutaneous needle for aspiration diagnosis and therapy. Combined with intravenous antibiotics, this method of abscess drainage has been reported as being successful in curing abscesses without surgery (Gerzof et al., 1978). A so-called "rind-sign" has been described with such psoas abscesses (Gerzof et al., 1978).

ILIACUS HEMATOMA. An iliacus hematoma has likewise been demonstrated by CT analysis in a patient who was taking anticoagulant medication (Korobkin and Palubinskas, 1978).

LYMPHOGENOUS AND SOFT TISSUE TUMORS. Computed tomography has been utilized in the staging and management of the malignant lymphomas, especially Hodgkin's disease. Of course, lymph node tumor replacement without enlargement cannot be recognized on computed tomography.

Once the disease is established and staged, it can be followed after therapy to gauge response.

Lymphoceles and cystic lesions have also been diagnosed within the pelvis (Sagel et al., 1978).

MASS LESIONS OF THE GENITOURINARY ORGANS. Mass lesions of the genitourinary organs will cause a displacement of adjoining organs and may have different attenuation values. These include carcinoma of the prostate and involvement of the seminal vesicles. With prostatic carcinoma, for example, a mass may be demonstrated posterior to a thick-walled invaded urinary bladder that will extend down and distort the adjoining seminal vesicle. Likewise the carcinoma may be staged in respect to the lateral wall of the pelvis. Unfortunately, differentiation of carcinoma from benign prostatic hypertrophy by computed tomography alone has not been demonstrated (Korobkin and Palubinskas, 1978).

A study of the urinary bladder lends itself particularly well to this modality. Not only does the CT scan show the mass in relation to its involvement of the urinary bladder lumen, but its posterior invasion or spread to adjoining pelvic soft tissues may accurately be evaluated (Levitt et al., 1978).

On one occasion we were able to demonstrate metastatic destruction to the pubis from a lesion suspected clinically to have arisen from the prostate gland, but computed tomography demonstrated a normal prostate gland and thus excluded this as the origin of this metastatic site. At times abscesses in relation to Crohn's disease have been demonstrated (Levitt et al., 1978).

FOREIGN BODY LOCALIZATION AND REMOVAL UTILIZING COMPUTED AXIAL TOMOGRAPHY (Haaga et al., 1978). Computed tomography has offered guidance for instrumentation for diagnosis in many areas of the body besides the pelvis. It has also offered such guidance in allowing the safe and rapid removal of a metallic foreign body from paravesical soft tissues deep within the male pelvis.

SUMMARY. Computed tomography of the male pelvis is still in its infancy at this writing but augurs a great deal in relation to future diagnosis as well as to staging of therapy.

Chang, SF: Pear-shaped bladder caused by large iliopsoas muscles. Radiology 128:349–350, 1978.

Gerzof SG, Robbins AH, and Birkett DH: Computed tomography in the diagnosis and management of abdominal abscesses. Gastrointest Radiol 3:287–294, 1978.

Haaga JR, Stewart BH, and Alfidi RJ: Foreign body localization and removal utilizing computed axial tomography. Urology 11:306–307, 1978.

Korobkin, M and Palubinskas AJ: CT of the urinary tract. Appl Radiol 7:47–52, 1978.

Levitt RG, Sagel SS, Stanley RJ, and Evens RG: Computed tomography of the pelvis. Roentgenol 13:193–200, 1978.

Sagel SS, Stanley RJ, Levitt RG, and Geisse G: Computed tomography of the kidney. Radiology 124:359–370, 1977.

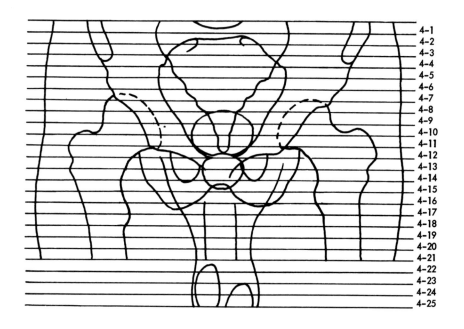

4-1
4-2
4-3
4-4
4-5
4-6
4-7
4-8
4-9
4-10
4-11
4-12
4-13
4-14
4-15
4-16
4-17
4-18
4-19
4-20
4-21
4-22
4-23
4-24
4-25

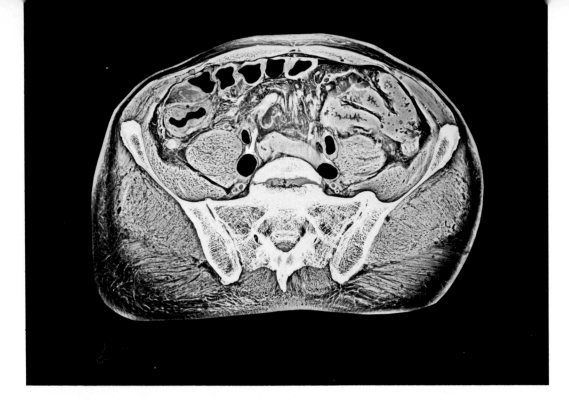

SECTION
4–1

Through the sacroiliac joint

Anatomic Considerations

The pelvic brim is bounded by the sacral promontory, arcuate line of the ilium, pectineal line of the pubis, pubic crest, and pubic symphysis. The opening of the pelvic inlet is reduced in size by the psoas major muscle, which overlaps the inlet. Lateral to the sacral promontory, the common iliac vessels reach the pelvic brim and divide into the external iliacs, which pass with the psoas major muscle, and the internal iliacs, into the pelvis.

In the following sections, some of the structures that pass from the abdominal cavity over the pelvic brim into the pelvis can be observed. From posterior to anterior, these are the lumbosacral trunk, sigmoid mesocolon (containing branches of the superior rectal arteries), internal iliac vessels, ureters, vas deferens, and middle umbilical ligament.

Clinical Considerations

Starting on the patient's right, the cecum is quite anteriorly situated but is highly variable in position; in some patients it is partially nonrotated, extending upward toward the right inferior margin of the liver, or hyperrotated, extending medially and upward toward the central portion of the lumbar spine. The appendix, therefore, is also variable in its relationship. There are two spaces created by the appendix and cecum, on the one hand, and the ileum and the mesentery for the small bowel, on the other. The spaces

surrounding the appendix and cecum become focal areas for the accumulation of exudative materials in the presence of a ruptured appendix and typhlitis (inflammation of the cecum); in the space for the small intestine between the cecum and the mesentery there is also a focus for accumulation of these materials, should inflammation of the ileum, cecum, or appendix occur.

The ileum is generally situated deep in the pelvis minor, extending upward in the abdomen to the right upper quadrant beneath the transverse colon; the ileal loops tend to be situated in the right half of the abdomen for the most part. The mesentery, as shown here, is a dividing zone between these two important elements of the small intestine. Often, when the mesentery becomes involved by a retroperitoneal inflammatory process, all of the small intestinal loops tend to accumulate to the left of it and inferiorly. If the root of the small bowel mesentery is inflamed, there is an obstruction to the lymphatics and other draining vessels of the small bowel mesentery so that swelling and edema of the small bowel loops become manifest on the plain radiograph of the abdomen.

The close relationship of the testicular artery and vein to the ureters is important. When these blood vessels are distended, the ureters take on an undulating appearance radiographically in excretory urography.

The ventral sacral foramina are closely applied to the sacral canal. This becomes important when expanding lesions, such as neural cysts involving the sacral foramina, erode the bone in this area and, on routine films of the pelvis, are readily recognizable as large areas of circumscribed bone destruction.

Lastly, the obliquity from the ventral to the dorsal aspect of the sacroiliac joints is noteworthy. In order to obtain a "through-and-through" demonstration of the sacroiliac joints, we must rotate the patient to approximately 30 to 45 degrees on the side opposite to the pertinent sacroiliac joint. This maneuver permits us to place the sacroiliac joint perpendicular to the x-ray film. A similar expedient may be employed with computed tomography.

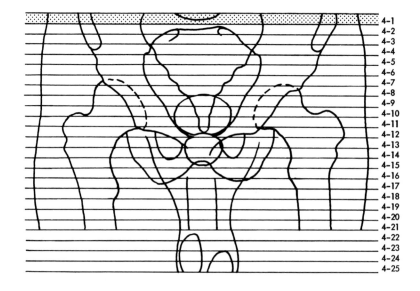

4–1
4–2
4–3
4–4
4–5
4–6
4–7
4–8
4–9
4–10
4–11
4–12
4–13
4–14
4–15
4–16
4–17
4–18
4–19
4–20
4–21
4–22
4–23
4–24
4–25

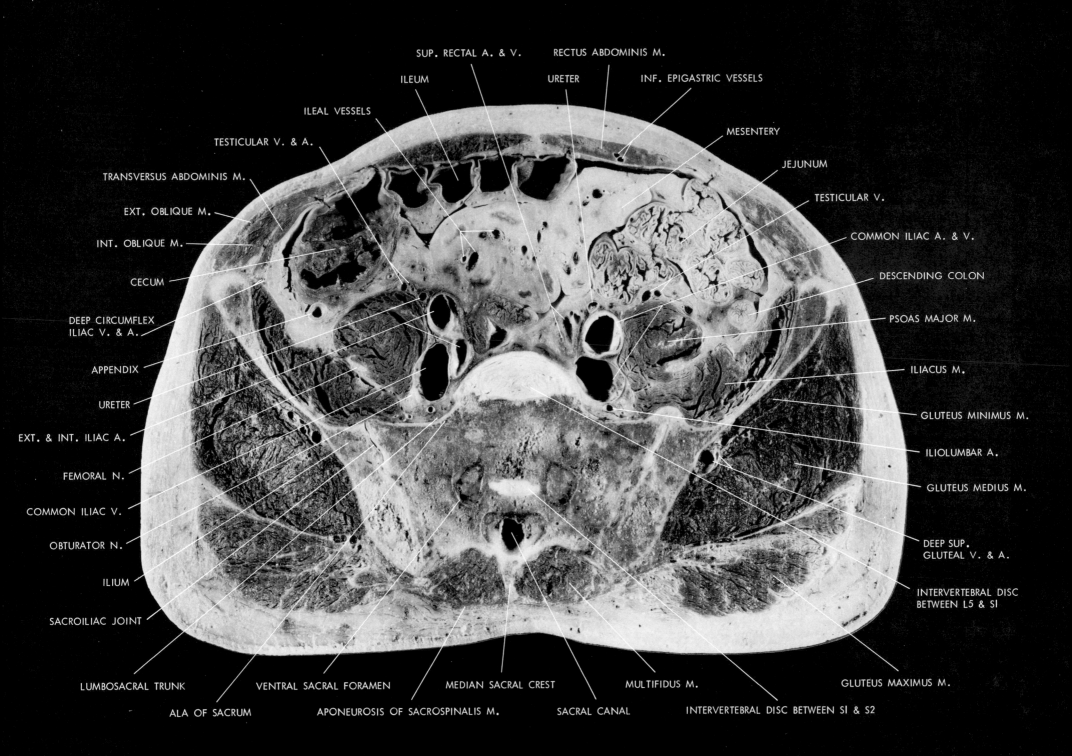

SUP. RECTAL A. & V.

RECTUS ABDOMINIS M.

ILEUM

URETER

INF. EPIGASTRIC VESSELS

ILEAL VESSELS

MESENTERY

TESTICULAR V. & A.

JEJUNUM

TRANSVERSUS ABDOMINIS M.

TESTICULAR V.

EXT. OBLIQUE M.

COMMON ILIAC A. & V.

INT. OBLIQUE M.

DESCENDING COLON

CECUM

PSOAS MAJOR M.

DEEP CIRCUMFLEX
ILIAC V. & A.

ILIACUS M.

APPENDIX

GLUTEUS MINIMUS M.

URETER

ILIOLUMBAR A.

EXT. & INT. ILIAC A.

GLUTEUS MEDIUS M.

FEMORAL N.

COMMON ILIAC V.

OBTURATOR N.

DEEP SUP.
GLUTEAL V. & A.

ILIUM

INTERVERTEBRAL DISC
BETWEEN L5 & S1

SACROILIAC JOINT

LUMBOSACRAL TRUNK

VENTRAL SACRAL FORAMEN

MEDIAN SACRAL CREST

MULTIFIDUS M.

GLUTEUS MAXIMUS M.

ALA OF SACRUM

APONEUROSIS OF SACROSPINALIS M.

SACRAL CANAL

INTERVERTEBRAL DISC BETWEEN S1 & S2

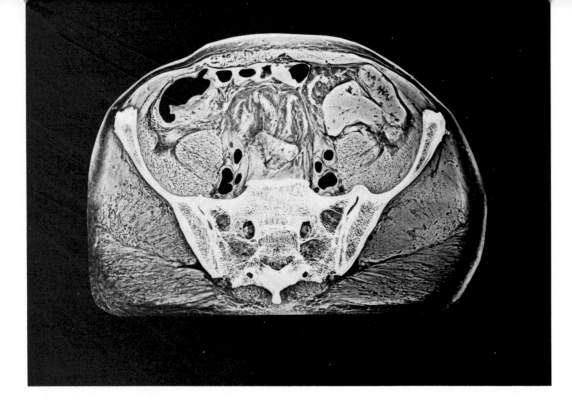

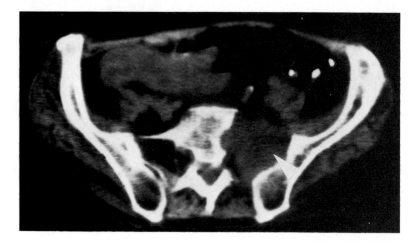

of the neural arch of the sacrum is involved in this destruction. (Courtesy of Dr. Neil Wolfman.)

The close relationship of the lumbosacral trunk to the ala of the sacrum and the adjoining sacroiliac joint has clinical implications when abnormalities of these adjoining structures are reflected by referred pain down the lumbosacral trunk. This becomes manifested clinically by pain in the thigh or by pain radiating from the pelvis to the lower extremities.

SECTION
4–2

Through the sacroiliac joint, 1 cm below the preceding section

Anatomic Considerations

The common iliac arteries, which are present in the preceding section, have divided into their terminal branches, the external and internal iliac arteries. As occurs in this specimen, the termination of the common iliac arteries usually takes place at the level of the lumbosacral articulation.

The external iliac artery has two branches, the inferior epigastric and deep circumflex iliac arteries. Both of these arteries can be seen in this illustration and in adjacent ones. The course of the external iliac artery can be followed progressively through Section 4–9. This artery is directly related to the psoas major muscle; as it progresses inferiorly, the external iliac artery becomes located in a more anterior direction. The external iliac artery becomes the femoral artery as it passes posterior to the inguinal ligament (Sections 4–9 and 4–10).

Clinical Considerations

This CT scan shows the pelvis of a patient with metastases from a renal carcinoma involving the soft tissues of the left pelvis minor and invading and destroying the left half of the sacrum (arrow). Note also that even a portion

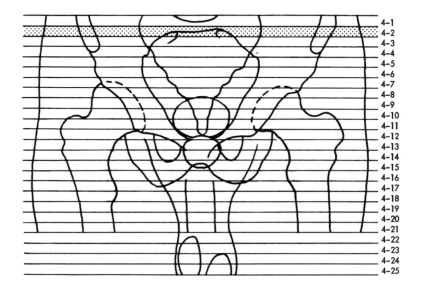

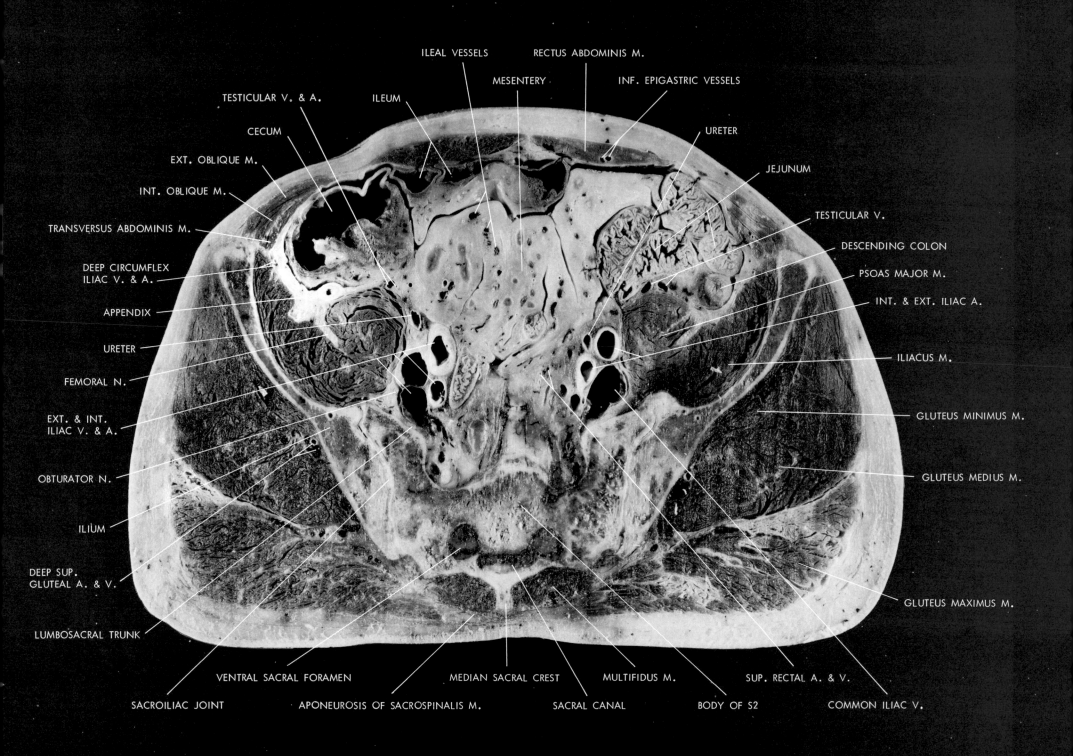

ILEAL VESSELS   RECTUS ABDOMINIS M.

MESENTERY   INF. EPIGASTRIC VESSELS

TESTICULAR V. & A.   ILEUM   URETER

CECUM   JEJUNUM

EXT. OBLIQUE M.   TESTICULAR V.

INT. OBLIQUE M.   DESCENDING COLON

TRANSVERSUS ABDOMINIS M.   PSOAS MAJOR M.

DEEP CIRCUMFLEX   INT. & EXT. ILIAC A.
ILIAC V. & A.

APPENDIX   ILIACUS M.

URETER

FEMORAL N.   GLUTEUS MINIMUS M.

EXT. & INT.
ILIAC V. & A.   GLUTEUS MEDIUS M.

OBTURATOR N.

ILIUM   GLUTEUS MAXIMUS M.

DEEP SUP.
GLUTEAL A. & V.

LUMBOSACRAL TRUNK

VENTRAL SACRAL FORAMEN   MEDIAN SACRAL CREST   MULTIFIDUS M.   SUP. RECTAL A. & V.

SACROILIAC JOINT   APONEUROSIS OF SACROSPINALIS M.   SACRAL CANAL   BODY OF S2   COMMON ILIAC V.

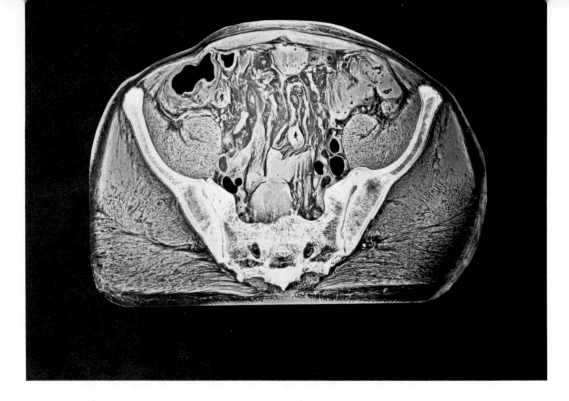

Clinical Considerations

The close relationship of the psoas major muscle and the iliacus muscle, with a minimal space between, is of clinical significance when an abscess descends from superior parts of the abdomen into this recess. The abscess may even invade the musculature to the underlying bony elements of the pelvis. Occasionally, destruction of the bony elements may occur. These accumulations produce a mass effect on plain films of the abdomen; they are readily apparent on computed tomography also. The latter method of examination has certain advantages in that the interfering gas shadows on plain films of the abdomen are no longer a problem in studying bony detail. In comparing the xeroradiographic appearance with the cross-sectional cut, it is interesting to note that the "edge effect" of the xeroradiograph enhances the separate muscular fasciculi as well as the adjoining fatty structures. (See Introduction for "edge enhancement" of xeroradiography.)

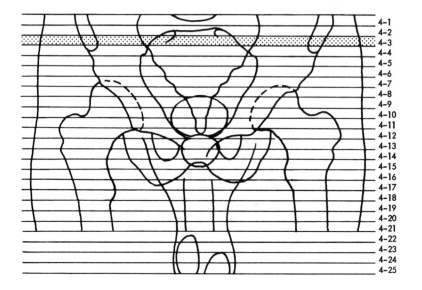

SECTION
4–3

*Through the
body of S2*

Anatomic Considerations

The sigmoid colon is first seen in this section and is visible through Section 4–9. It extends from the aperture of the lesser pelvis to the pelvic surface of the third sacral vertebra, where it becomes continuous with the rectum. The length of the sigmoid colon varies from 15 to 80 cm. When it is relatively short, it lies free in the lesser pelvis, but when long, it is coiled and may lie in many areas of the abdominal cavity. It normally forms one or two loops before terminating in the rectum. The peritoneum completely surrounds the sigmoid colon and is attached to the pelvic wall by the mesocolon. In this specimen, it formed several loops before terminating.

In this series of sections, the various relations of the sigmoid colon can be observed. To the left are the external iliac vessels, obturator vessels, vas deferens, and ureter. Ventrally, the sigmoid colon is separated from the urinary bladder by the coils of the ileum and the jejunum.

The sigmoid and superior rectal arteries supply the sigmoid colon.

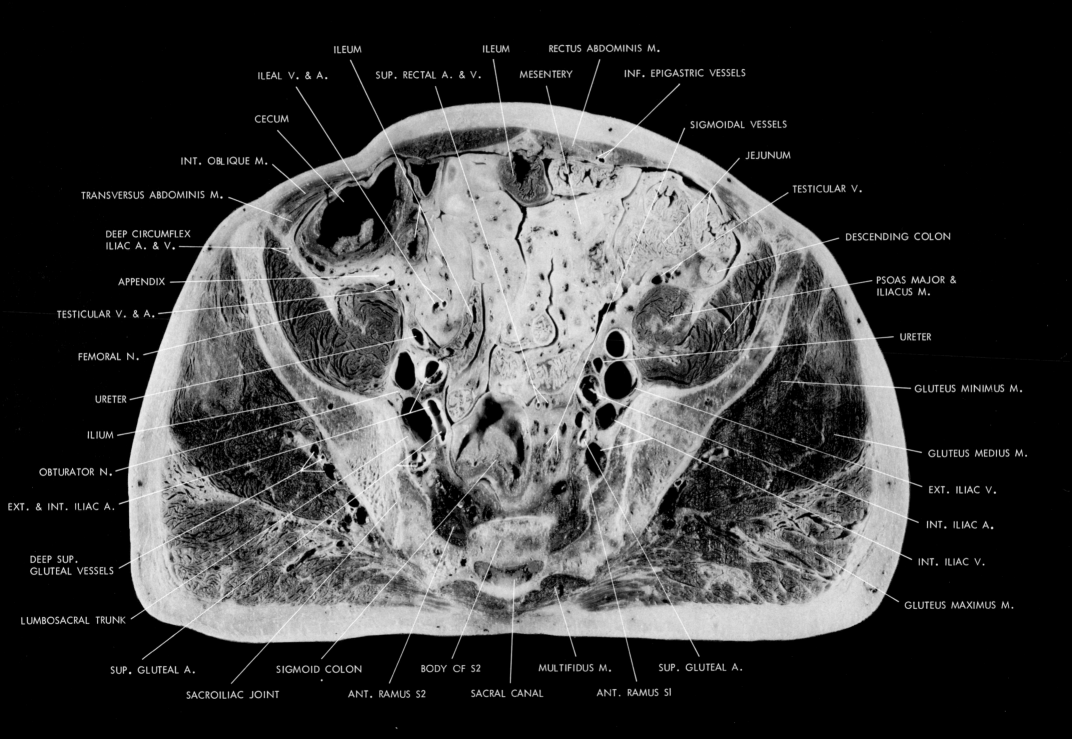

ILEUM   ILEUM   RECTUS ABDOMINIS M.

ILEAL V. & A.   SUP. RECTAL A. & V.   MESENTERY   INF. EPIGASTRIC VESSELS

CECUM   SIGMOIDAL VESSELS

INT. OBLIQUE M.   JEJUNUM

TRANSVERSUS ABDOMINIS M.   TESTICULAR V.

DEEP CIRCUMFLEX ILIAC A. & V.   DESCENDING COLON

APPENDIX   PSOAS MAJOR & ILIACUS M.

TESTICULAR V. & A.   URETER

FEMORAL N.   GLUTEUS MINIMUS M.

URETER   GLUTEUS MEDIUS M.

ILIUM   EXT. ILIAC V.

OBTURATOR N.   INT. ILIAC A.

EXT. & INT. ILIAC A.   INT. ILIAC V.

DEEP SUP. GLUTEAL VESSELS   GLUTEUS MAXIMUS M.

LUMBOSACRAL TRUNK

SUP. GLUTEAL A.   SIGMOID COLON   BODY OF S2   MULTIFIDUS M.   SUP. GLUTEAL A.

SACROILIAC JOINT   ANT. RAMUS S2   SACRAL CANAL   ANT. RAMUS S1

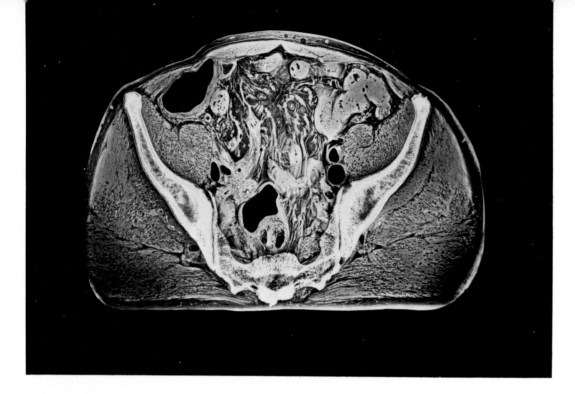

Note that in this section the descending colon is more anteriorly situated and is almost at the same level as the cecum. The space between the descending colon and the adjoining parietal peritoneum is very small, however.

In this section, the perirectal fat, which contains the blood vessels of the rectum, is wider to the left of the rectum than to the right, as is often the case. When perirenal air insufflation must be carried out to visualize the various structures in the retroperitoneum, especially surrounding the kidneys and the suprarenal glands, the left perirectal fossa is the preferred choice for insufflation. Great care must be exercised at the time of insufflation, however, so that the gaseous medium introduced does not enter a blood vessel; otherwise, gas emboli may be formed, which would become extremely hazardous to the patient, particularly if the gas is air.

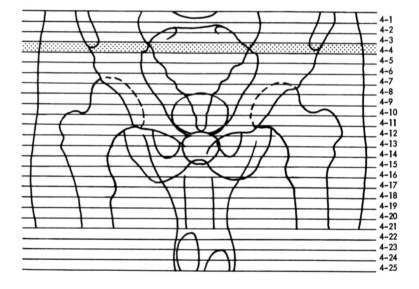

4-1
4-2
4-3
4-4
4-5
4-6
4-7
4-8
4-9
4-10
4-11
4-12
4-13
4-14
4-15
4-16
4-17
4-18
4-19
4-20
4-21
4-22
4-23
4-24
4-25

SECTION
4-4

Through the body of S3

Anatomic Considerations

The internal iliac (hypogastric) artery, the most variable artery in the body, supplies the pelvis, perineum, and gluteal area. This artery often divides into an anterior and a posterior division a short distance from its origin from the common iliac artery. The superior gluteal artery, one of the largest branches from the posterior division of the internal iliac artery, can be observed in this illustration. The superior gluteal artery usually passes between the lumbosacral trunk and first sacral nerve and, with the superior gluteal vein and nerve, exits the pelvis above the piriformis through the greater sciatic foramen. Shortly after it exits the pelvis, the superior gluteal artery divides into a deep branch that courses between the gluteus medius and minimus muscles and a superficial branch that lies deep to the gluteus maximus muscle.

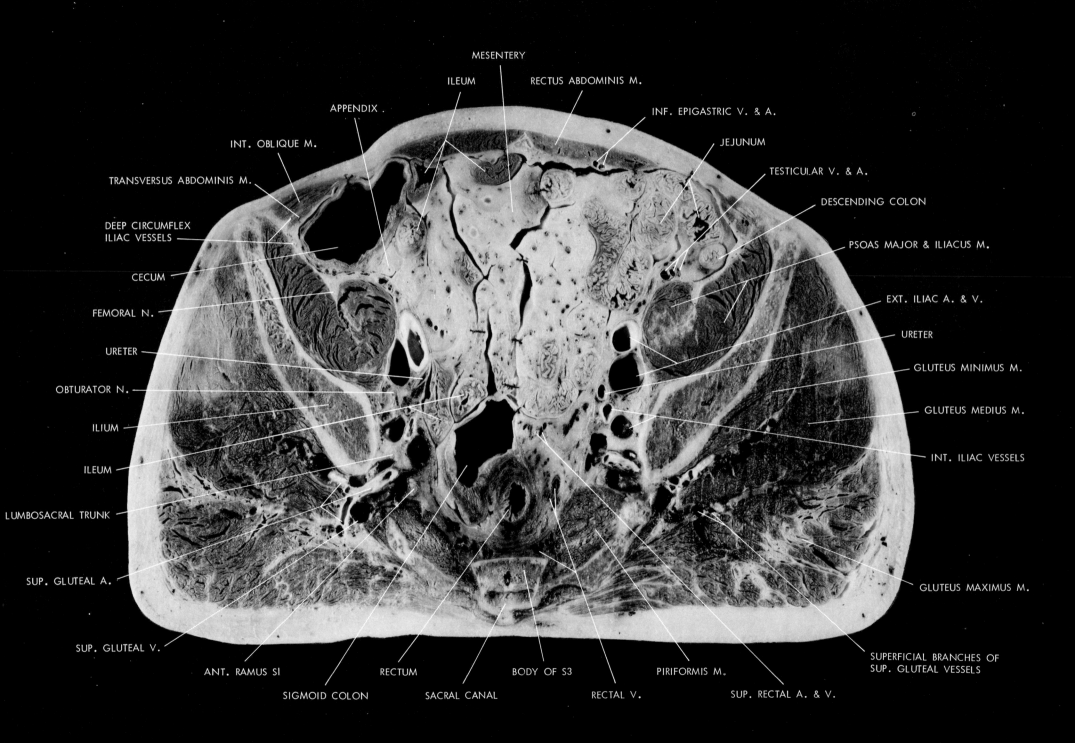

MESENTERY

ILEUM   RECTUS ABDOMINIS M.

APPENDIX .   INF. EPIGASTRIC V. & A.

INT. OBLIQUE M.   JEJUNUM

TRANSVERSUS ABDOMINIS M.   TESTICULAR V. & A.

DEEP CIRCUMFLEX   DESCENDING COLON
ILIAC VESSELS

CECUM   PSOAS MAJOR & ILIACUS M.

FEMORAL N.   EXT. ILIAC A. & V.

URETER   URETER

OBTURATOR N.   GLUTEUS MINIMUS M.

ILIUM   GLUTEUS MEDIUS M.

ILEUM   INT. ILIAC VESSELS

LUMBOSACRAL TRUNK

SUP. GLUTEAL A.   GLUTEUS MAXIMUS M.

SUP. GLUTEAL V.   SUPERFICIAL BRANCHES OF
                                          SUP. GLUTEAL VESSELS

ANT. RAMUS S1   RECTUM   BODY OF S3   PIRIFORMIS M.

SIGMOID COLON   SACRAL CANAL   RECTAL V.   SUP. RECTAL A. & V.

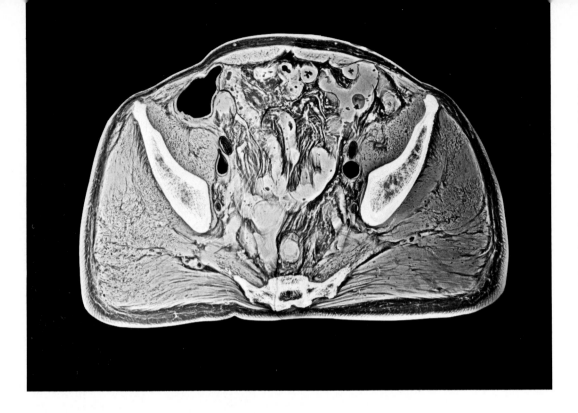

Clinical Considerations

In this section, the sigmoid colon may be seen just over the midline and primarily to its right; this relationship is common in the adult. When the entire sigmoid colon is identified to the left of the midline, one may usually suspect a mass lesion displacing it. On the other hand, if the mass lesion originates in the sigmoid colon, such as by inflammation of diverticuli of the sigmoid colon, it may be displaced ventrally or to the right, surrounding the adjoining abscess thus created. Moreover, this same inflammatory process will often displace the ileal loops ventrally and invade the mesentery of the small intestine, often going beyond the mesentery into the fatty layers and serosa surrounding the ileal loops and causing a displacement or separation, or both, of these loops.

In the presence of an enveloping inflammatory process, the ileal loops become very matted together and virtually impossible to move outside of the pelvis minor by external means. Their separation and individual examination by conventional radiographic contrast-enhanced techniques is very difficult.

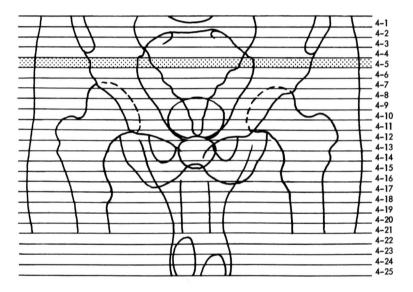

4-1
4-2
4-3
4-4
4-5
4-6
4-7
4-8
4-9
4-10
4-11
4-12
4-13
4-14
4-15
4-16
4-17
4-18
4-19
4-20
4-21
4-22
4-23
4-24
4-25

SECTION
4–5

Through the body of S4

Anatomic Considerations

In this illustration the sciatic nerve is seen for the first time. This nerve is the largest branch of the sacral plexus, which is formed by the lumbosacral trunk and the anterior divisions of spinal nerves S1, S2, and S3. Several branches of the sacral plexus can be found in some of the sections of the lower extremity as well as in these of the pelvis. The branches of the sacral plexus are the sciatic nerve, the superior and inferior gluteal nerves, the posterior femoral cutaneous nerve, and the nerves to the quadratus femoris, obturator internus, and piriformis.

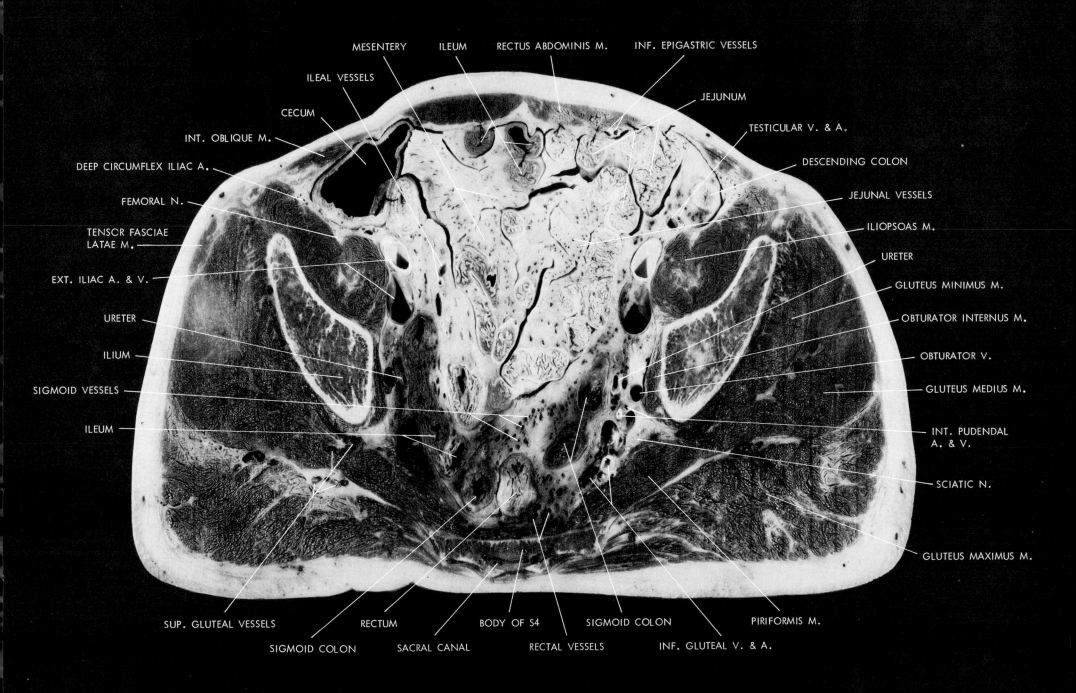

MESENTERY   ILEUM   RECTUS ABDOMINIS M.   INF. EPIGASTRIC VESSELS

ILEAL VESSELS

CECUM   JEJUNUM

INT. OBLIQUE M.   TESTICULAR V. & A.

DEEP CIRCUMFLEX ILIAC A.   DESCENDING COLON

FEMORAL N.   JEJUNAL VESSELS

TENSOR FASCIAE LATAE M.   ILIOPSOAS M.

EXT. ILIAC A. & V.   URETER

ILEUM   GLUTEUS MINIMUS M.

URETER   OBTURATOR INTERNUS M.

ILIUM   OBTURATOR V.

SIGMOID VESSELS   GLUTEUS MEDIUS M.

ILEUM   INT. PUDENDAL A. & V.

SCIATIC N.

GLUTEUS MAXIMUS M.

SUP. GLUTEAL VESSELS   RECTUM   BODY OF S4   SIGMOID COLON   PIRIFORMIS M.

SIGMOID COLON   SACRAL CANAL   RECTAL VESSELS   INF. GLUTEAL V. & A.

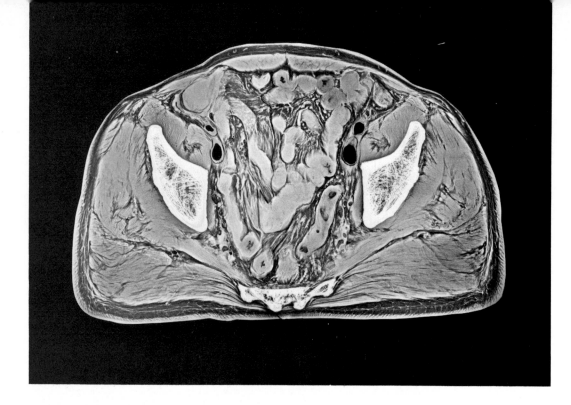

The internal pudendal vessels, pudendal nerve, and nerve to the obturator internus also enter the gluteal region below the piriformis but course over the spine of the ischium to enter the ischiorectal fossa by passing through the lesser sciatic foramen.

Clinical Considerations

In this section, the rectum retains its relatively midline position, whereas now there are sigmoid loops of bowel identified somewhat more to the left than to the right. The deep situation of the ileum, prior to its rise to join the cecum at the ileocecal junction, is well defined.

The perirectal fat and vessels are more numerous to the left of and anterior to the rectum, a point of some significance if one is to insufflate the perirectal fat with a gaseous medium, such as air.

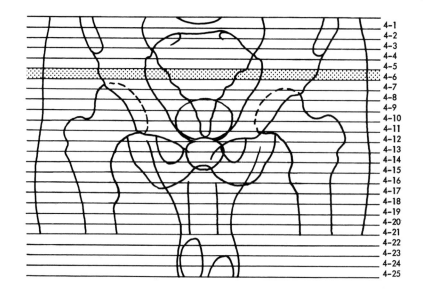

SECTION 4-6

Through the sacrum, 1 cm below the preceding section

Anatomic Considerations

The greater and lesser sciatic notches are converted into foramina by the sacrospinous and sacrotuberous ligaments. Several structures pass through these foramina, which serve as communications between the pelvis and lower extremity. The piriformis exits the greater sciatic foramen, and the tendon of the obturator internus passes through the lesser sciatic foramen. The piriformis is a key to the identification of the structures in the gluteal region: the superior gluteal nerve and vessels exit above the muscle (Section 4-4); the sciatic nerve, posterior femoral cutaneous nerve, nerve to the quadratus femoris, and inferior gluteal nerve and vessels all exit below the piriformis.

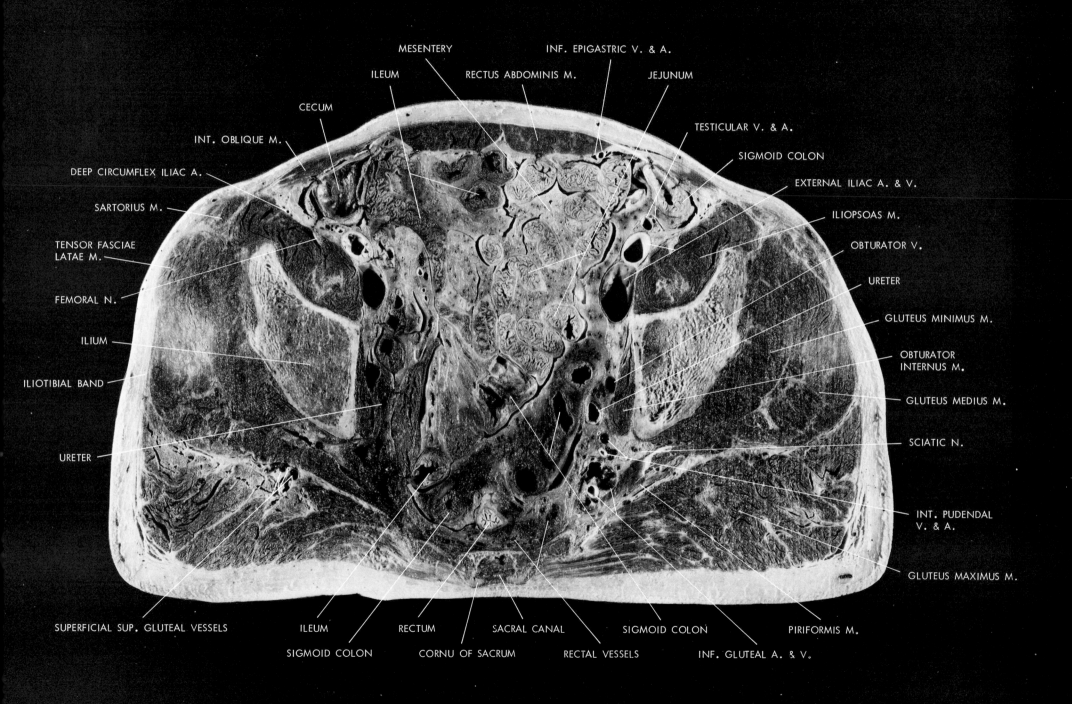

MESENTERY   INF. EPIGASTRIC V. & A.

ILEUM   RECTUS ABDOMINIS M.   JEJUNUM

CECUM

TESTICULAR V. & A.

INT. OBLIQUE M.

SIGMOID COLON

DEEP CIRCUMFLEX ILIAC A.

EXTERNAL ILIAC A. & V.

SARTORIUS M.

ILIOPSOAS M.

TENSOR FASCIAE LATAE M.

OBTURATOR V.

FEMORAL N.

URETER

GLUTEUS MINIMUS M.

ILIUM

OBTURATOR INTERNUS M.

ILIOTIBIAL BAND

GLUTEUS MEDIUS M.

SCIATIC N.

URETER

INT. PUDENDAL V. & A.

GLUTEUS MAXIMUS M.

SUPERFICIAL SUP. GLUTEAL VESSELS   ILEUM   RECTUM   SACRAL CANAL   SIGMOID COLON   PIRIFORMIS M.

SIGMOID COLON   CORNU OF SACRUM   RECTAL VESSELS   INF. GLUTEAL A. & V.

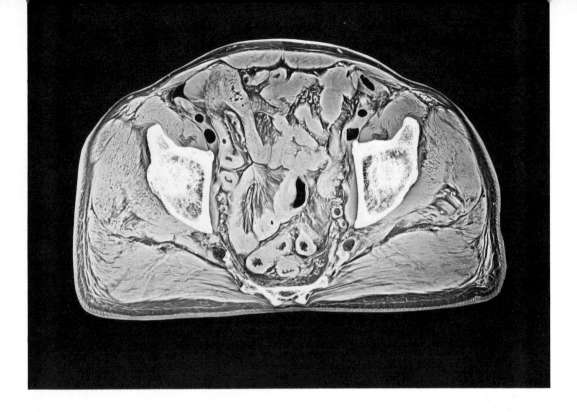

Clinical Considerations

Note the persistence of the posterior relationship of the ileum in close contiguity with the sigmoid colon. This becomes clinically important in inflammatory processes such as regional enteritis, in which the ileum is very frequently involved, and sigmoidal colitis resulting from diverticulitis, in which the sigmoid is involved. Because of this contiguity of ileum and sigmoid, inflammatory exudate may extend in either direction from inflammatory processes involving either organ.

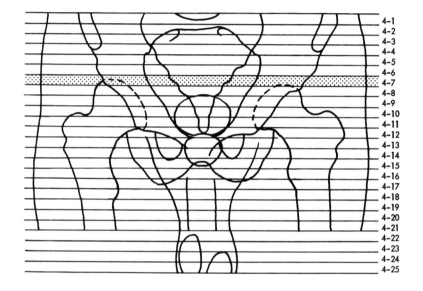

SECTION
4–7

Through the upper portion of the head of the femur

Anatomic Considerations

The three portions of the innominate, or hip, bone can be seen in this illustration; the pubis, ilium, and ischium fuse with each other at the time of puberty. This site of union of the three bones is the acetabulum, which is the depression that articulates with the head of the femur.

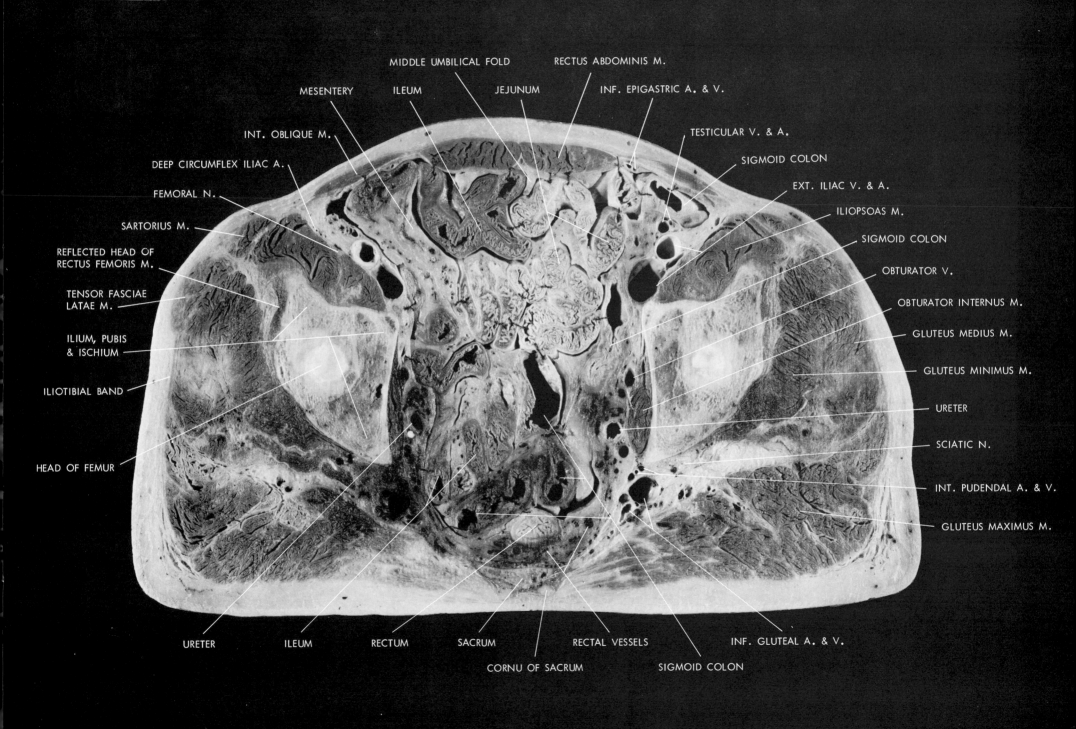

MIDDLE UMBILICAL FOLD

RECTUS ABDOMINIS M.

MESENTERY

ILEUM

JEJUNUM

INF. EPIGASTRIC A. & V.

INT. OBLIQUE M.

TESTICULAR V. & A.

DEEP CIRCUMFLEX ILIAC A.

SIGMOID COLON

FEMORAL N.

EXT. ILIAC V. & A.

SARTORIUS M.

ILIOPSOAS M.

REFLECTED HEAD OF
RECTUS FEMORIS M.

SIGMOID COLON

TENSOR FASCIAE
LATAE M.

OBTURATOR V.

OBTURATOR INTERNUS M.

ILIUM, PUBIS
& ISCHIUM

GLUTEUS MEDIUS M.

GLUTEUS MINIMUS M.

ILIOTIBIAL BAND

URETER

SCIATIC N.

HEAD OF FEMUR

INT. PUDENDAL A. & V.

GLUTEUS MAXIMUS M.

URETER

ILEUM

RECTUM

SACRUM

RECTAL VESSELS

INF. GLUTEAL A. & V.

CORNU OF SACRUM

SIGMOID COLON

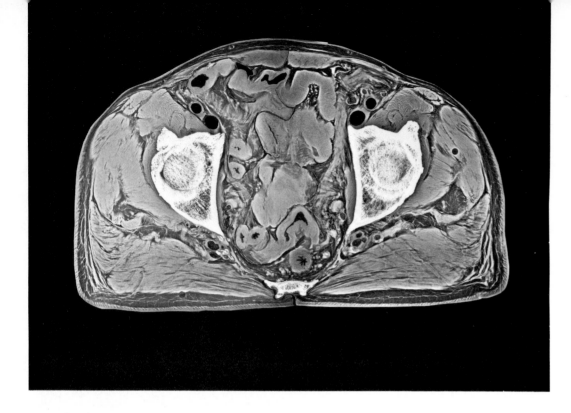

Anteriorly, the upper two thirds are related to the ileum and sigmoid colon; the lower third is separated from the bladder by the seminal vesicles and vas deferens and is directly related to the prostate. Laterally, the rectum is related to the levator ani muscles.

Five rectal arteries — the superior, a pair of middle, and a pair of inferior — supply the rectum. The rectal venous plexuses are drained by the superior, middle, and inferior rectal veins. The superior is part of the portal system; the middle and inferior are systemic veins. The plexus forms a link between the portal and systemic veins.

Clinical Considerations

The ureters near the ureterovesical junction and the base plate of the urinary bladder have a triangular relationship with the vesicourethral orifice ("bladder trigone"). The base plate of the urinary bladder is important in micturition.

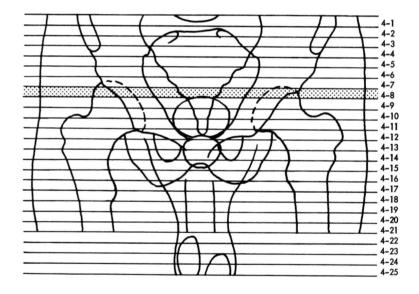

SECTION
4-8

Through the head of the femur, 1 cm below the preceding section

Anatomic Considerations

The rectum can be observed in Sections 4-4 to 4-14. The rectum is approximately 10 to 15 cm long. It commences anterior to the third segment of the sacrum, proceeds with a curve conforming to the curve of the sacrum and coccyx, and, at the level of the apex of the prostate, becomes the anal canal. Proximally, the rectum has the same diameter as the sigmoid colon; distally, it widens to form the ampulla, which narrows to the anal canal. Besides the anteroposterior curve, the rectum has three flexures: the upper and lower are concave toward the left, the middle one toward the right. The upper third of the rectum has peritoneum on its front and sides, the middle third has it only on the front; the lower third is devoid of peritoneum.

By following Sections 4-4 to 4-14 some of the relations of the rectum can be observed. Posterior to the rectum are the sacrum, coccyx, and rectal vessels.

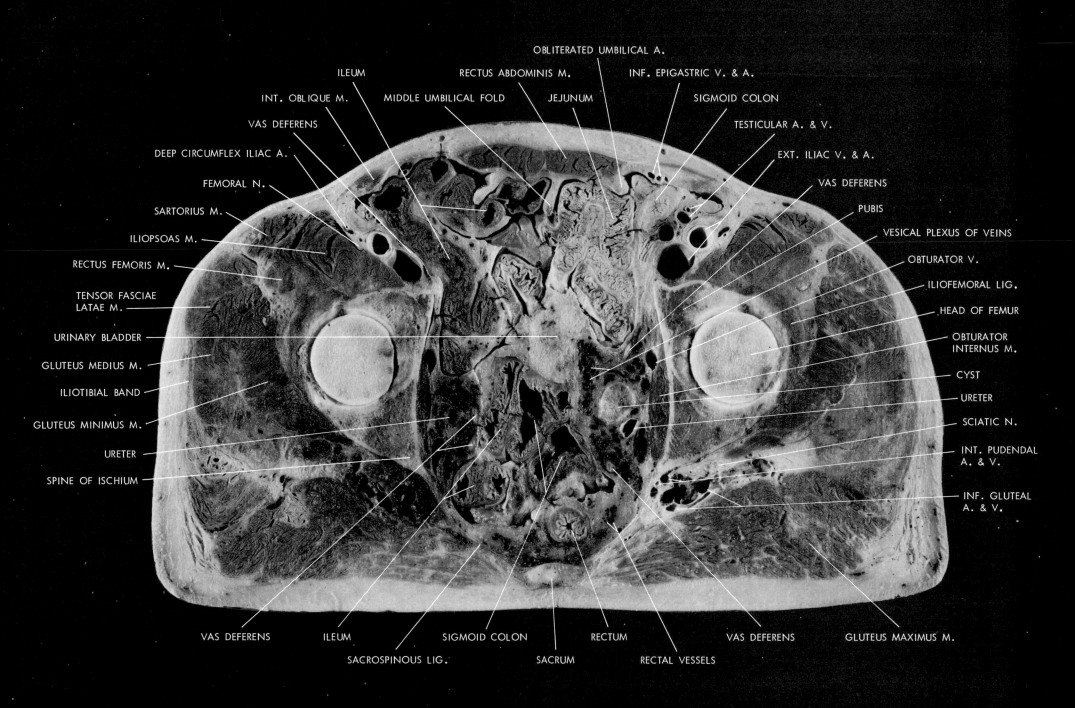

OBLITERATED UMBILICAL A.

ILEUM

RECTUS ABDOMINIS M.

INF. EPIGASTRIC V. & A.

INT. OBLIQUE M.

MIDDLE UMBILICAL FOLD

JEJUNUM

SIGMOID COLON

VAS DEFERENS

TESTICULAR A. & V.

DEEP CIRCUMFLEX ILIAC A.

EXT. ILIAC V. & A.

FEMORAL N.

VAS DEFERENS

SARTORIUS M.

PUBIS

ILIOPSOAS M.

VESICAL PLEXUS OF VEINS

RECTUS FEMORIS M.

OBTURATOR V.

ILIOFEMORAL LIG.

TENSOR FASCIAE LATAE M.

HEAD OF FEMUR

URINARY BLADDER

OBTURATOR INTERNUS M.

GLUTEUS MEDIUS M.

CYST

ILIOTIBIAL BAND

URETER

GLUTEUS MINIMUS M.

SCIATIC N.

URETER

INT. PUDENDAL A. & V.

SPINE OF ISCHIUM

INF. GLUTEAL A. & V.

VAS DEFERENS

ILEUM

SIGMOID COLON

RECTUM

VAS DEFERENS

GLUTEUS MAXIMUS M.

SACROSPINOUS LIG.

SACRUM

RECTAL VESSELS

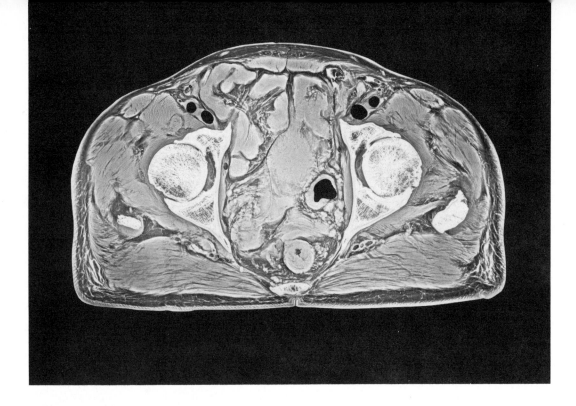

dilated and forms the ampulla. It then narrows and joins the duct of the seminal vesicle to form the ejaculatory duct. In the accompanying Sections (4–8 to 4–12), it is possible to observe the relations of the vas deferens in the lesser pelvis to the ureters, seminal vesicles, urinary bladder, sigmoid colon, and rectum. The relationship of the vas deferens to the external iliac vessels can be seen in Sections 4–8 and 4–9.

Clinical Considerations

In this section, the urachus is a closed, bandlike structure, still identified by its attachment to the urinary bladder, which in its fetal state is widely patent. It may remain patent after birth, forming a "urachal cyst" or even a communication between the urinary bladder and the anterior abdominal wall.

The medial umbilical fold, visible in this section, is sometimes apparent in the newborn in the presence of pneumoperitoneum, forming a foldlike structure in this lower abdominal relationship, even as does the ligamentum teres in the region of the liver. These become important signs in the diagnosis of pneumoperitoneum of the newborn.

Note the rather large space between the rectum and the urinary bladder, in which sigmoid colon happens to be situated in this section. There is therefore more space for the exudate from inflammatory processes to collect in the male than in the female, in whom the space is occupied by the uterus, its adjoining ligaments, and tissues.

SECTION 4–9

Through the head of the femur, 1 cm below the preceding section

Anatomic Considerations

The spermatic cord consists of structures that pass to and from the testes. It begins at the deep inguinal ring and ends at the superior pole of the testis. In the abdominal wall, it passes obliquely through the inguinal canal to the superficial inguinal ring and then descends into the scrotum. The left spermatic cord is usually longer than the right.

The structures of the spermatic cord — vas deferens, arteries to the vas deferens and testes, pampiniform plexus of veins, lymph vessels, and nerves — are invested with three layers of fascia. From outside inward they are the external spermatic fascia, the cremasteric muscle and fascia, and the internal spermatic fascia. These are derived from the external oblique muscle, the internal oblique muscle, and the transversalis fascia, respectively.

The vas deferens can be observed in Sections 4–8 through 4–25 in various locations. It begins in continuity with the lower pole of the epididymis and ascends by passing along the medial border of the epididymis, posterior to the testis, in the posterior part of the spermatic cord to the deep inguinal ring. It then crosses the pelvic brim, continues deep to the peritoneum along the lateral wall of the pelvis to the ischial spine, and passes medially to the posterior surface of the bladder. Near the terminal end, the vas deferens is

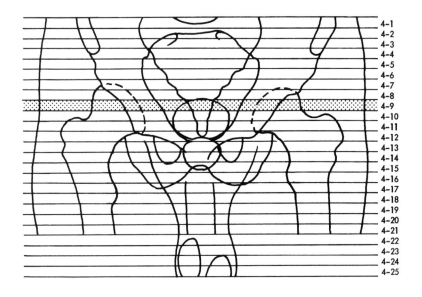

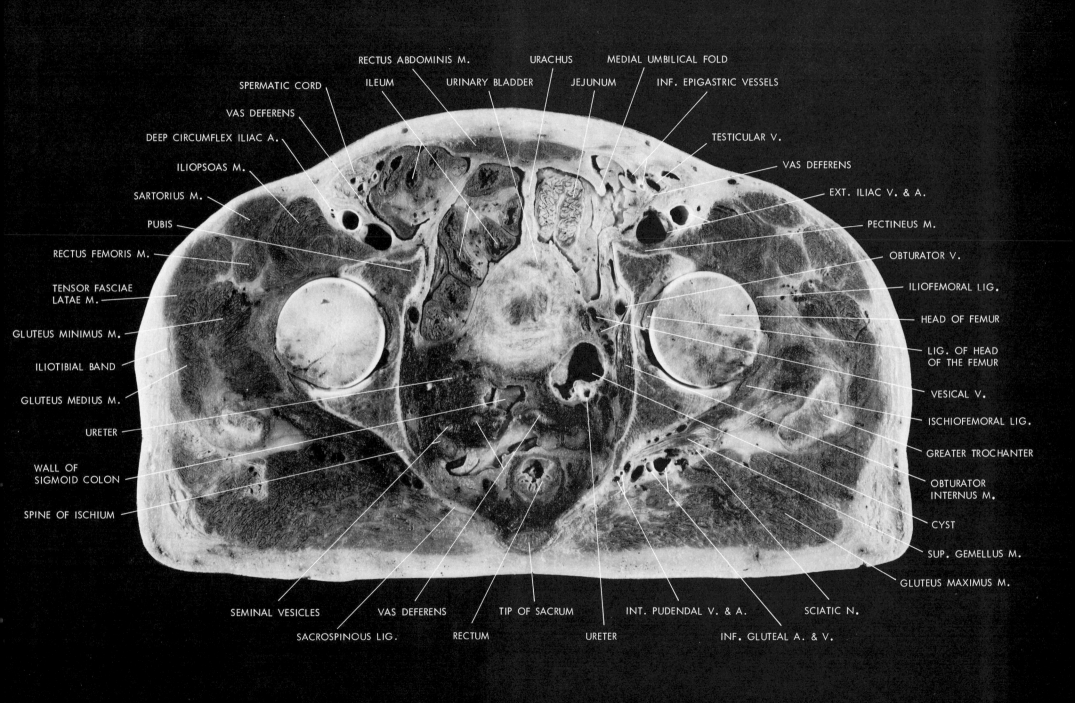

RECTUS ABDOMINIS M.   URACHUS   MEDIAL UMBILICAL FOLD

SPERMATIC CORD   ILEUM   URINARY BLADDER   JEJUNUM   INF. EPIGASTRIC VESSELS

VAS DEFERENS   TESTICULAR V.

DEEP CIRCUMFLEX ILIAC A.   VAS DEFERENS

ILIOPSOAS M.   EXT. ILIAC V. & A.

SARTORIUS M.   PECTINEUS M.

PUBIS   OBTURATOR V.

RECTUS FEMORIS M.   ILIOFEMORAL LIG.

TENSOR FASCIAE   HEAD OF FEMUR
LATAE M.

GLUTEUS MINIMUS M.   LIG. OF HEAD
OF THE FEMUR

ILIOTIBIAL BAND   VESICAL V.

GLUTEUS MEDIUS M.   ISCHIOFEMORAL LIG.

URETER   GREATER TROCHANTER

WALL OF   OBTURATOR
SIGMOID COLON   INTERNUS M.

SPINE OF ISCHIUM   CYST

SUP. GEMELLUS M.

GLUTEUS MAXIMUS M.

SEMINAL VESICLES   VAS DEFERENS   TIP OF SACRUM   INT. PUDENDAL V. & A.   SCIATIC N.

SACROSPINOUS LIG.   RECTUM   URETER   INF. GLUTEAL A. & V.

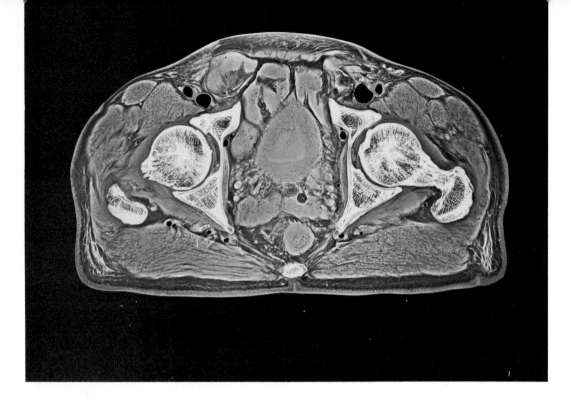

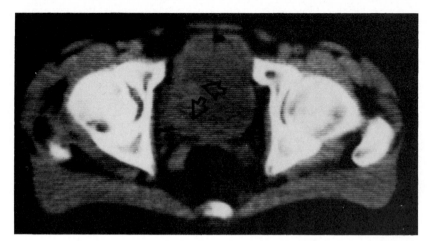

Clinical Considerations

The CT scan shows a filling defect on the right wall of the urinary bladder (see arrows) due to a tumor that has invaded the wall of the organ and extended by growth to the pelvic wall. The most likely cause would be an advanced carcinoma, allowing for appropriate staging and treatment of this disease. The right seminal vesicle is displaced downward, by comparison with the left, although clearly demarcated. The rectum is clearly demonstrated in its presacral position by its gas content.

Because the seminal vesicles are close to the rectum, they can be palpated on rectal examination.

Infection from the bladder may pass along the ejaculatory duct and either along the vas deferens to the epididymis or else to the seminal vesicles.

SECTION

4–10

*Through the
mid-portion of
the acetabulum
and coccyx*

Anatomic Considerations

Portions of the urinary bladder are shown in Sections 4–8 through 4–11. The relations of the urinary bladder depend on the amount of distention: In the contracted state, it is located in the true or lesser pelvis; when distended, it expands superiorly and anteriorly into the abdominal cavity.

Several relations of the bladder can be seen in these illustrations. Anteriorly, the apex of the bladder is continuous with the median umbilical ligament, which is the remnant of the urachus. The superior surface is covered by peritoneum and is related to coils of the ileum and the sigmoid colon. Posteriorly, the peritoneum continues and covers the ureters, the vas deferens, and the superior portions of the seminal vesicles. It then passes inferiorly to form the rectovesical pouch before continuing on to the anterior surface of the rectum. The inferolateral surfaces are related to the levator ani and internal obturator muscles. The bladder receives its blood supply primarily by the superior and inferior vesical arteries. The superior vesical artery arises from the umbilical artery, which is a branch of the internal iliac, and the inferior vesical artery arises for the most part from the internal iliac artery.

The articulation between the head of the femur and the cup-shaped acetabulum is a ball-and-socket synovial joint. Most of the head of the femur is encompassed by the acetabulum. This type of morphologic structure does not allow as much free movement at the hip joint as does the shoulder joint.

The xeroradiograph clearly defines the trabecular pattern of the bony structures. The seminal vesicles appear more clustered and less discrete because of the "through and through" section depicted by the radiograph. The lumina of the major blood vessels have been intensified for ease of formulating the teaching comparison. The xeroradiograph gives another dimension in understanding the intimate and yet discrete relationships of all labelled structures.

*MALE PELVIS
AND
PERINEUM*

182

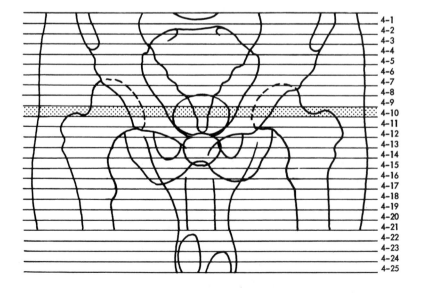

4–1
4–2
4–3
4–4
4–5
4–6
4–7
4–8
4–9
4–10
4–11
4–12
4–13
4–14
4–15
4–16
4–17
4–18
4–19
4–20
4–21
4–22
4–23
4–24
4–25

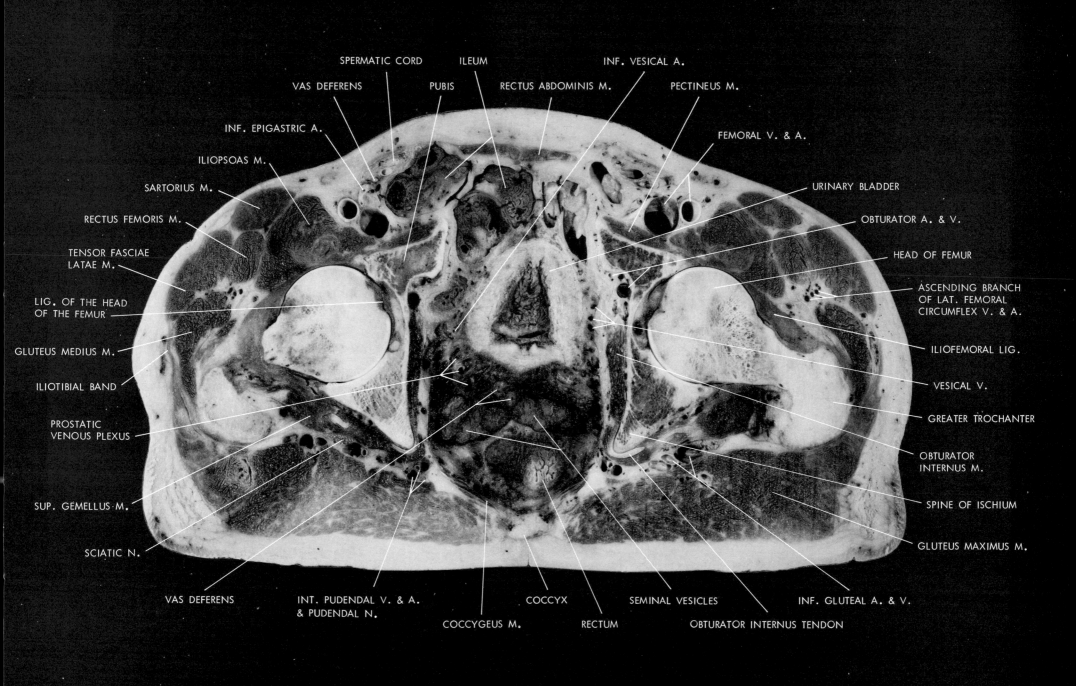

SPERMATIC CORD   ILEUM   INF. VESICAL A.

VAS DEFERENS   PUBIS   RECTUS ABDOMINIS M.   PECTINEUS M.

INF. EPIGASTRIC A.   FEMORAL V. & A.

ILIOPSOAS M.   URINARY BLADDER

SARTORIUS M.   OBTURATOR A. & V.

RECTUS FEMORIS M.   HEAD OF FEMUR

TENSOR FASCIAE   ASCENDING BRANCH
LATAE M.   OF LAT. FEMORAL
    CIRCUMFLEX V. & A.

LIG. OF THE HEAD   ILIOFEMORAL LIG.
OF THE FEMUR

GLUTEUS MEDIUS M.   VESICAL V.

ILIOTIBIAL BAND   GREATER TROCHANTER

PROSTATIC   OBTURATOR
VENOUS PLEXUS   INTERNUS M.

SUP. GEMELLUS M.   SPINE OF ISCHIUM

SCIATIC N.   GLUTEUS MAXIMUS M.

VAS DEFERENS   INT. PUDENDAL V. & A.   COCCYX   SEMINAL VESICLES   INF. GLUTEAL A. & V.
    & PUDENDAL N.

COCCYGEUS M.   RECTUM   OBTURATOR INTERNUS TENDON

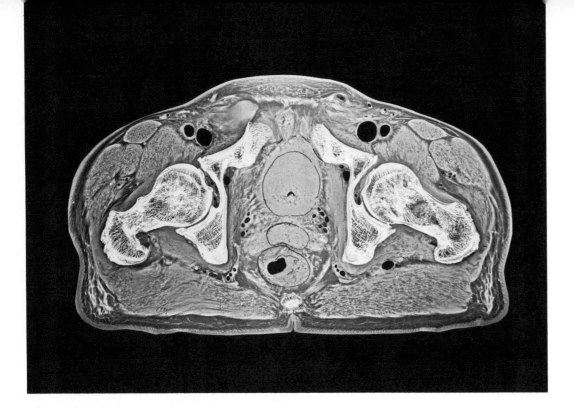

Clinical Considerations

The normal angle between the neck and shaft of the femur is approximately 130 degrees. This is particularly important in the analysis of the anteversion of infants and children, which at times must be corrected by orthopedic measures.

The perirectal fat is the immediate plane for dissection of perirectal air when applied diagnostically. The prostate, seminal vesicles, and prostatic urethra are important signposts of potential disease. The fatty planes surrounding the obturator internus muscle become a fertile field for invasion by contiguous neoplasms, and their clear definition on this section is most important in the staging of pelvic disease.

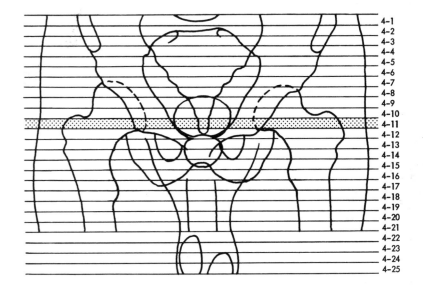

SECTION
4–11

Through the superior ramus of the pubis and tip of the coccyx

Anatomic Considerations

In this and the preceding sections the seminal vesicles can be observed. They are paired sacculated tubes (5 to 7 cm long) that are found between the fundus of the bladder and the rectum. They are separated from the rectum by the fascia of Denonvillier. Each ends superiorly in a cul-de-sac; the lower ends are constricted to form small narrow ducts that join the termination of the vas deferens to form the ejaculatory ducts. The medial margin of each vesicle is related to the ampulla of the vas deferens; the lateral margin is related to the prostatic plexus of veins.

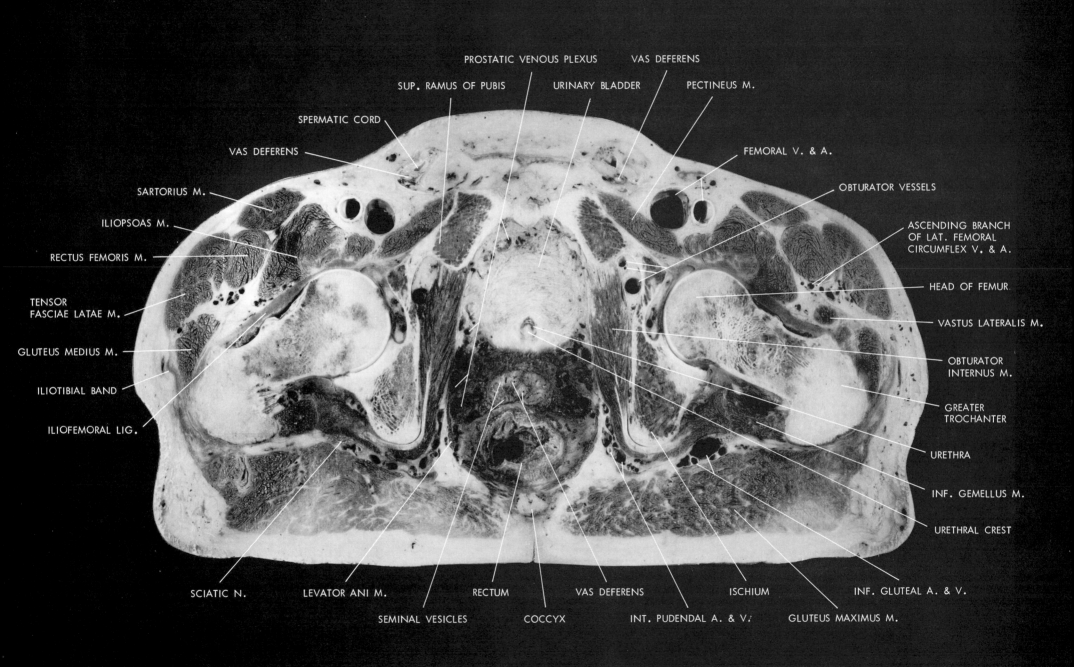

PROSTATIC VENOUS PLEXUS

VAS DEFERENS

SUP. RAMUS OF PUBIS

URINARY BLADDER

PECTINEUS M.

SPERMATIC CORD

VAS DEFERENS

FEMORAL V. & A.

SARTORIUS M.

OBTURATOR VESSELS

ILIOPSOAS M.

ASCENDING BRANCH
OF LAT. FEMORAL
CIRCUMFLEX V. & A.

RECTUS FEMORIS M.

HEAD OF FEMUR

TENSOR
FASCIAE LATAE M.

VASTUS LATERALIS M.

GLUTEUS MEDIUS M.

OBTURATOR
INTERNUS M.

ILIOTIBIAL BAND

GREATER
TROCHANTER

ILIOFEMORAL LIG.

URETHRA

INF. GEMELLUS M.

URETHRAL CREST

SCIATIC N.

LEVATOR ANI M.

RECTUM

VAS DEFERENS

ISCHIUM

INF. GLUTEAL A. & V.

SEMINAL VESICLES

COCCYX

INT. PUDENDAL A. & V.

GLUTEUS MAXIMUS M.

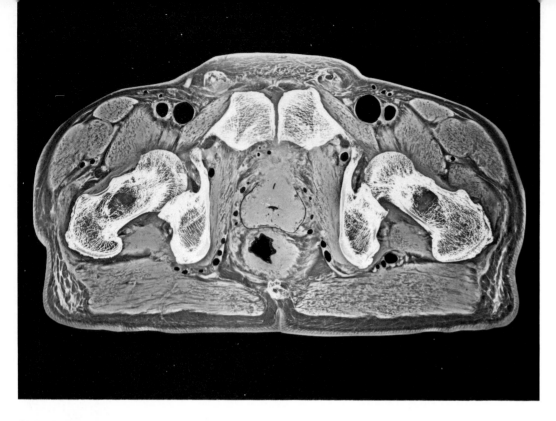

The gland has a distinct capsule that is made up of fibrous tissue and smooth muscle. In addition, the prostate has a distinct fibrous sheath that is continous with the parietal layer of the surrounding fascia. Between the fibrous sheath and the capsule, a plexus of veins surrounds the sides and base of the gland. This prostatic plexus of veins receives the dorsal vein of the penis and communicates with the vesical plexus of veins, vertebral plexus of veins, and internal iliac veins. The arteries to the prostate arise from the internal pudendal, inferior vesical, and middle rectal arteries.

The sciatic nerve exits the pelvis *via* the greater sciatic foramen at a point midway between the posterior superior iliac spine and ischial tuberosity and passes inferiorly through a point midway between the tuberosity of the ischium and greater trochanter of the femur. The nerve from superior to inferior is related anteriorly to the tendon of the obturator internus, and to the superior gemellus, inferior gemellus, and quadratus femoris muscles.

Clinical Considerations

On rectal examination, hypertrophy of the prostate can be detected. This section and Section 4–11 have very similar clinical importance in relation to the prostate, seminal vesicles, and perirectal fat, particularly.

SECTION
4–12

Through the superior portion of the symphysis pubis

Anatomic Considerations

The prostate is located in the pelvis between the urinary bladder and the urogenital diaphragm, posterior to the symphysis pubis and pubic arch and anterior to the ampulla of the rectum. The gland presents for examination a base, apex, and three surfaces. The base of the prostate is united to the neck of the bladder by muscular tissue at the orifice of the urethra. A vesical groove separates the rounded border of the base from the bladder. The apex is in contact with the deep fascia of the urogenital diaphragm. The anterior surface, which is approximately 2 cm posterior to the pubic symphysis, extends from the base to the apex and is connected to the pubic bones by the median puboprostatic ligament and to the arcus tendinous by the lateral puboprostatic ligaments. The urethra emerges from this surface just superior and anterior to the apex of the gland. The posterior surface is approximately 4 cm from the anus. The two ejaculatory ducts enter through this surface and divide the gland into two portions. The small superior portion, which is bounded by the two ejaculatory ducts and the urethra anteriorly, forms the median lobe. The large inferior portion is divided into the right and left lobes by a small depression. These lateral lobes form the main mass of the gland and are located posterior to the urethra. The inferolateral surfaces are prominent areas that are related to the levator ani muscles.

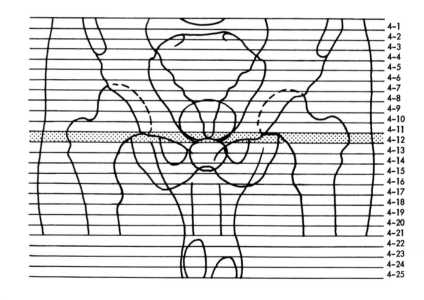

4–1
4–2
4–3
4–4
4–5
4–6
4–7
4–8
4–9
4–10
4–11
4–12
4–13
4–14
4–15
4–16
4–17
4–18
4–19
4–20
4–21
4–22
4–23
4–24
4–25

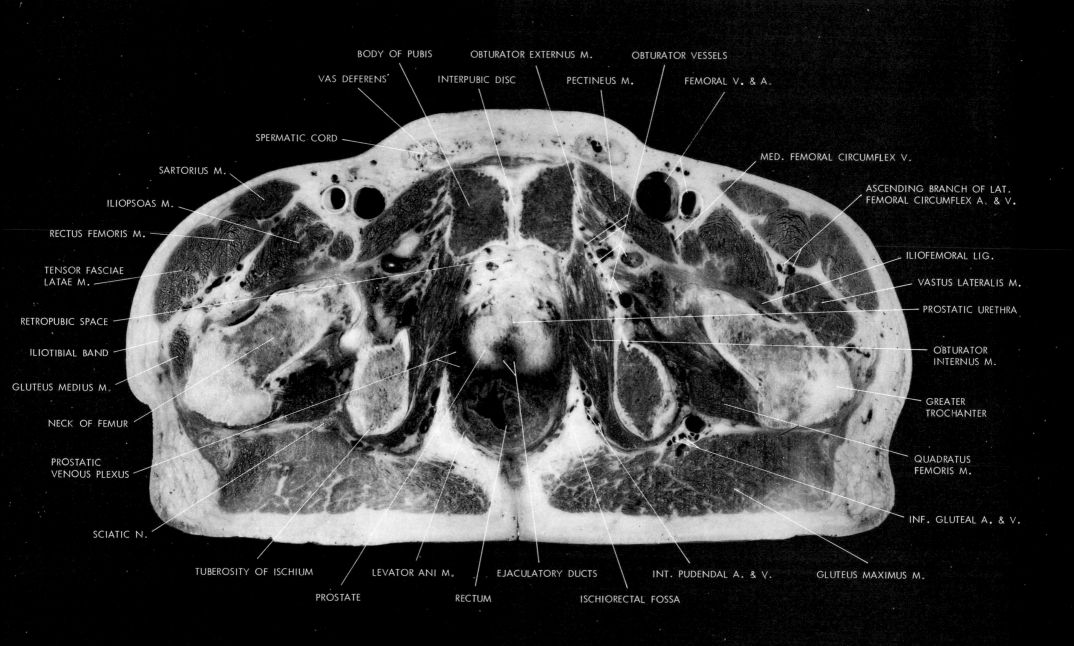

BODY OF PUBIS   OBTURATOR EXTERNUS M.   OBTURATOR VESSELS

VAS DEFERENS   INTERPUBIC DISC   PECTINEUS M.   FEMORAL V. & A.

SPERMATIC CORD

MED. FEMORAL CIRCUMFLEX V.

SARTORIUS M.

ASCENDING BRANCH OF LAT.
FEMORAL CIRCUMFLEX A. & V.

ILIOPSOAS M.

RECTUS FEMORIS M.

ILIOFEMORAL LIG.

TENSOR FASCIAE
LATAE M.

VASTUS LATERALIS M.

PROSTATIC URETHRA

RETROPUBIC SPACE

ILIOTIBIAL BAND

OBTURATOR
INTERNUS M.

GLUTEUS MEDIUS M.

GREATER
TROCHANTER

NECK OF FEMUR

PROSTATIC
VENOUS PLEXUS

QUADRATUS
FEMORIS M.

INF. GLUTEAL A. & V.

SCIATIC N.

TUBEROSITY OF ISCHIUM   LEVATOR ANI M.   EJACULATORY DUCTS   INT. PUDENDAL A. & V.   GLUTEUS MAXIMUS M.

PROSTATE   RECTUM   ISCHIORECTAL FOSSA

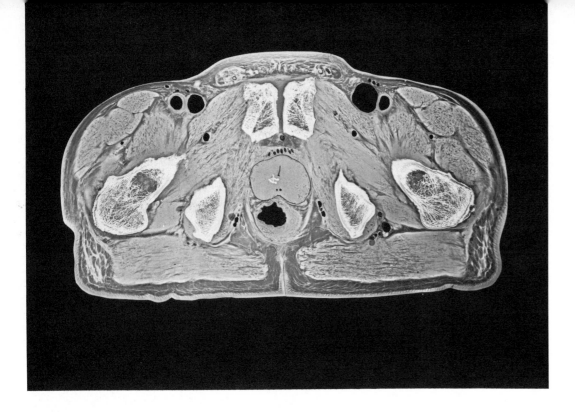

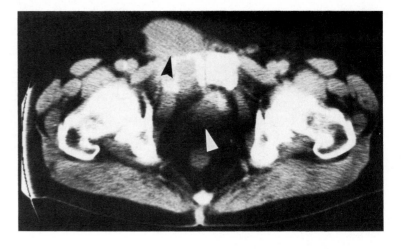

The dorsal vein of the penis and its relation to the prostatic plexus of veins can be observed. The plexus of veins drains into the internal iliac vein; some of the venous drainage is to the vertebral plexus of veins. This communication may explain the readiness with which carcinoma of the prostate spreads to the vertebrae.

The encapsulated appearance of the prostate and the importance of the integrity of this capsule are basic to an understanding of prostatic malignancy and its spread and release of acid phosphatase.

SECTION

4–13

Through the inferior portion of the symphysis pubis

Anatomic Considerations

The two ejaculatory ducts are evident in this section. They are formed by the union of the lower ends of the seminal vesicles and the terminal portion of the vas deferens. The ducts are approximately 2 cm long, beginning at the base of the prostate gland and passing between the median and lateral lobes. They terminate by opening on each side of the prostatic utricle on the colliculus seminalis.

Clinical Considerations

This CT scan shows the pelvis with a large undifferentiated carcinoma (black arrow) metastatic to the right pubis, destroying the bone of the right pubis and impressing itself upon the urinary bladder. The prostate is identified (white arrow). This prostate was considered abnormal by ultrasonography, but the computed tomographic scan showed it to be normal. The exact origin of this lesion was not identified, but a biopsy of the prostate revealed it to be normal. (Courtesy of Dr. Neil Wolfman.)

The xeroradiograph demonstrates prostatic calculi that are not observed in the gross specimen.

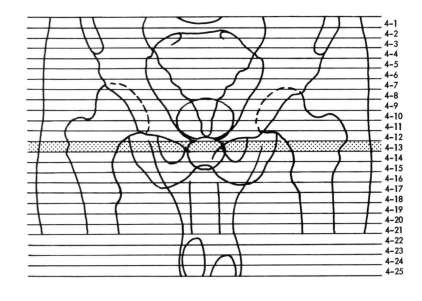

4–1
4–2
4–3
4–4
4–5
4–6
4–7
4–8
4–9
4–10
4–11
4–12
4–13
4–14
4–15
4–16
4–17
4–18
4–19
4–20
4–21
4–22
4–23
4–24
4–25

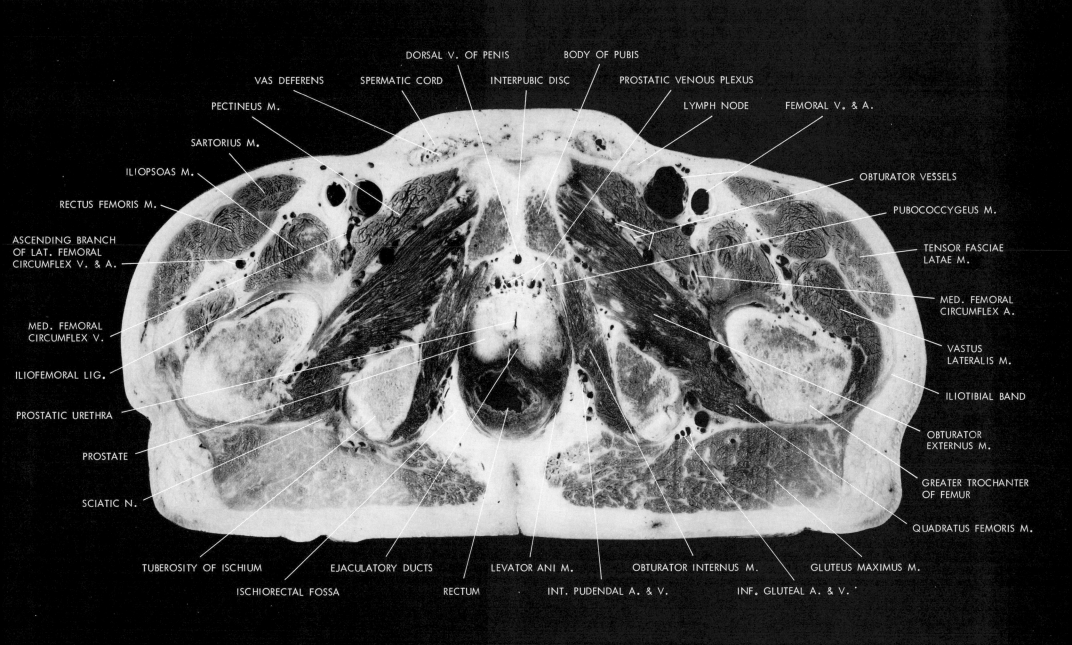

DORSAL V. OF PENIS   BODY OF PUBIS

VAS DEFERENS   SPERMATIC CORD   INTERPUBIC DISC   PROSTATIC VENOUS PLEXUS

PECTINEUS M.   LYMPH NODE   FEMORAL V. & A.

SARTORIUS M.

ILIOPSOAS M.   OBTURATOR VESSELS

RECTUS FEMORIS M.   PUBOCOCCYGEUS M.

ASCENDING BRANCH
OF LAT. FEMORAL
CIRCUMFLEX V. & A.   TENSOR FASCIAE
LATAE M.

MED. FEMORAL
CIRCUMFLEX A.

MED. FEMORAL
CIRCUMFLEX V.   VASTUS
LATERALIS M.

ILIOFEMORAL LIG.   ILIOTIBIAL BAND

PROSTATIC URETHRA   OBTURATOR
EXTERNUS M.

PROSTATE   GREATER TROCHANTER
OF FEMUR

SCIATIC N.   QUADRATUS FEMORIS M.

TUBEROSITY OF ISCHIUM   EJACULATORY DUCTS   LEVATOR ANI M.   OBTURATOR INTERNUS M.   GLUTEUS MAXIMUS M.

ISCHIORECTAL FOSSA   RECTUM   INT. PUDENDAL A. & V.   INF. GLUTEAL A. & V.

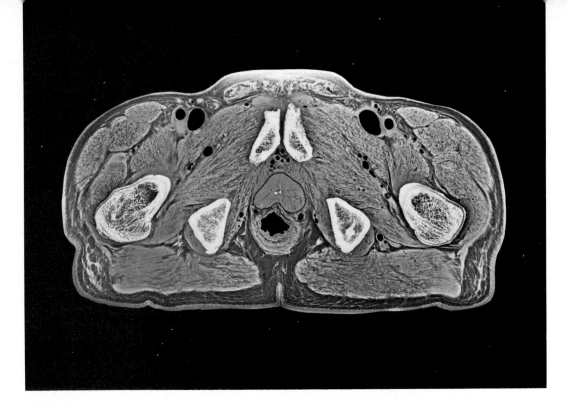

internus muscle, medially by the fascia of the levator ani and sphincter ani externus muscles, anteriorly by the posterior borders of the transverse perinei superficialis and profundus muscles, and posteriorly by the fascia over the gluteus maximus muscle and the sacrotuberous ligament. The fossa contains a great amount of lobulated fat and the inferior rectal vessels and nerves.

Clinical Considerations

The ischiorectal fossae communicate with each other behind the anus; therefore, infection in one fossa can readily pass to the other. Infections of the anal canal and the perianal sweat glands spread easily to the ischiorectal fossa.

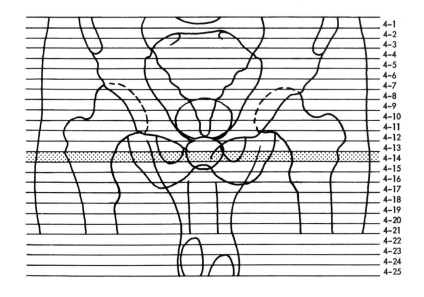

SECTION
4-14

Through the inferior ramus of the pubis

Anatomic Considerations

Alcock's canal is located in the lateral wall of the ischiorectal fossa. The canal is formed by a splitting of the fascia of the obturator internus muscle and contains the internal pudendal vessels and nerve. The inferior rectal vessels and nerve arise within the canal.

The ischiorectal fossa is bounded laterally by the fascia of the obturator

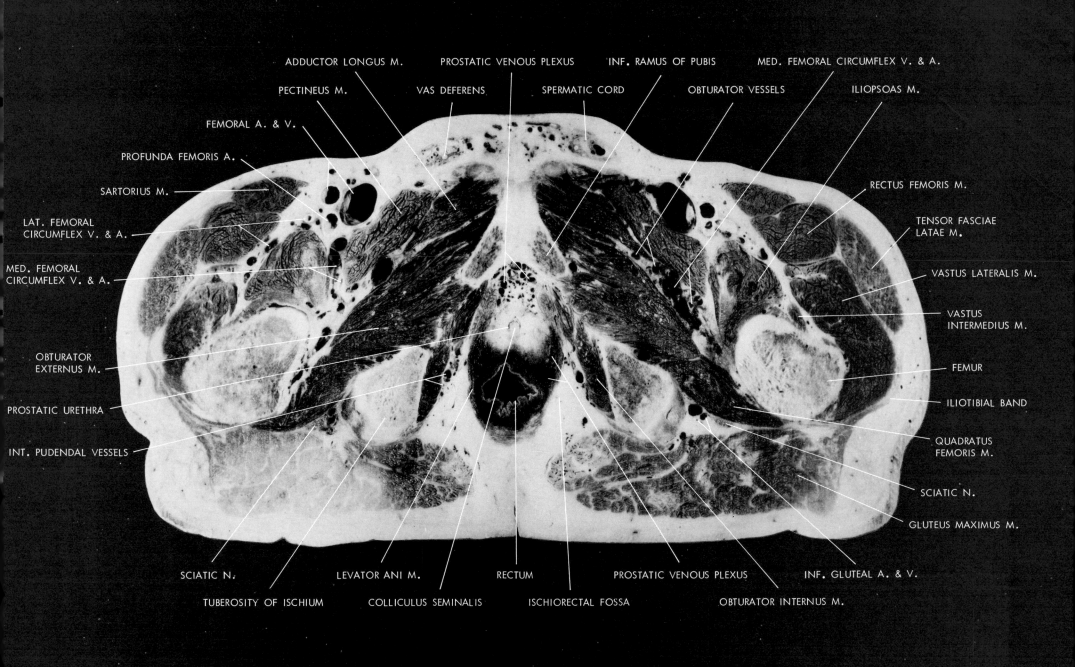

ADDUCTOR LONGUS M.

PROSTATIC VENOUS PLEXUS

INF. RAMUS OF PUBIS

MED. FEMORAL CIRCUMFLEX V. & A.

PECTINEUS M.

VAS DEFERENS

SPERMATIC CORD

OBTURATOR VESSELS

ILIOPSOAS M.

FEMORAL A. & V.

PROFUNDA FEMORIS A.

RECTUS FEMORIS M.

SARTORIUS M.

TENSOR FASCIAE LATAE M.

LAT. FEMORAL CIRCUMFLEX V. & A.

VASTUS LATERALIS M.

MED. FEMORAL CIRCUMFLEX V. & A.

VASTUS INTERMEDIUS M.

OBTURATOR EXTERNUS M.

FEMUR

PROSTATIC URETHRA

ILIOTIBIAL BAND

INT. PUDENDAL VESSELS

QUADRATUS FEMORIS M.

SCIATIC N.

GLUTEUS MAXIMUS M.

SCIATIC N.

LEVATOR ANI M.

RECTUM

PROSTATIC VENOUS PLEXUS

INF. GLUTEAL A. & V.

TUBEROSITY OF ISCHIUM

COLLICULUS SEMINALIS

ISCHIORECTAL FOSSA

OBTURATOR INTERNUS M.

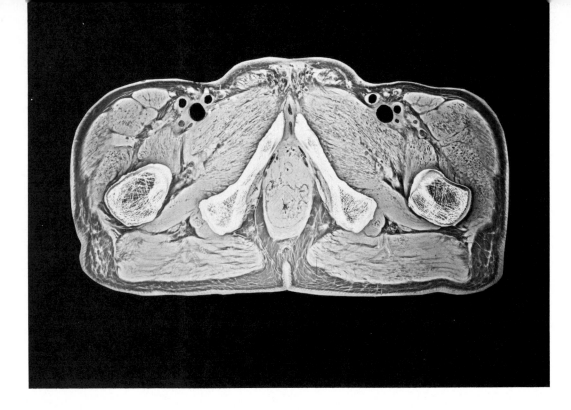

The deep pouch is found between the two layers of the urogenital diaphragm, which is located between the rami of the pubis and ischium of the two sides. In addition to the structures mentioned previously, the deep pouch contains the deep transverse perinei muscles, branches of the pudendal nerve, internal pudendal vessels, and Cowper's glands. The homologous glands in the female (greater vestibular or Bartholin's glands) are found in the superficial pouch.

Clinical Considerations

Here the triangular relationship of the pubis anteriorly, the tuberosity of the ischium posteriorly, and the anal canal between the two ischial tuberosities is well demonstrated for localization purposes in computed tomography.

A superficial inguinal lymph node is pointed out. These lymph nodes are so variable in size in the groin region that they cannot take on serious significance in most lymphangiography for staging or diagnosis of malignancy. On the other hand, more cephalad in the pelvis, lymphangiography is increasingly important in the diagnosis of many of the malignant lymphomas or metastases from testicular tumors. In such cases, size is perhaps of lesser importance than architecture and filling defects from metastases contained within the lymph node.

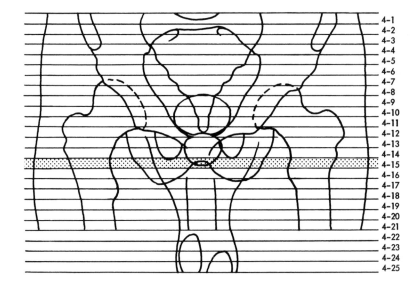

SECTION
4–15

Through the tuberosity of the ischium

Anatomic Considerations

The muscles present in the lesser pelvis are the obturator internus, piriformis, levator ani, and coccygeus. The first two muscles form part of the lateral wall of the pelvis; the last two form the pelvic diaphragm, which closes the pelvic outlet. The piriformis and obturator muscles pass out of the pelvis through the greater and lesser sciatic foramina, respectively, into the gluteal area. The obturator internus forms the lateral wall of the ischiorectal fossa. The coccygeus is a small muscle that forms the most posterior part of the pelvic diaphragm. Because the levator ani forms most of the pelvic diaphragm, it is responsible for the support of the pelvic viscera. It is divided into two major components, the pubococcygeus and the iliococcygeus. The portion of the pubococcygeus associated with the prostate is called the levator prostatae, and the portion that is associated with the rectum is called the puborectalis muscle. The pelvic diaphragm can be observed from Sections 4–10 to 4–15.

In this section some of the contents of the deep pouch of the perineum, such as the membranous urethra and sphincter urethrae muscle, can be observed.

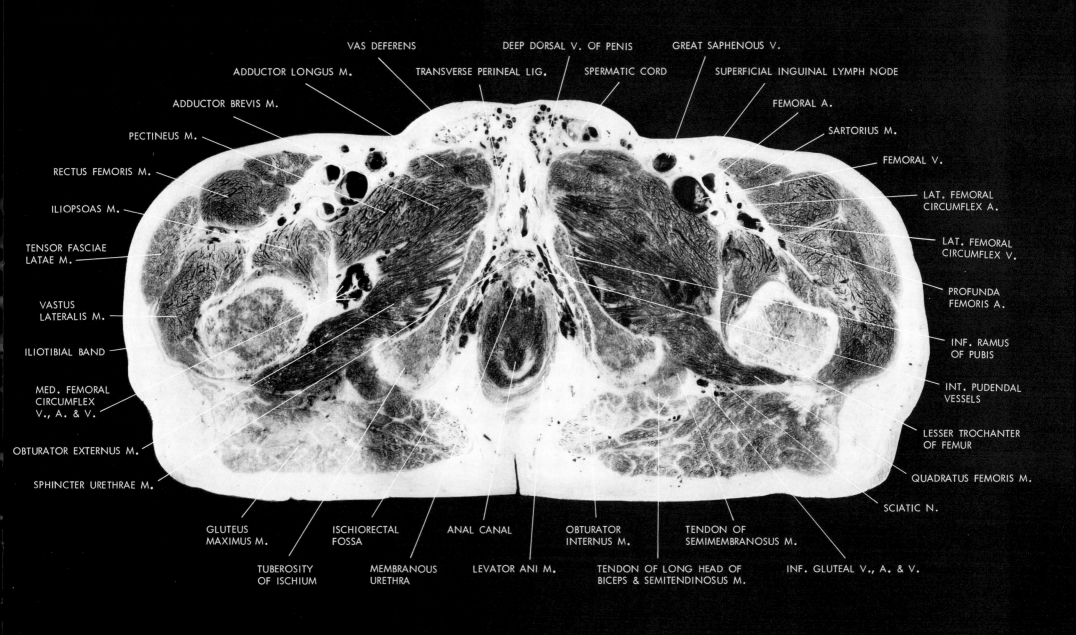

VAS DEFERENS

DEEP DORSAL V. OF PENIS

GREAT SAPHENOUS V.

ADDUCTOR LONGUS M.

TRANSVERSE PERINEAL LIG.

SPERMATIC CORD

SUPERFICIAL INGUINAL LYMPH NODE

ADDUCTOR BREVIS M.

FEMORAL A.

PECTINEUS M.

SARTORIUS M.

RECTUS FEMORIS M.

FEMORAL V.

ILIOPSOAS M.

LAT. FEMORAL
CIRCUMFLEX A.

TENSOR FASCIAE
LATAE M.

LAT. FEMORAL
CIRCUMFLEX V.

VASTUS
LATERALIS M.

PROFUNDA
FEMORIS A.

ILIOTIBIAL BAND

INF. RAMUS
OF PUBIS

MED. FEMORAL
CIRCUMFLEX
V., A. & V.

INT. PUDENDAL
VESSELS

OBTURATOR EXTERNUS M.

LESSER TROCHANTER
OF FEMUR

SPHINCTER URETHRAE M.

QUADRATUS FEMORIS M.

SCIATIC N.

GLUTEUS
MAXIMUS M.

ISCHIORECTAL
FOSSA

ANAL CANAL

OBTURATOR
INTERNUS M.

TENDON OF
SEMIMEMBRANOSUS M.

TUBEROSITY
OF ISCHIUM

MEMBRANOUS
URETHRA

LEVATOR ANI M.

TENDON OF LONG HEAD OF
BICEPS & SEMITENDINOSUS M.

INF. GLUTEAL V., A. & V.

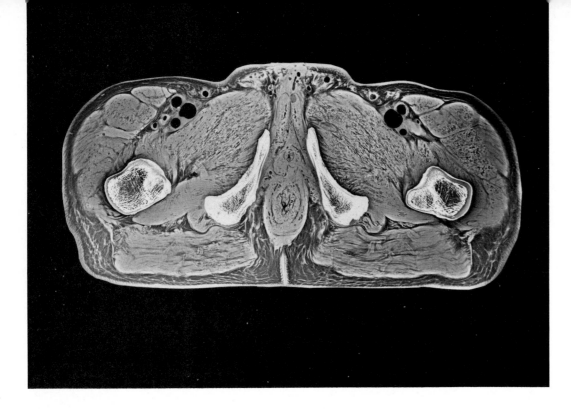

deep dorsal vein of the penis in retrograde fashion that originally demonstrated the continuity, without intervening valves, between this structure and the deep pelvic veins going posteriorly to the region of the sacrum and greater sciatic notch and thereafter cephalad along the perivertebral plexus to the base of the skull. This relationship was extremely well dissected and demonstrated by Batson in his important revelation of the continuity of venous structures from the deep dorsal vein of the penis, on the one hand, to the deep veins of the pelvis, lumbar spine, and even skull, on the other. He postulated quite correctly that this was a frequent route for the metastasis of prostate malignancies.

A continuation of the musculature and the perivascular fascial planes, perhaps better demonstrated by xeroradiography, forms the so-called capsular visualization surrounding the hip joints. Actually, this so-called capsule is not indeed the joint capsule but really the equivalent thereof as delineated by these muscle fascial planes and their attachments.

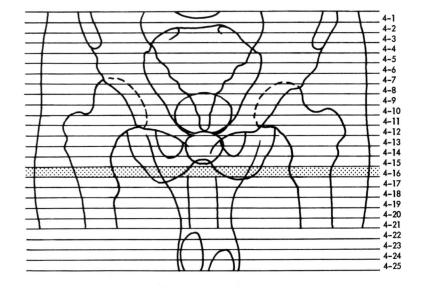

SECTION
4–16

Through the tuberosity of the ischium, 1 cm below the preceding section

Anatomic Considerations

The superficial pouch of the perineum is bounded superiorly by the perineal membrane (inferior fascial layer of the urogenital diaphragm) and inferiorly by Colles' fascia. This and adjacent illustrations show some of the contents of the superficial pouch. In the male, it contains the crura and bulb of the penis; the ischiocavernosus, bulbocavernosus, and superficial transverse perineus muscles; the posterior scrotal branches of the perineal artery; and the medial and lateral posterior scrotal nerves.

Clinical Considerations

In this section, the deep dorsal vein of the penis, far anteriorly situated, and its relationship to the crus of the penis are clearly seen. It was the injection of the

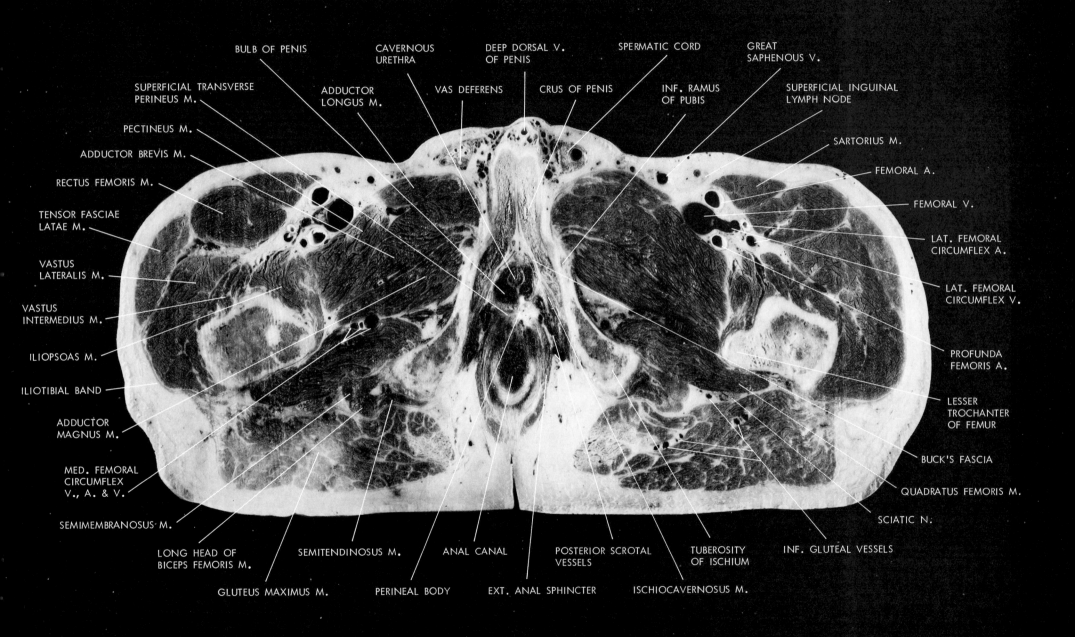

BULB OF PENIS

CAVERNOUS
URETHRA

DEEP DORSAL V.
OF PENIS

SPERMATIC CORD

GREAT
SAPHENOUS V.

SUPERFICIAL TRANSVERSE
PERINEUS M.

ADDUCTOR
LONGUS M.

VAS DEFERENS

CRUS OF PENIS

INF. RAMUS
OF PUBIS

SUPERFICIAL INGUINAL
LYMPH NODE

PECTINEUS M.

SARTORIUS M.

ADDUCTOR BREVIS M.

FEMORAL A.

RECTUS FEMORIS M.

FEMORAL V.

TENSOR FASCIAE
LATAE M.

LAT. FEMORAL
CIRCUMFLEX A.

VASTUS
LATERALIS M.

LAT. FEMORAL
CIRCUMFLEX V.

VASTUS
INTERMEDIUS M.

ILIOPSOAS M.

PROFUNDA
FEMORIS A.

ILIOTIBIAL BAND

LESSER
TROCHANTER
OF FEMUR

ADDUCTOR
MAGNUS M.

BUCK'S FASCIA

MED. FEMORAL
CIRCUMFLEX
V., A. & V.

QUADRATUS FEMORIS M.

SCIATIC N.

SEMIMEMBRANOSUS M.

LONG HEAD OF
BICEPS FEMORIS M.

SEMITENDINOSUS M.

ANAL CANAL

POSTERIOR SCROTAL
VESSELS

TUBEROSITY
OF ISCHIUM

INF. GLUTEAL VESSELS

GLUTEUS MAXIMUS M.

PERINEAL BODY

EXT. ANAL SPHINCTER

ISCHIOCAVERNOSUS M.

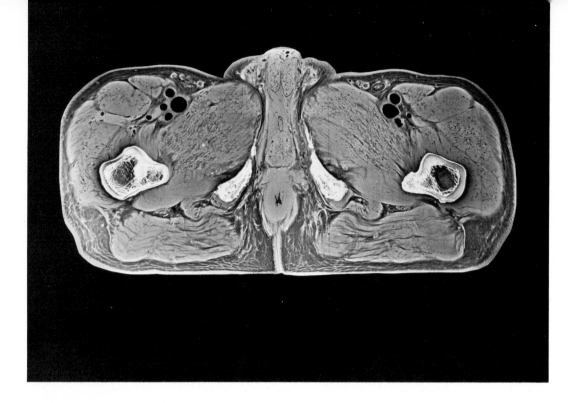

The blood supply is derived from the middle and inferior rectal arteries. The venous return is by the portal and systemic circulation.

Clinical Considerations

The midline relationships of the corpora cavernosa, cavernous urethra, gracilis muscle, bulbocavernosus muscle, superficial transverse perineus muscle, and anal canal should be carefully studied and delineated in this section. They form a separate column by a thick fascial plane separable from muscles that will take part extensively in more distal portions of the body, especially the thigh.

The pampiniform plexus of vessels in their close relationship to the corpora cavernosa vessels likewise should be carefully delineated, particularly since these structures may be visualized by contrast enhancement during computed axial tomography.

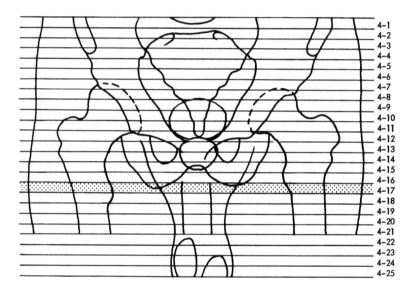

SECTION
4–17

Through the lesser trochanter of the femur

Anatomic Considerations

The anal canal is seen in Sections 4–15 to 4–18. It is the terminal portion of the large intestine and begins at the level of the apex of the prostate and ends at the anus. The length varies from 2.5 to 4 cm. The anal canal has no peritoneal covering but is surrounded by the sphincter ani internus muscle and supported by the levator ani and sphincter ani externus muscles.

Posterior to it is the anococcygeal body; anterior to it, but separated by the perineal body, are the membranous portions of the urethra, the bulb of the penis, and the transverse perineal muscles. The upper half of the anal canal is related on each side to the levator ani, and the lower part to the ischiorectal fossa.

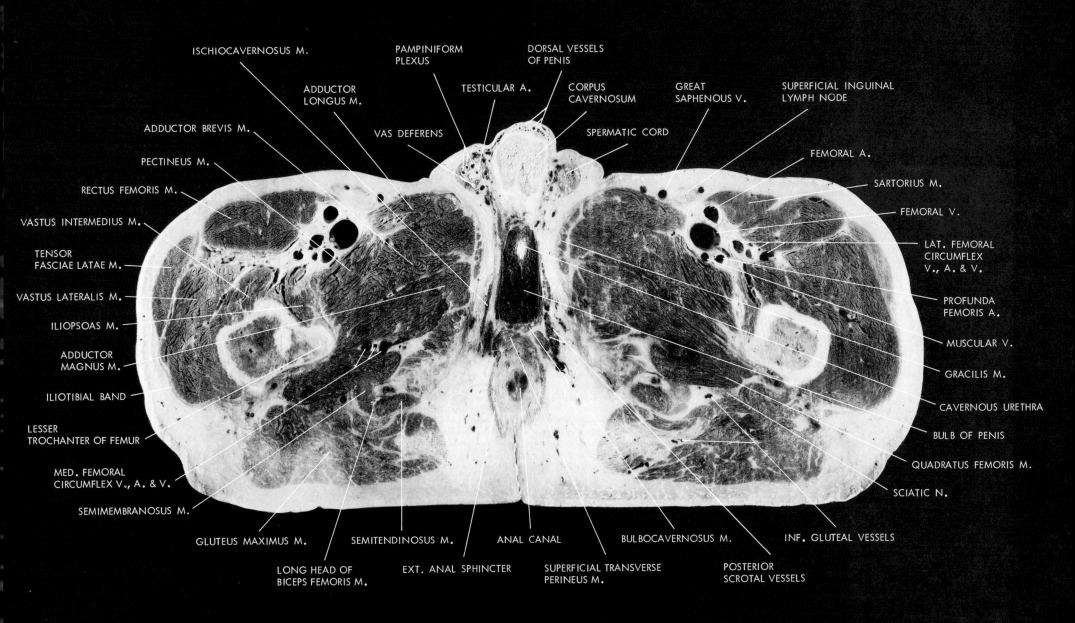

ISCHIOCAVERNOSUS M.

PAMPINIFORM PLEXUS

DORSAL VESSELS OF PENIS

ADDUCTOR LONGUS M.

TESTICULAR A.

CORPUS CAVERNOSUM

GREAT SAPHENOUS V.

SUPERFICIAL INGUINAL LYMPH NODE

ADDUCTOR BREVIS M.

VAS DEFERENS

SPERMATIC CORD

PECTINEUS M.

FEMORAL A.

RECTUS FEMORIS M.

SARTORIUS M.

VASTUS INTERMEDIUS M.

FEMORAL V.

TENSOR FASCIAE LATAE M.

LAT. FEMORAL CIRCUMFLEX V., A. & V.

VASTUS LATERALIS M.

PROFUNDA FEMORIS A.

ILIOPSOAS M.

MUSCULAR V.

ADDUCTOR MAGNUS M.

GRACILIS M.

ILIOTIBIAL BAND

CAVERNOUS URETHRA

LESSER TROCHANTER OF FEMUR

BULB OF PENIS

MED. FEMORAL CIRCUMFLEX V., A. & V.

QUADRATUS FEMORIS M.

SEMIMEMBRANOSUS M.

SCIATIC N.

GLUTEUS MAXIMUS M.

SEMITENDINOSUS M.

ANAL CANAL

BULBOCAVERNOSUS M.

INF. GLUTEAL VESSELS

LONG HEAD OF BICEPS FEMORIS M.

EXT. ANAL SPHINCTER

SUPERFICIAL TRANSVERSE PERINEUS M.

POSTERIOR SCROTAL VESSELS

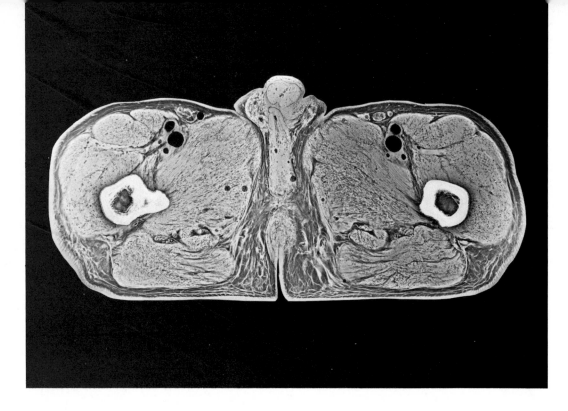

The profunda femoris artery arises from the femoral artery in the femoral triangle. Both the medial and lateral femoral circumflex arteries originate from either the femoral or profunda femoris in the femoral triangle. In this specimen, the medial femoral circumflex arises from the femoral (Section 4-13), and the lateral femoral circumflex stems from the profunda femoris at its origin (Section 4-14).

Clinical Considerations

Note the more anterior relationship of the femoral artery in respect to the femoral vein. In performance of direct needle puncture, prior to catheterization in the Seldinger technique, the needle initially penetrates both walls of the femoral artery and sometimes even both walls of the femoral vein. When the needle is withdrawn to the lumen of the femoral artery, the pulsatory effect of the opened needle in the artery can be recognized. Catheterization may then proceed in its appropriate sequence. It can readily be understood, however, why hemorrhage may occasionally occur as a complication of this procedure.

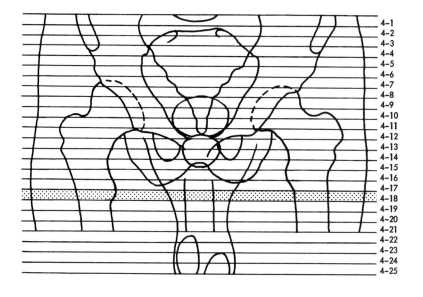

SECTION
4-18

Through the upper portion of the shaft of the femur

Anatomic Considerations

The femoral triangle is bounded by the inguinal ligament superiorly, the sartorius muscle laterally, and the lateral border of the adductor longus muscle medially. As can be seen in the illustration, the iliopsoas and pectineus muscles form the floor of this triangle. The femoral triangle contains the femoral artery, vein, and some of their branches and lymphatics. The femoral nerve is not actually in the triangle *per se*, since it lies deep to the fascia covering the iliopsoas muscle. The relationships of these structures to each other are constant. At the base of the triangle (Section 4-10), the femoral artery lies between the femoral nerve, which is lateral, and the femoral vein, which is medial; the lymphatics lie medial to the femoral vein. As the femoral vessels descend in the femoral triangle, their relationship to each other changes. As can be seen in this section, the femoral artery lies anterior to the vein.

MALE PELVIS AND PERINEUM

198

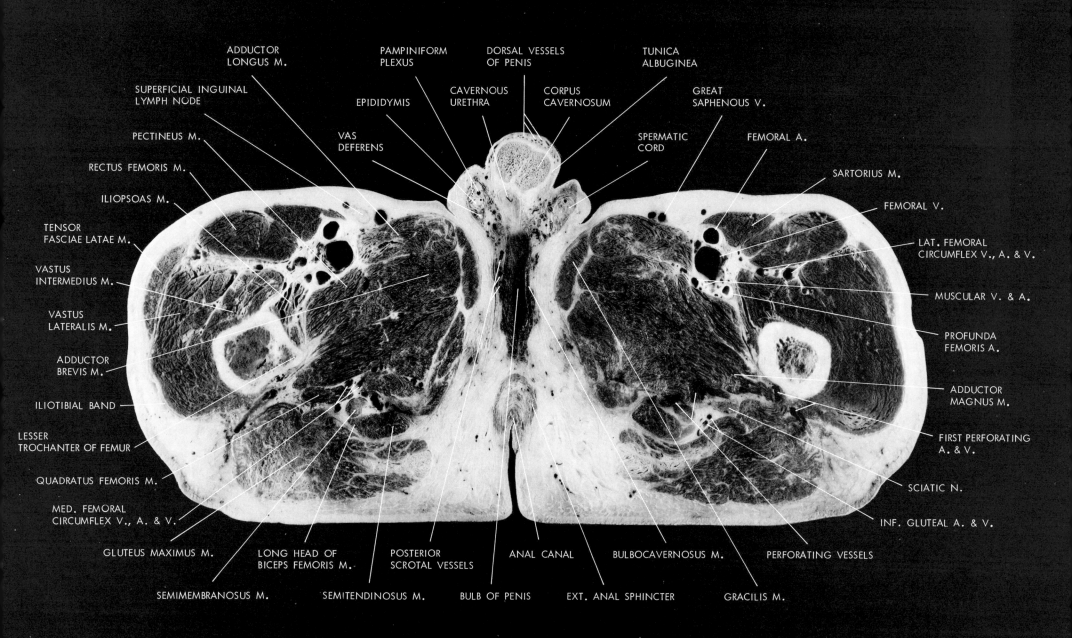

ADDUCTOR LONGUS M.

PAMPINIFORM PLEXUS

DORSAL VESSELS OF PENIS

TUNICA ALBUGINEA

SUPERFICIAL INGUINAL LYMPH NODE

EPIDIDYMIS

CAVERNOUS URETHRA

CORPUS CAVERNOSUM

GREAT SAPHENOUS V.

PECTINEUS M.

VAS DEFERENS

SPERMATIC CORD

FEMORAL A.

RECTUS FEMORIS M.

SARTORIUS M.

ILIOPSOAS M.

FEMORAL V.

TENSOR FASCIAE LATAE M.

LAT. FEMORAL CIRCUMFLEX V., A. & V.

VASTUS INTERMEDIUS M.

MUSCULAR V. & A.

VASTUS LATERALIS M.

PROFUNDA FEMORIS A.

ADDUCTOR BREVIS M.

ADDUCTOR MAGNUS M.

ILIOTIBIAL BAND

LESSER TROCHANTER OF FEMUR

FIRST PERFORATING A. & V.

QUADRATUS FEMORIS M.

SCIATIC N.

MED. FEMORAL CIRCUMFLEX V., A. & V.

INF. GLUTEAL A. & V.

GLUTEUS MAXIMUS M.

LONG HEAD OF BICEPS FEMORIS M.

POSTERIOR SCROTAL VESSELS

ANAL CANAL

BULBOCAVERNOSUS M.

PERFORATING VESSELS

SEMIMEMBRANOSUS M.

SEMITENDINOSUS M.

BULB OF PENIS

EXT. ANAL SPHINCTER

GRACILIS M.

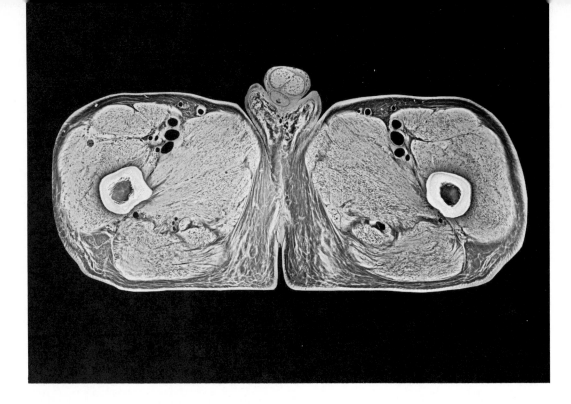

tered smooth muscle fibers. The dartos tunic is continuous with Colles' fascia in the perineum and with Scarpa's fascia on the anterior abdominal wall.

Clinical Considerations

In this section it will be noted that the base of the penis and the scrotum are in themselves beginning to be defined and that the relationships of the vascular structures of the penis and the tributaries of the pampiniform plexus can readily be described.

Likewise, the relationships of the femoral artery and vein, and the profunda femoris vein and artery are more clearly defined in their direct ventrodorsal relationship.

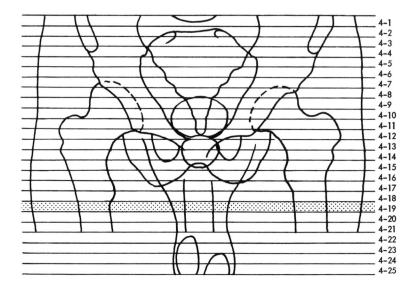

SECTION
4–19

Through the shaft of the femur, 1 cm below the preceding section

Anatomic Considerations

The scrotum can be seen in this photograph and in the following six illustrations. The scrotum is the cutaneous sac that contains the testes, epididymis, and parts of the spermatic cords. It is divided into two lateral parts by a median raphe that is continuous anteriorly on the penis and posteriorly to the anus. The scrotum is composed of two layers: the skin, which is thin and pigmented, and the dartos tunic, which is superficial fascia containing scat-

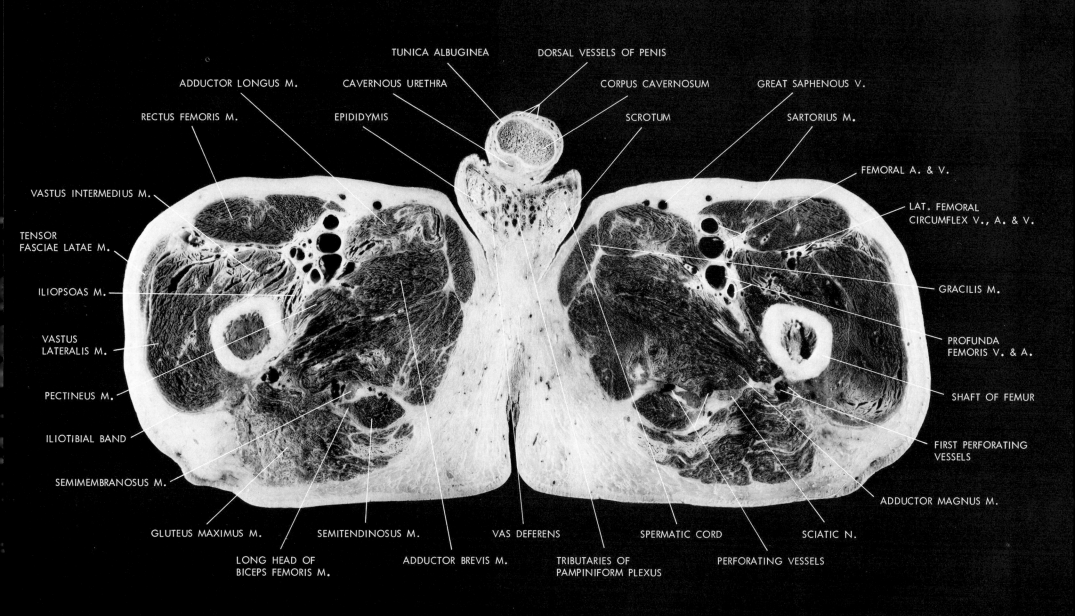

TUNICA ALBUGINEA

DORSAL VESSELS OF PENIS

ADDUCTOR LONGUS M.

CAVERNOUS URETHRA

CORPUS CAVERNOSUM

GREAT SAPHENOUS V.

RECTUS FEMORIS M.

EPIDIDYMIS

SCROTUM

SARTORIUS M.

FEMORAL A. & V.

VASTUS INTERMEDIUS M.

LAT. FEMORAL CIRCUMFLEX V., A. & V.

TENSOR FASCIAE LATAE M.

ILIOPSOAS M.

GRACILIS M.

VASTUS LATERALIS M.

PROFUNDA FEMORIS V. & A.

PECTINEUS M.

SHAFT OF FEMUR

ILIOTIBIAL BAND

FIRST PERFORATING VESSELS

SEMIMEMBRANOSUS M.

ADDUCTOR MAGNUS M.

GLUTEUS MAXIMUS M.

SEMITENDINOSUS M.

VAS DEFERENS

SPERMATIC CORD

SCIATIC N.

LONG HEAD OF BICEPS FEMORIS M.

ADDUCTOR BREVIS M.

TRIBUTARIES OF PAMPINIFORM PLEXUS

PERFORATING VESSELS

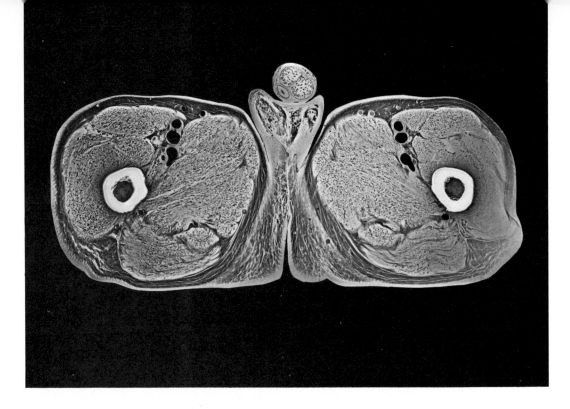

artery pierces the fibrous capsule of the penis, especially toward the distal end of the organ. The venous drainage of the penis is to the prostatic plexus of veins via the deep dorsal vein of the penis and to the external pudendal vein *via* the superficial dorsal vein of the penis.

Clinical Considerations

In this section, apart from the anatomic considerations described in respect to the penis and scrotum, note the compartmental relationships of the muscular groups surrounding the femur. The large vascular structures of the femoral artery and vein and the profunda femoris vein and artery form a band extending down to the medial aspect of the shaft of the femur, separating the more lateral group of muscles from those that are medial. The band of vasculature can be intensified by contrast enhancement techniques in computed axial tomography.

It is interesting at this point to relate that in patients with renal insufficiency, there is bone resorption at the points of adductor insertion of the various muscles throughout the body. This pertains not only to the thigh but also to the humerus and the hands. Just why this should be so is not clear.

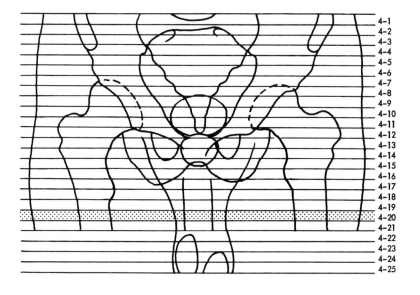

SECTION
4–20

Through the shaft of the femur, 1 cm below the preceding section

Anatomic Considerations

The penis, which can be seen in this and adjacent sections, is composed of three fibroelastic cylinders: the right and left corpora cavernosa and the corpus spongiosum. The corpora cavernosa fuse with each other in the median plane except posteriorly, where as the crura, they separate to attach to the pubic arch. As can be seen in the sections, the urethra traverses the corpus spongiosum. The proximal swollen portion of the corpus spongiosum is the bulb of the penis; the distal swollen portion is the glans penis. The deep fascia of the penis (Buck's fascia) invests the penile shaft, crura, and bulb. This fascia attaches with the crura and bulb to the ischiopubic rami and superficial layer of the urogenital diaphragm.

Blood is supplied to the penis by the terminal branches of the internal pudendal artery: the deep and dorsal arteries of the penis. The deep artery of the penis exits the deep pouch of the perineum by piercing the perineal membrane and enters the crus of the penis in the superficial pouch. The dorsal

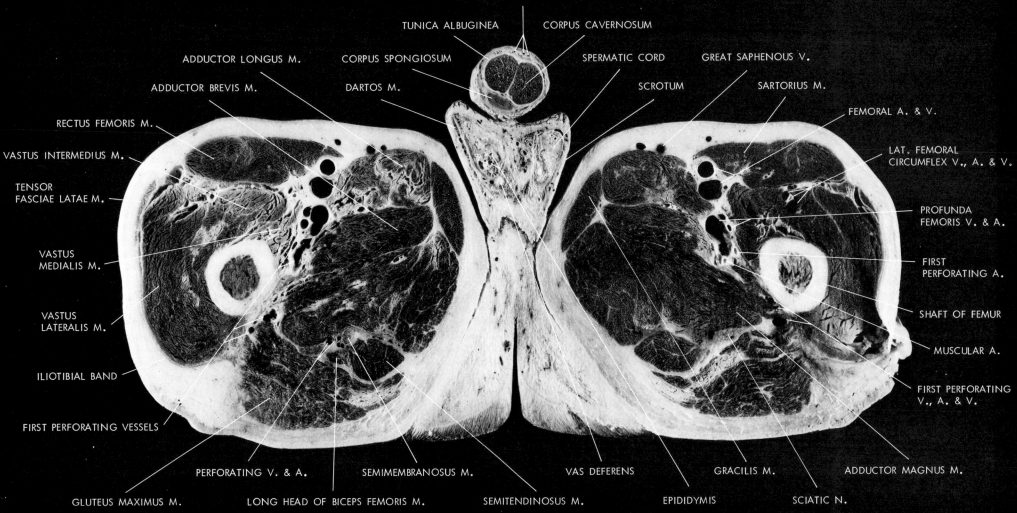

DORSAL VESSELS OF PENIS

TUNICA ALBUGINEA   CORPUS CAVERNOSUM

ADDUCTOR LONGUS M.   CORPUS SPONGIOSUM   SPERMATIC CORD   GREAT SAPHENOUS V.

ADDUCTOR BREVIS M.   DARTOS M.   SCROTUM   SARTORIUS M.

RECTUS FEMORIS M.   FEMORAL A. & V.

VASTUS INTERMEDIUS M.   LAT. FEMORAL
                                                                              CIRCUMFLEX V., A. & V.

TENSOR
FASCIAE LATAE M.   PROFUNDA
                                                                              FEMORIS V. & A.

VASTUS
MEDIALIS M.   FIRST
                                                                              PERFORATING A.

VASTUS
LATERALIS M.   SHAFT OF FEMUR

                                                                              MUSCULAR A.

ILIOTIBIAL BAND   FIRST PERFORATING
                                                                              V., A. & V.

FIRST PERFORATING VESSELS

PERFORATING V. & A.   SEMIMEMBRANOSUS M.   VAS DEFERENS   GRACILIS M.   ADDUCTOR MAGNUS M.

GLUTEUS MAXIMUS M.   LONG HEAD OF BICEPS FEMORIS M.   SEMITENDINOSUS M.   EPIDIDYMIS   SCIATIC N.

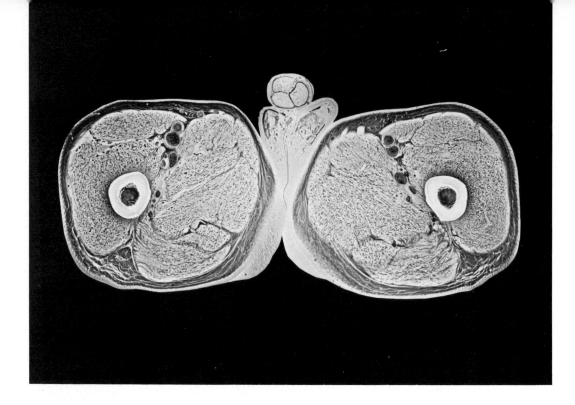

Clinical Considerations

In this section the scrotal contents and the compartments of the penis also can be identified. At times, clinically, it becomes important to identify the entire contents of the scrotum, especially when the vital structures contained therein may be surrounded by either fluid-containing mass structures or solid tumors, especially those pertaining to one of the testes. Such fluid- and solid-containing masses are readily palpable clinically, but their points of origin are not readily discerned at times. Secondary ionizing radiation should be carefully considered prior to computed axial tomography of this area; at times, the benefits to be obtained for the patient far outweigh the relatively minimal effects of the radiation under these circumstances.

SECTION 4-21

Through the shaft of the femur, 1 cm below the preceding section

Anatomic Considerations

The epididymis is an elongated structure on the lateral part of the posterior border of the testis. The upper end is called the head, which is connected to the testis by the efferent ducts. The body and tail are connected to the gland only by connective tissue. The efferent ducts unite to form the canal of the epididymis, which is highly coiled and emerges from the tail as the vas deferens.

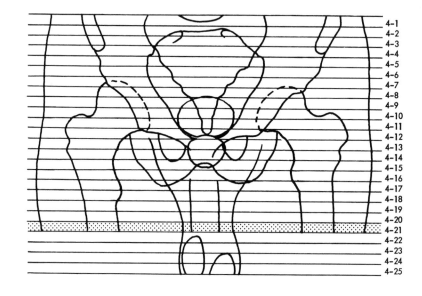

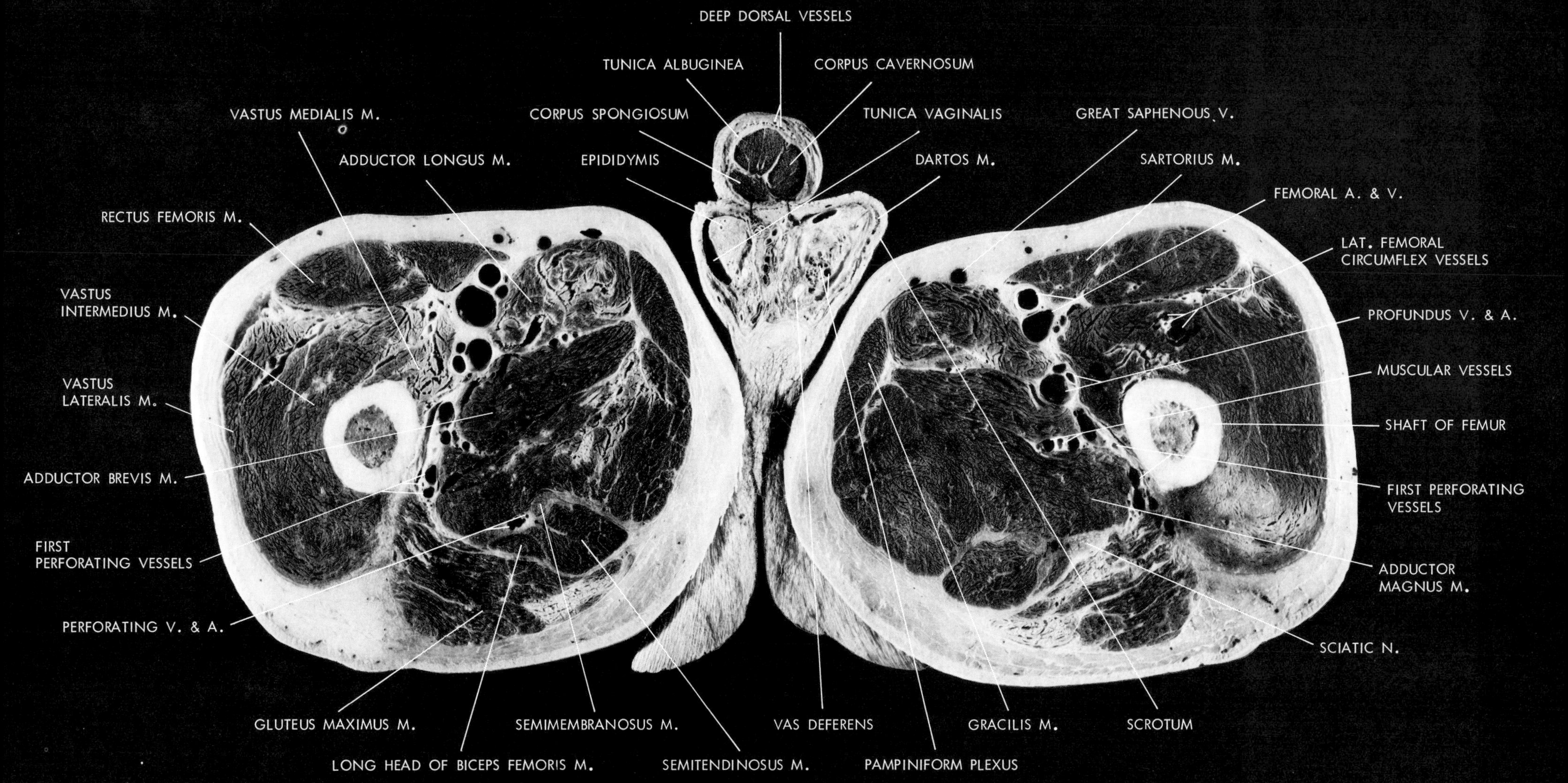

DEEP DORSAL VESSELS

TUNICA ALBUGINEA

CORPUS CAVERNOSUM

VASTUS MEDIALIS M.

CORPUS SPONGIOSUM

TUNICA VAGINALIS

GREAT SAPHENOUS V.

ADDUCTOR LONGUS M.

EPIDIDYMIS

DARTOS M.

SARTORIUS M.

RECTUS FEMORIS M.

FEMORAL A. & V.

LAT. FEMORAL
CIRCUMFLEX VESSELS

VASTUS
INTERMEDIUS M.

PROFUNDUS V. & A.

MUSCULAR VESSELS

VASTUS
LATERALIS M.

SHAFT OF FEMUR

ADDUCTOR BREVIS M.

FIRST PERFORATING
VESSELS

FIRST
PERFORATING VESSELS

ADDUCTOR
MAGNUS M.

PERFORATING V. & A.

SCIATIC N.

GLUTEUS MAXIMUS M.

SEMIMEMBRANOSUS M.

VAS DEFERENS

GRACILIS M.

SCROTUM

LONG HEAD OF BICEPS FEMORIS M.

SEMITENDINOSUS M.

PAMPINIFORM PLEXUS

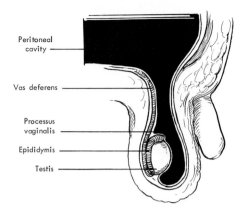

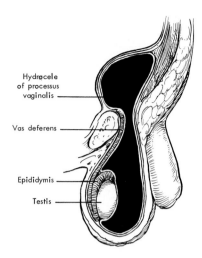

Peritoneal cavity

Vas deferens

Processus vaginalis

Epididymis

Testis

Hydrocele of processus vaginalis

Vas deferens

Epididymis

Testis

A. Relation of the testis to the processus vaginalis prior to its closure from the peritoneal cavity.

B. A congenital hydrocele. The processus vaginalis has sealed off at its proximal end from the peritoneal cavity.

SECTIONS
4–22 to 4–25

Through the scrotum, 1 cm apart

Anatomic Considerations

The testes are paired structures suspended in the scrotum by the spermatic cords. The left testis lies at a lower level than does the right. The superior and posterolateral surfaces of the testis are related to the epididymis. The testis is covered by a capsule of dense fibrous tissue, the tunica albuginea. Septa pass into the testis from this capsule and divide it into lobes that contain the seminiferous tubules. The seminiferous tubules communicate with the head of the epididymis by a series of tubules — straight tubules, rete testis, and efferent ducts.

The testis contains additional coverings external to the tunica albuginea. From external to internal they are the external spermatic fascia, which is a continuation of the external oblique muscle; the cremasteric muscle and the fascia that is derived from the internal oblique muscle; the internal spermatic fascia, which is a continuation of the transversalis fascia; and the tunica vaginalis, derived from the peritoneum (processus vaginalis). The tunica vaginalis is a serous sac that consists of visceral and parietal layers. The visceral layer covers the front and sides of the testis and epididymis and is continuous with the parietal layer near the posterior border of the testis. The parietal layer lines a portion of the internal spermatic fascia. As can be seen from the illustrations, the tunica vaginalis does not completely surround the testis and epididymis. Normally, only a small amount of fluid occupies the space between the visceral and parietal layers; in this specimen the space is enlarged because of the accumulation of fluid.

The testicular arteries arise from the abdominal aorta. Veins from the testis and epididymis form the pampiniform plexus, which drains on the left into the renal vein and on the right into the inferior vena cava. The lymphatic drainage of the testes is to nodes along the abdominal aorta near the kidneys; the scrotum drains into the superficial inguinal lymph nodes.

Clinical Considerations

In these sections, the testis is for the most part separable from the epididymis by a scrotal septum. This separation is of clinical significance in defining

lesions of the testes, as contrasted with those that concern primarily the pathology of the epididymis. Benign tumors of the testis are rare. Malignant tumors are much more frequent, though fortunately not common. They are divided into three main groups: (1) the seminoma, which has a relatively good prognosis; (2) the embryonal carcinoma; and (3) the teratoma, which is of intermediate malignancy. The majority of malignant testicular tumors do not secrete hormones, but such secretion may occur with embryonic carcinoma, in which gonadotropins may be demonstrated as being similar to those secreted in the urine by women with a chorionepithelioma of the placenta. (A fourth category of testicular tumor is the "mixed type.")

Among the other abnormalities that could be detected with sections of the scrotum are (1) a hydrocele, which is a circumscribed collection of fluid found especially in the tunica vaginalis of the testicle; (2) a congenital hydrocele in the unobliterated canal between the peritoneal cavity and that of the tunica vaginalis; (3) a diffused hydrocele, which is a collection of fluid diffused in the loose connective tissue of the spermatic cord; (4) a Dupuytren's hydrocele, which is a bilocular hydrocele of the tunica vaginalis testis; (5) an encysted hydrocele, which occurs in cysts outside the cavity of the tunica vaginalis testis; (6) a funicular hydrocele, which is a hydrocele of the tunica vaginalis of the spermatic cord in a space closed toward the testes and open toward the peritoneal cavity; (7) a Gibbon's hydrocele, which is a hydrocele associated with a large hernia; (8) a hernial hydrocele, which is a distention of a hernia sac with a fluid in the scrotum; and (9) a scrotal hydrocele, which is a circumscribed collection of fluid in the scrotum itself.

The general anatomy in longitudinal section of a hydrocele as related to the peritoneal pouch on the one hand and the spermatic cord and testicle on the other is indicated by diagram.

Occasionally, inflammation of both the epididymis and the testes occurs simultaneously, in which case the condition is called epididymo-orchitis.

One of the common inflammations of the epididymis is tuberculosis, which must not be confused with a testicular tumor.

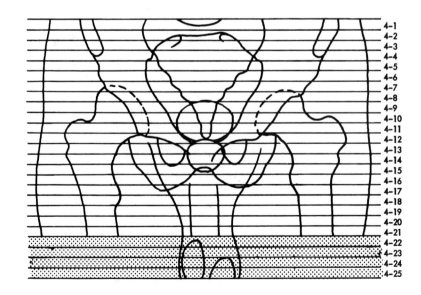

4–1
4–2
4–3
4–4
4–5
4–6
4–7
4–8
4–9
4–10
4–11
4–12
4–13
4–14
4–15
4–16
4–17
4–18
4–19
4–20
4–21
4–22
4–23
4–24
4–25

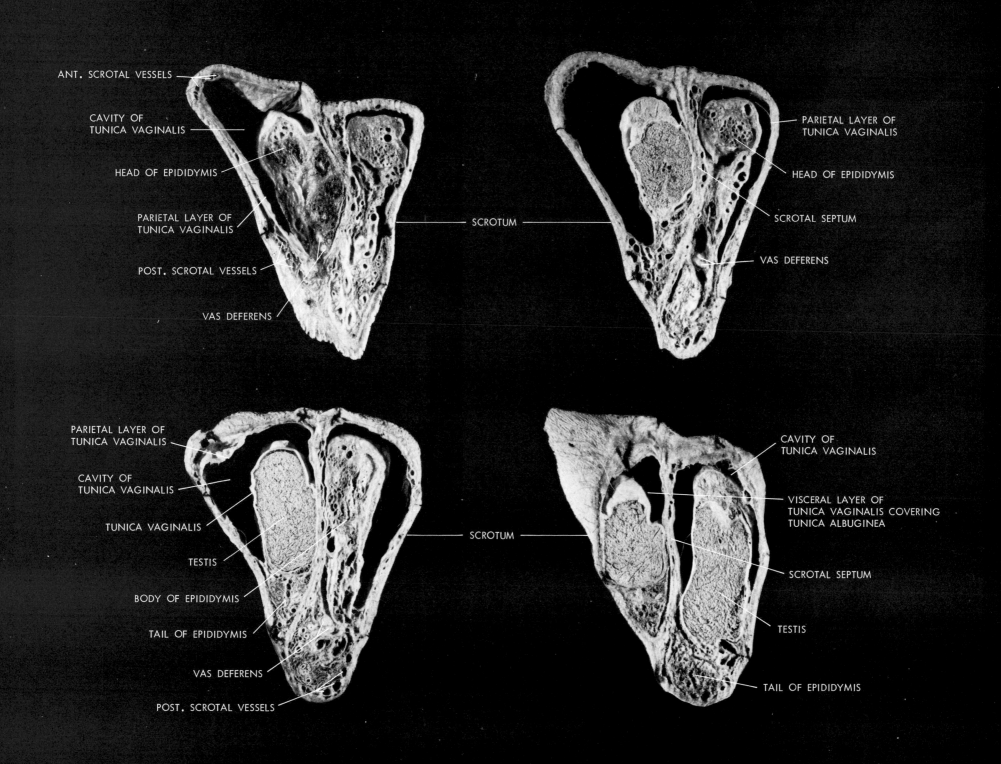

ANT. SCROTAL VESSELS

CAVITY OF
TUNICA VAGINALIS

HEAD OF EPIDIDYMIS

PARIETAL LAYER OF
TUNICA VAGINALIS

POST. SCROTAL VESSELS

VAS DEFERENS

PARIETAL LAYER OF
TUNICA VAGINALIS

HEAD OF EPIDIDYMIS

SCROTAL SEPTUM

VAS DEFERENS

SCROTUM

PARIETAL LAYER OF
TUNICA VAGINALIS

CAVITY OF
TUNICA VAGINALIS

TUNICA VAGINALIS

TESTIS

BODY OF EPIDIDYMIS

TAIL OF EPIDIDYMIS

VAS DEFERENS

POST. SCROTAL VESSELS

CAVITY OF
TUNICA VAGINALIS

VISCERAL LAYER OF
TUNICA VAGINALIS COVERING
TUNICA ALBUGINEA

SCROTAL SEPTUM

TESTIS

TAIL OF EPIDIDYMIS

SCROTUM

5

Female Pelvis and Perineum

The sections of this region extend from the superior pole of the ovary through the external genitalia and therefore include sections of the thigh. The sections were taken from a nulliparous female approximately 20 years of age. This specimen was selected because the relationships of the intact reproductive organs were normal.

Conventional radiography has made great advances in the clinical investigation of the female pelvis. These have been described or referenced in considerable detail by Meschan, 1975.

Imaging Applications in the Pediatric and Child-Bearing Years

ULTRASONOGRAPHY. Ultrasonography has the serious limitations of gas interference, bone rebound, and relatively low resolution. Nevertheless, this modality has been found useful for general diagnosis of masses in the pediatric patient (including differentiation of cystic from solid structures); specific evaluation of pelvic anatomy and aberrations thereof (Haller et al., 1977); diagnosis of certain endocrine disorders (Lippe and Sample, 1978); studies of ambiguous genitalia; and evaluations of children with precocious puberty or adolescents with amenorrhea, hirsutism, or virilization.

The urinary bladder is also particularly well suited to ultrasonic evaluation because it is a cystic mass directly beneath the anterior abdominal wall. In fact, in the infant, the urinary bladder is more abdominal than pelvic. The normal vesical wall produces a rather crisp echo in contrast to rather fuzzy pictures obtained when there is trabeculation or inflammation of the wall of the urinary bladder.

Because of the absence of ionizing radiation, ultrasonography is at this time considered the modality of choice for pregnant patients. Early pregnancy may be visualized by the fifth or sixth week and may be routinely seen by the seventh week. Gestational age may be determined from fairly accurate graphs by visualizing and measuring the gestational sac. The fetal heart may be recorded by the Doppler effect after the eighth week. The placenta may be visualized by the ninth or tenth week. Unfortunately the detection of the gestational sac is not a certainty after the 13th week, but then cephalometry becomes helpful in determination of fetal age. Multiple pregnancies may be detected as early as in the third month.

Later in pregnancy, the head and rump of the fetus may be observed by the 13th to 15th week. Somewhat later still, some of the internal organs of the fetus and the extremities may be visualized. Fetal crown and rump measurements allow the obstetrician to evaluate growth rate, placental function, and cephalopelvic disproportion.

Abnormalities that may be suspected in early pregnancy include threatened abortion; abnormal gestational sac; incomplete abortion (where there is no demonstrable gestational sac or fetus); missed abortion; and hydatidiform mole, which is a highly malignant tumor that may simulate a pregnancy. Ectopic pregnancy is rarely diagnosable.

The placenta is not always easy to demarcate, but hydropic degenerative changes in the placenta previa, premature separation, or implantation are usually demonstrable.

Fetal anomalies readily detected are hydramnios (an excess of amniotic fluid), hydrocephalus, or anencephaly.

Since the cavity of the uterus is seen in the puerperal period, it is possible to determine whether the cavity remains unusually large. Fibroids of the uterus are usually demonstrable, since their demarcation lines are diffuse, unlike cysts, which are more sharply defined. Degeneration within fibroids may also be diagnosed on occasion (Miyamoto, 1977).

Unfortunately, abscesses, hematoma, and necrotic tumors may overlap somewhat, and differentiation among these entities is not always feasible.

COMPUTED TOMOGRAPHY. Unfortunately, the exposure of the patient to x-radiation precludes the use of computed tomography in obstetric and often gynecologic evaluations in young individuals, except in dire circumstances.

Computed tomography of the abdomen and pelvis (Leonidas et al., 1978) in infants and children may demonstrate such tumors as the ovarian dermoid, ureteropelvic junction obstruction, and neural crest tumors. Computed tomography also offers specific and valuable information regarding both the intraperitoneal and the extraperitoneal tissues. It shows small differences in x-ray absorption and allows identification of masses in or adjacent to other structures not otherwise definable, differentiation of cystic from solid structures, and visualization of minute calcifications within masses.

Computed Tomographic Studies of the Adult Female Pelvis

Evaluation of the genital tract in adult females encompasses anomalies of the genital tract, pelvic tumors, intrauterine devices, pelvic inflammatory disease, and pregnancy. After a pelvic mass has been detected in routine examination, it should first be documented with ultrasonography. Thereafter, ovarian tumors, which are specifically difficult to palpate, may be studied by computed tomography. Pelvic calcifications are likewise well demonstrated. In the female, typical anomalies include ipsilateral agenesis of the uterine horn and duplication of the uterus, cervix, and vagina. Patients with duplicated genital tracts may have obstruction of one tract, resulting in a hydrometros or hydrocolpos. Diverticula of the urinary bladder or ureteroceles may appear as cystic masses in the pelvis also.

Lymph nodes can be visualized by both computed tomography and ultrasound, although the value of ultrasound in this application is limited. In a patient with a malignant lymphoma, the x-radiation is quite tolerable, and the presence and size of the lesion can be accurately delineated. Contrast enhancement of adjacent organs when feasible further increases the accuracy of this technology.

Ordinarily in a pelvic scan the patient is placed in the scanning gantry, and the first scan is done at the level of the pubic symphysis with sections being made either at 1.3- or 2-cm intervals, moving cephalad. Contrast in the urinary bladder as well as in the blood vessels and the gastrointestinal tract may be helpful. Glucagon may be administered to diminish bowel peristalsis, which may cause motion artifacts.

Fortunately, in computed tomography most of the organs are enhanced by the fat that surrounds them. The urethra, of course, can be further identified when a catheter is in place. The levator ani and obturator muscles and the base of the urinary bladder are all well demonstrated. The uterus is seen on cuts done 3 to 6 cm above the pubic symphysis, even though the position of the uterus is variable. The normal ovary may not be seen routinely. The rectosigmoid is present on all lower cuts, and loops of bowel are demonstrated especially well when Gastrografin has been administered. The bony structures of the acetabulum, the sacrum, and the iliac wings as well as the musculature medial to the iliac wings are all symmetrically disposed and well demonstrated. The lymph nodes may be difficult to detect unless they are enlarged, calcified, or opacified by Ethiodol.

A point to be emphasized is that clinical staging of a tumor of the urinary bladder or uterus has always offered a distinct problem when exquisite accuracy is desired. Cystoscopy, by its direct visualization of the mucosa of the urinary bladder, can adequately delineate the intraluminal tumor, but the extension beyond the bladder wall has been difficult to detect. Computed tomography can be used to follow the effect of radiation therapy in bladder carcinoma.

The uterus has a range of normal sizes, depending upon the age of the patient. Unfortunately, there are no good guidelines to use in judging size. The uterus unaffected by malignancy is first better examined by gray scale ultrasound, but occasionally evaluation must be accomplished with CT scanning when the patient cannot distend the urinary bladder. Staging of endometrial or cervical carcinoma may be advanced significantly by demonstration of adenopathy or direct extension of the tumor beyond the confines of the uterus itself.

Occasionally, ovaries of normal size are demonstrated just lateral to the uterus by CT scanning, but they are not routinely seen. Ultrasound is probably the primary diagnostic technique used to evaluate enlargement of the ovaries (amplified by pelvic pneumography) and to distinguish between cystic and solid ovarian masses. Computed tomography can add considerable information about the distant spread of malignant ovarian tumors. It can also demonstrate the position of the ureters (enhanced with contrast agent) in relation to a complex ovarian mass. This may be particularly valuable to the surgeon who must bypass these vital structures.

CT study of orthopedic tumors of the pelvis and lower extremities is also valuable (Weis et al., 1978). Whenever a surgeon contemplates very extensive *en bloc* resection of a bony mass lesion, computed tomography offers a number of factors particularly useful in planning the surgical approach: (1) precise size of the mass; (2) location and relationship of the mass to muscle bundles and fascia; (3) marginal definition of the mass; (4) relationship to the neural and vascular structures, particularly if the vascular structures are intensified by contrast agent; and (5) relation to other bony structures as well. The complete removal of a musculoskeletal malignancy remains the basis for most curative approaches to therapy for these lesions. Prostheses have been developed for replacement of removed bony structures.

Haller JO, Schneider M, Kassner G, Staiano SJ, Noyes MB, Campos EM, and McPherson H: Ultrasonography in pediatrics, gynecology and obstetrics. AJR 128:423–429, 1977.

Leonidas JC, Carter BL, Leape LL, Ramenofsky ML, and Schwartz AM: Computed tomography in diagnosis of abdominal masses in infancy and childhood, comparison with excretory urography. Arch Dis Child 53.2:120–125, 1978.

Lippe BM and Sample WF: Pelvic ultrasonography in endocrine disorders. J Pediatr 92:897–902, 1978.

Meschan I: An Atlas of Anatomy Basic to Radiology. Philadelphia, W. B. Saunders, 1975.

Miyamoto AT: Diagnostic ultrasound in obstetrics. In Robbins, Laurence L. (editor): Golden's Diagnostic Radiology. Section 10. Obstetrical Radiology (John A. Campbell, editor). Williams and Wilkins Co., Baltimore, 1977.

Weis L, Heelan RT and Watson RC: Computed tomography of orthopedic tumors of the pelvis and lower extremities. In Urist, M. R. (editor): Clinical Orthopedics and Related Research. J. B. Lippincott Co., Philadelphia, 130:254–259, 1978.

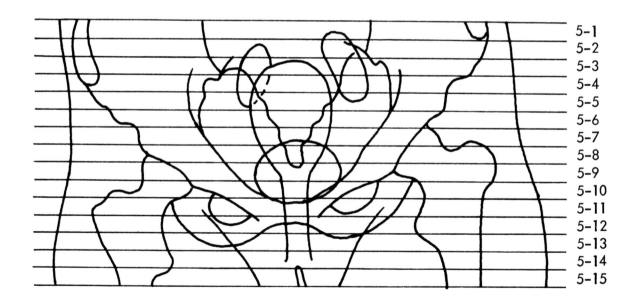

5-1
5-2
5-3
5-4
5-5
5-6
5-7
5-8
5-9
5-10
5-11
5-12
5-13
5-14
5-15

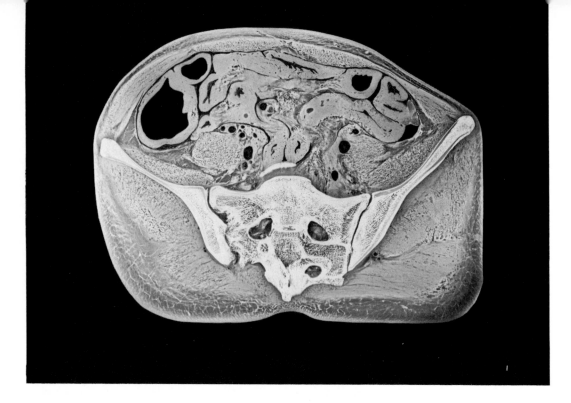

Clinical Considerations

The striking visibility of the bony structures of the pelvis with computed tomography is very important, particularly if extension of a neoplastic or inflammatory mass into the bone *per se* is suspected.

The cecum is a freely mesenterized organ and may or may not be visualized at this level, depending upon its exact location within the body. Clinically, the cecum is highly mobile and may be either hyper-rotated, nonrotated, or in a rather variable position irrespective of rotation. Visualization of the wall and lumen of the cecum is readily accomplished by conventional radiographic techniques, such as high density double contrast radiography. Occasionally, however, it might be desirable to examine a CT scan of the pericecal region, as in the event of associated inflammation from a periappendiceal abscess or perityphlitis. Such inflammations may accompany chronic granulomatous processes, especially of the tuberculosis or actinomycosis variety.

Generally, the ileum is quite well visualized by conventional radiographic techniques, particularly with the advent of enteroclysis. The introduction of barium under direct radiographic visualization gives one a very accurate concept of the mucosal pattern of the ileum, as well as the small intestinal loops proximal to this. On occasion, however, the visualization of matted lymph nodes or infiltration and ulcerative processes of the wall of the ileum gives rise to abscesses adjoining it. This is assisted considerably by computed tomography and even ultrasound on occasion.

SECTION 5-1

Through the superior aspect of the left ovary

Anatomic Considerations

The pelvis is the funnel-shaped portion of the trunk located inferoposterior to the abdominal cavity. The true, or minor, pelvic cavity lies below the brim of the pelvis; the false, or major, pelvis is located between the iliac fossae and is part of the abdominal cavity.

The bony pelvis of the female differs from that of the male in several respects: The superior aperture or inlet of the female pelvis is larger because the ilia flare out laterally, the sacrum is wider and less curved, and the anterior iliac spines and the ischial tuberosities are more widely separated.

The pelvic inlet can be classified into four major types. The inlet of the gynecoid pelvis is circular or slightly oval. The inlet of the anthropoid pelvis is relatively long in an anteroposterior direction and has a short transverse diameter. The platypelloid pelvis has an elongated transverse diameter and a short anteroposterior one. The android pelvis has masculine characteristics.

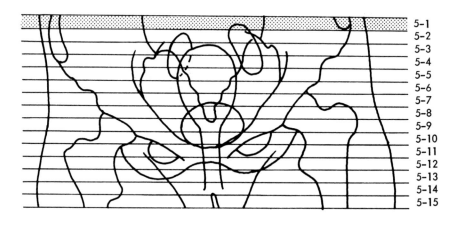

5-1
5-2
5-3
5-4
5-5
5-6
5-7
5-8
5-9
5-10
5-11
5-12
5-13
5-14
5-15

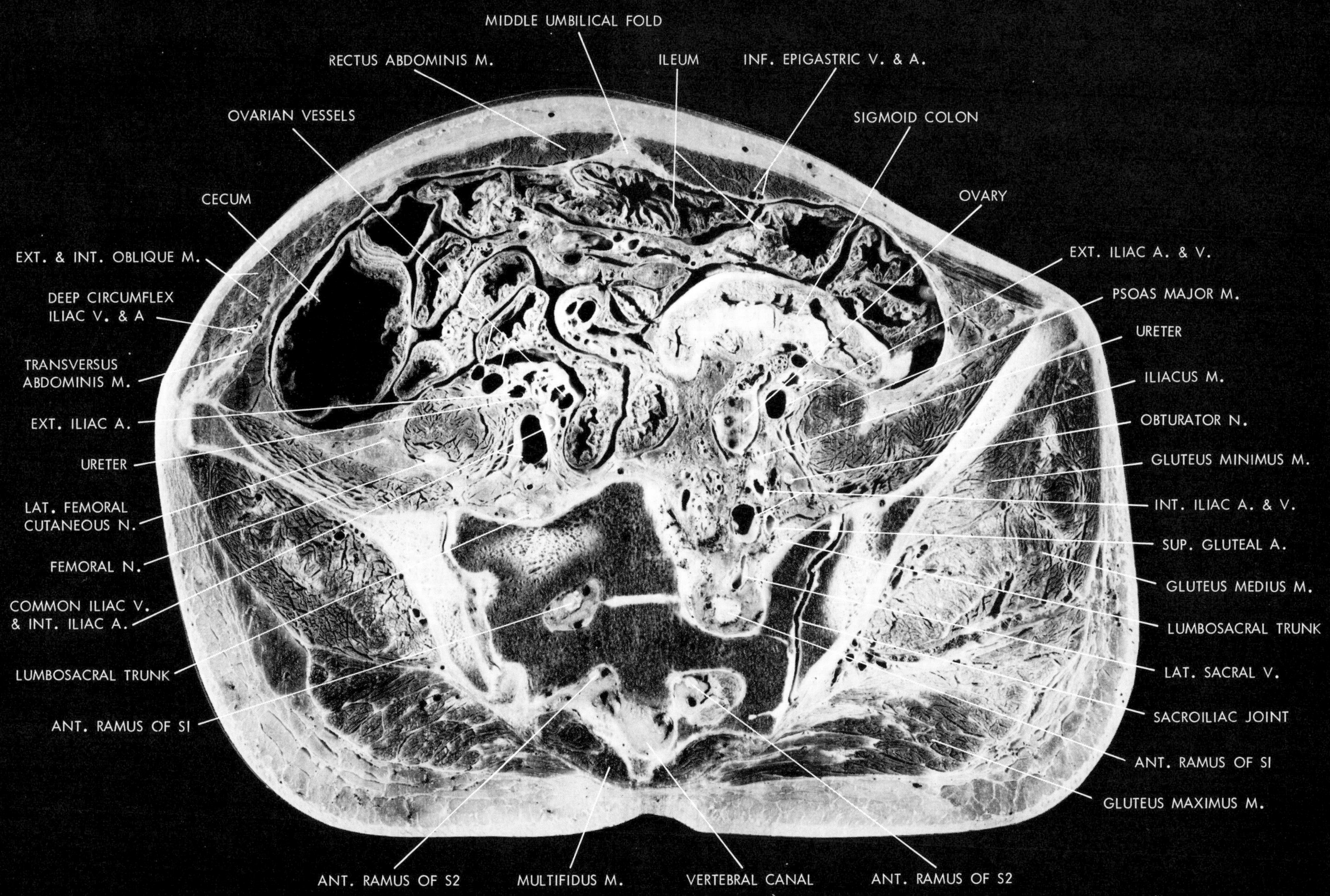

MIDDLE UMBILICAL FOLD

RECTUS ABDOMINIS M.　　　ILEUM　　INF. EPIGASTRIC V. & A.

OVARIAN VESSELS　　　　　　　　　　　　　　SIGMOID COLON

CECUM　　　　　　　　　　　　　　　OVARY

EXT. & INT. OBLIQUE M.　　　　　　　　　　　　　EXT. ILIAC A. & V.

DEEP CIRCUMFLEX　　　　　　　　　　　　　　PSOAS MAJOR M.
ILIAC V. & A

TRANSVERSUS　　　　　　　　　　　　　　URETER
ABDOMINIS M.
　　　　　　　　　　　　　　　　　　　　ILIACUS M.
EXT. ILIAC A.
　　　　　　　　　　　　　　　　　　　　OBTURATOR N.
URETER
　　　　　　　　　　　　　　　　　　　　GLUTEUS MINIMUS M.
LAT. FEMORAL
CUTANEOUS N.　　　　　　　　　　　　　　INT. ILIAC A. & V.

FEMORAL N.　　　　　　　　　　　　　　　SUP. GLUTEAL A.

COMMON ILIAC V.　　　　　　　　　　　　　GLUTEUS MEDIUS M.
& INT. ILIAC A.
　　　　　　　　　　　　　　　　　　　　LUMBOSACRAL TRUNK
LUMBOSACRAL TRUNK
　　　　　　　　　　　　　　　　　　　　LAT. SACRAL V.
ANT. RAMUS OF SI
　　　　　　　　　　　　　　　　　　　　SACROILIAC JOINT

　　　　　　　　　　　　　　　　　　　　ANT. RAMUS OF SI

　　　　　　　　　　　　　　　　　　　　GLUTEUS MAXIMUS M.

ANT. RAMUS OF S2　　MULTIFIDUS M.　　VERTEBRAL CANAL　　ANT. RAMUS OF S2

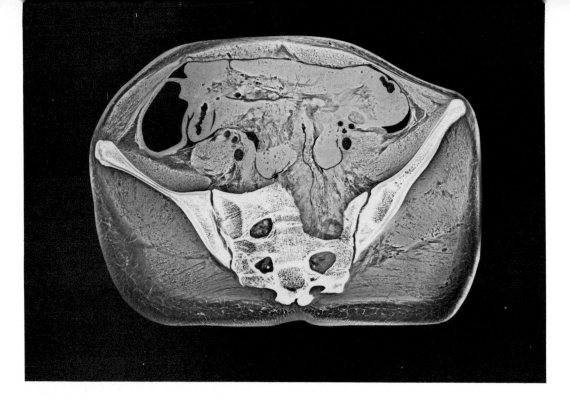

Clinical Considerations

Although both ovaries are visible anatomically in this slice at times it may be difficult to visualize them by either computed tomography or ultrasound. When the ovary becomes cystic or enlarged, possibly even in relation to neoplasia contained within it, it becomes readily distinguishable. It is only when it is very significantly involved that it may be seen with ultrasound.

The iliacus and psoas muscles are avenues for the spread of inflammatory disease from the retroperitoneal tissues and vertebral column contained within the abdomen to the region of the pelvis. It is not unusual, therefore, to see masses contiguous with the iliacus muscle; hence, its identification becomes clinically significant.

Although the ureters appear very small in this slice, they can often be visualized when contrast agents such as the ditrazoates are utilized by excretory urography.

The sigmoid colon is the most frequent site in the large intestine for diverticular formation, particularly in those adults beyond age 40. In the more elderly, these diverticula are very subject to inflammation and abscess formation. The identification of such abscesses is readily obtained by computed tomography, even when fistulization or even diverticulum demonstration is not apparent by conventional x-ray techniques.

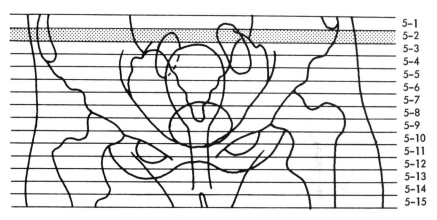

SECTION
5–2

Through the ovaries

Anatomic Considerations

The ovaries in this section are located in the ovarian fossae. The fossa is bounded by the external iliac vessels, the ureter, and the obturator nerve. In the multiparous and occasionally in the nulliparous female, however, the ovaries may be located in the pouch of Douglas.

The ovary is attached to the back of the broad ligament by the mesovarium, to the lateral pelvic wall by the suspensory ligament, and to the uterus by the ovarian ligament.

The ovarian vessels enter the hilus of the ovary in the suspensory ligament. The ovarian artery arises from the abdominal aorta at approximately the level of the second lumbar vertebra. The ovary also receives blood from the uterine artery. The right and left ovarian veins terminate in the inferior vena cava and left renal vein, respectively.

The sigmoid colon is located primarily in the lesser pelvis and is closely related to the left ovary and to the coils of the ileum that extend into the pelvic cavity.

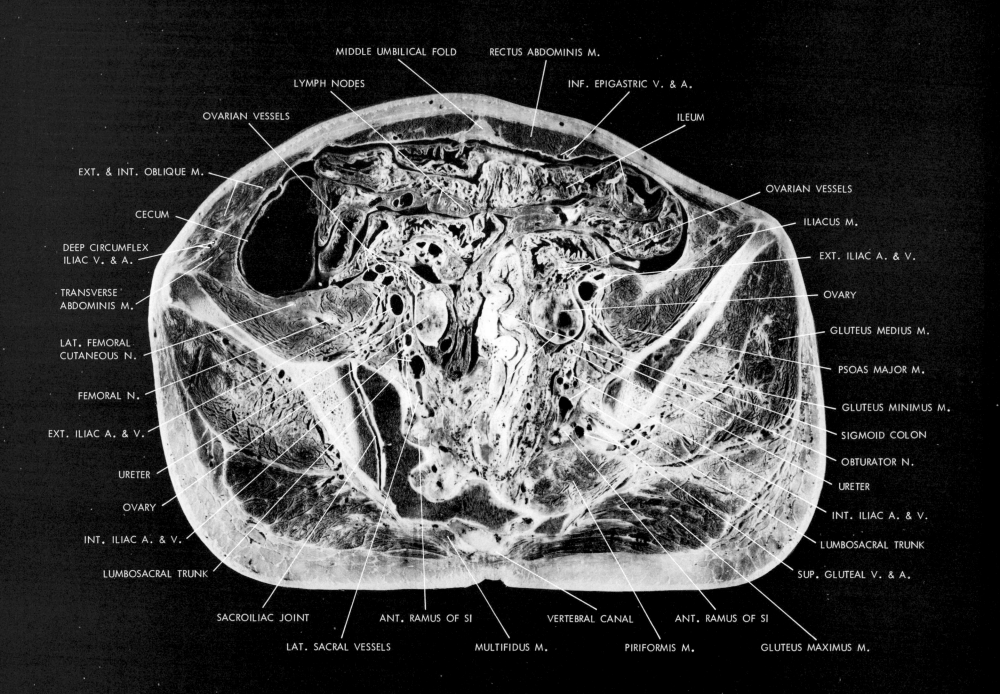

MIDDLE UMBILICAL FOLD

RECTUS ABDOMINIS M.

LYMPH NODES

INF. EPIGASTRIC V. & A.

OVARIAN VESSELS

ILEUM

EXT. & INT. OBLIQUE M.

OVARIAN VESSELS

CECUM

ILIACUS M.

DEEP CIRCUMFLEX
ILIAC V. & A.

EXT. ILIAC A. & V.

TRANSVERSE
ABDOMINIS M.

OVARY

LAT. FEMORAL
CUTANEOUS N.

GLUTEUS MEDIUS M.

PSOAS MAJOR M.

FEMORAL N.

GLUTEUS MINIMUS M.

EXT. ILIAC A. & V.

SIGMOID COLON

OBTURATOR N.

URETER

URETER

OVARY

INT. ILIAC A. & V.

INT. ILIAC A. & V.

LUMBOSACRAL TRUNK

LUMBOSACRAL TRUNK

SUP. GLUTEAL V. & A.

SACROILIAC JOINT

ANT. RAMUS OF SI

VERTEBRAL CANAL

ANT. RAMUS OF SI

LAT. SACRAL VESSELS

MULTIFIDUS M.

PIRIFORMIS M.

GLUTEUS MAXIMUS M.

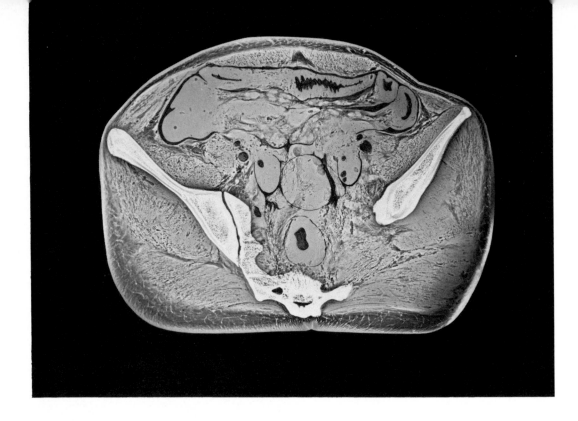

Clinical Considerations

The oviduct, when patent, is more readily apparent radiographically by hysterosalpingography. The oviduct is the only direct communication from the exterior into the peritoneal cavity and serves as a potential pathway for infection.

The oviduct is a common site for an ectopic pregnancy. During a tubal pregnancy, the blastocyst usually implants in the ampullary region. The oviduct often ruptures during the first trimester of gestation, resulting in severe internal hemorrhaging.

The rectum is very clearly visualized by conventional high-density double contrast barium enema techniques as well as by endoscopy; hence, the cross-sectional techniques for study are not apt to be utilized. For visualization of the space between the uterus and the rectum, however, this slice is particularly useful. At times a malignancy of the uterus invades this space and can thereby be detected, whereas the more conventional methods of radiography fail to reveal such invasion. The space between the uterus and the rectum is often referred to as the pouch of Douglas. This space is frequently occupied by inflammatory or neoplastic disease. As noted from this slice, the uterus is so closely contiguous with the rectum that involvement of this space becomes exceedingly important, even to a minimal degree, if it can be detected by computed tomographic techniques.

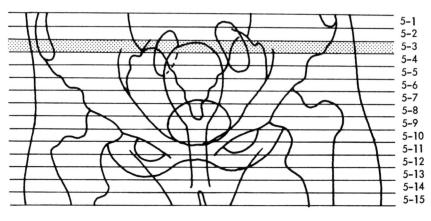

SECTION
5–3

Through the ovaries, 1 cm below the preceding section

Anatomic Considerations

The oviducts are paired tubes approximately 10 to 12 cm long that convey ova from the peritoneal cavity and sperm from the uterus. The oviduct or uterine tube is divided into three portions: The isthmus is the short medial segment that is continuous with the uterus, the ampulla is the dilated and longest portion of the oviduct and is usually the site of fertilization, and the infundibulum is the portion of the uterine tube that opens directly into the peritoneal cavity. The blood supply to the oviduct is from tubal branches from both the ovarian and the uterine arteries; the veins accompany the arteries.

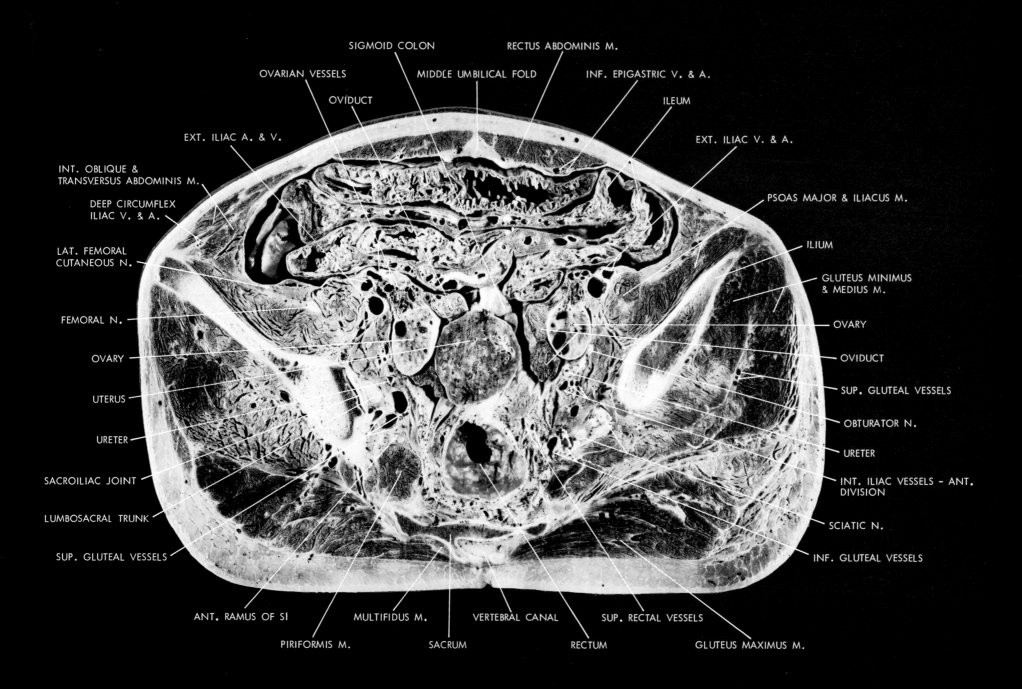

SIGMOID COLON

RECTUS ABDOMINIS M.

OVARIAN VESSELS

MIDDLE UMBILICAL FOLD

INF. EPIGASTRIC V. & A.

OVIDUCT

ILEUM

EXT. ILIAC A. & V.

EXT. ILIAC V. & A.

INT. OBLIQUE &
TRANSVERSUS ABDOMINIS M.

PSOAS MAJOR & ILIACUS M.

DEEP CIRCUMFLEX
ILIAC V. & A.

ILIUM

LAT. FEMORAL
CUTANEOUS N.

GLUTEUS MINIMUS
& MEDIUS M.

FEMORAL N.

OVARY

OVARY

OVIDUCT

UTERUS

SUP. GLUTEAL VESSELS

URETER

OBTURATOR N.

URETER

SACROILIAC JOINT

INT. ILIAC VESSELS - ANT.
DIVISION

LUMBOSACRAL TRUNK

SCIATIC N.

SUP. GLUTEAL VESSELS

INF. GLUTEAL VESSELS

ANT. RAMUS OF SI

MULTIFIDUS M.

VERTEBRAL CANAL

SUP. RECTAL VESSELS

PIRIFORMIS M.

SACRUM

RECTUM

GLUTEUS MAXIMUS M.

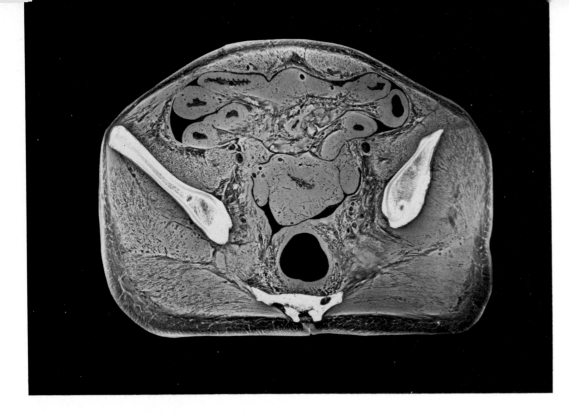

The vesicular surface of the uterus is nearly flat and is related to the bladder. The intestinal surface is convex and is separated from the rectum by the upper part of the rectouterine pouch and by the coils of the ileum. Laterally, the broad ligament attaches to the side walls of the pelvis. The muscular floor of the pelvis, the uterosacral ligaments, and the lateral cervical (cardinal) ligaments give major support to the uterus.

Clinical Considerations

For demonstration of the uterine cavity, hysterosalpingography is probably the radiographic technique of choice. At times it is difficult to determine the cause of a filling defect contained within the uterine cavity, and computed tomographic cross-sectional techniques may prove helpful to the radiologist. The uterus in relation to its cavity may at times be occupied by either endometrial polyps, fibromata, or malignancy.

In this section, the ureters can still be seen and could be visualized if excretory urography were employed in the course of computed tomography.

The visualization of the ileac loops in this portion of the pelvis is extremely variable and only in the presence of either thickening of the wall of the ileum or replacement of these loops by a solid, cystic, or inflammatory mass does visualization of this slice become important.

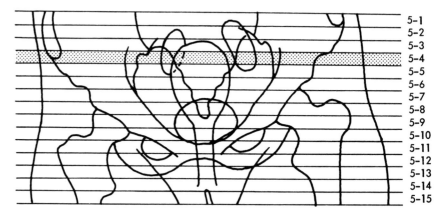

5-1
5-2
5-3
5-4
5-5
5-6
5-7
5-8
5-9
5-10
5-11
5-12
5-13
5-14
5-15

SECTION 5-4

Through the uterus

Anatomic Considerations

The uterus is an unpaired organ situated between two layers of the broad ligament. It communicates above with the oviduct and inferiorly with the vagina and is divided into the fundus, the body, the isthmus, and the cervix.

Although it lies in the middle of the pelvis, it is seldom median in position. The uterus is at right angles to the vagina and pelvic brim. When it is inclined forward from the vertical axis of the trunk, the uterus is in the position of anteversion. Between the cervix and body, the uterus is normally bent forward (anteflexed). Under certain conditions the uterus may be found backward (retroverted) or doubled back on itself (retroflexed) at the junction of the body and cervix.

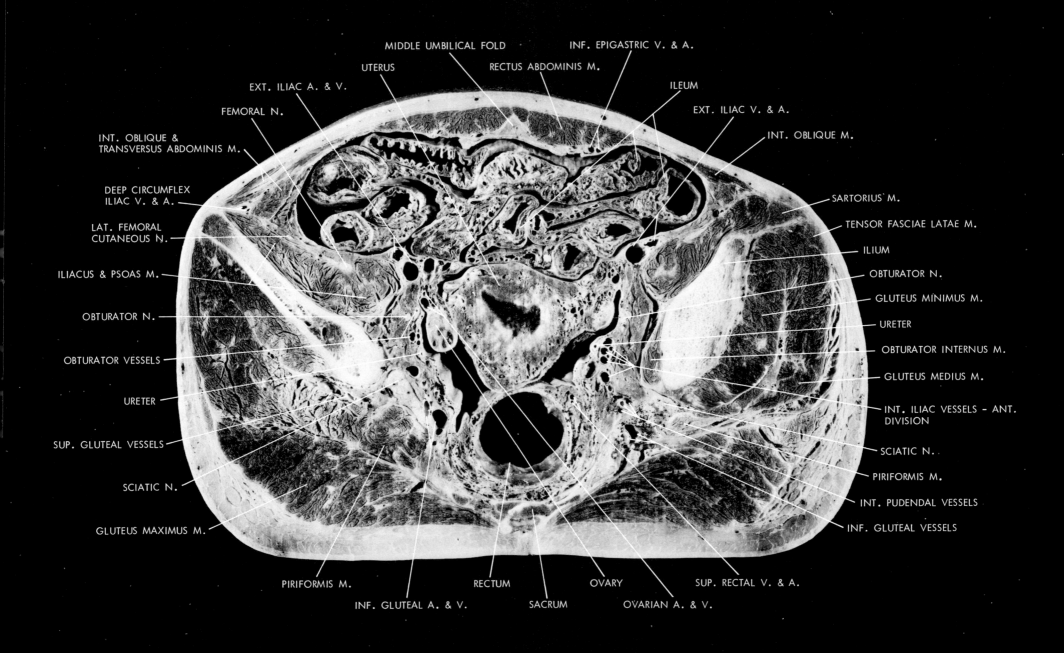

MIDDLE UMBILICAL FOLD

INF. EPIGASTRIC V. & A.

UTERUS

RECTUS ABDOMINIS M.

EXT. ILIAC A. & V.

ILEUM

FEMORAL N.

EXT. ILIAC V. & A.

INT. OBLIQUE &
TRANSVERSUS ABDOMINIS M.

INT. OBLIQUE M.

DEEP CIRCUMFLEX
ILIAC V. & A.

SARTORIUS M.

TENSOR FASCIAE LATAE M.

LAT. FEMORAL
CUTANEOUS N.

ILIUM

ILIACUS & PSOAS M.

OBTURATOR N.

GLUTEUS MINIMUS M.

OBTURATOR N.

URETER

OBTURATOR VESSELS

OBTURATOR INTERNUS M.

GLUTEUS MEDIUS M.

URETER

INT. ILIAC VESSELS - ANT.
DIVISION

SUP. GLUTEAL VESSELS

SCIATIC N.

SCIATIC N.

PIRIFORMIS M.

INT. PUDENDAL VESSELS

GLUTEUS MAXIMUS M.

INF. GLUTEAL VESSELS

PIRIFORMIS M.

RECTUM

OVARY

SUP. RECTAL V. & A.

INF. GLUTEAL A. & V.

SACRUM

OVARIAN A. & V.

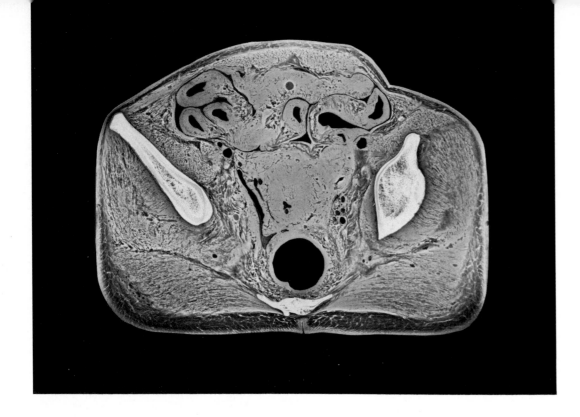

version process, which the uterus may at times undergo. It may be either anteverted, in which case it is bent on itself anteriorly, or retroverted. In any case, visualization of the uterine cavity, including the cervical canal, is best accomplished radiologically by more conventional techniques such as hystero-salpingography, if at all possible.

The position of the ureters in respect to the uterus is important to note. Surgically panhysterectomy, or total removal of the uterus, must be accomplished without transection or injury to the ureters. In this respect, the anatomic relationship of the ureters to the uterus must be carefully documented at the time of surgery and the ureters avoided.

The close association of the venous plexuses in relation to the ureter, oviducts, and uterus gives rise to a syndrome clinically known as the "ovarian vein syndrome." In this syndrome, pressure from the ovary or its contiguous structures on the uterine veins may give rise to dilatation of these veins, a rather "corkscrew" appearance of the ureters on excretory urography, and even a partial blockage of the ureters, giving rise to the so-called dilated ureter, or hydroureter.

The close association between the uterine cervix and the rectum is once again noted. It can be seen that carcinomas or other malignancies of the uterine cervix may readily invade the wall of the rectum or the tissues contained between these two structures. Invasion of the rectum occurring with a carcinoma of the cervix immediately establishes it as a Stage 4, a very advanced carcinoma with a very poor prognosis.

SECTION 5–5

Through the uterus, 1 cm below the preceding section

Anatomic Considerations

The uterine veins are the chief drainage vessels of the vaginal and uterine plexuses of veins. They are formed lateral to the cervix from descending branches from the uterus and ascending branches from the vagina. The veins pass laterally in the lateral cervical ligaments, and terminate in the internal iliac veins. The venous plexus communicates with the ovarian and rectal veins. The communication between the uterine and rectal veins allows uterine blood to enter the portal circulation.

Clinical Considerations

The fact that the uterine fundus as well as the cervical canal is visualized in this single section is an indication of the importance of understanding the

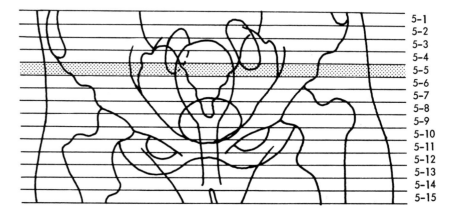

5–1
5–2
5–3
5–4
5–5
5–6
5–7
5–8
5–9
5–10
5–11
5–12
5–13
5–14
5–15

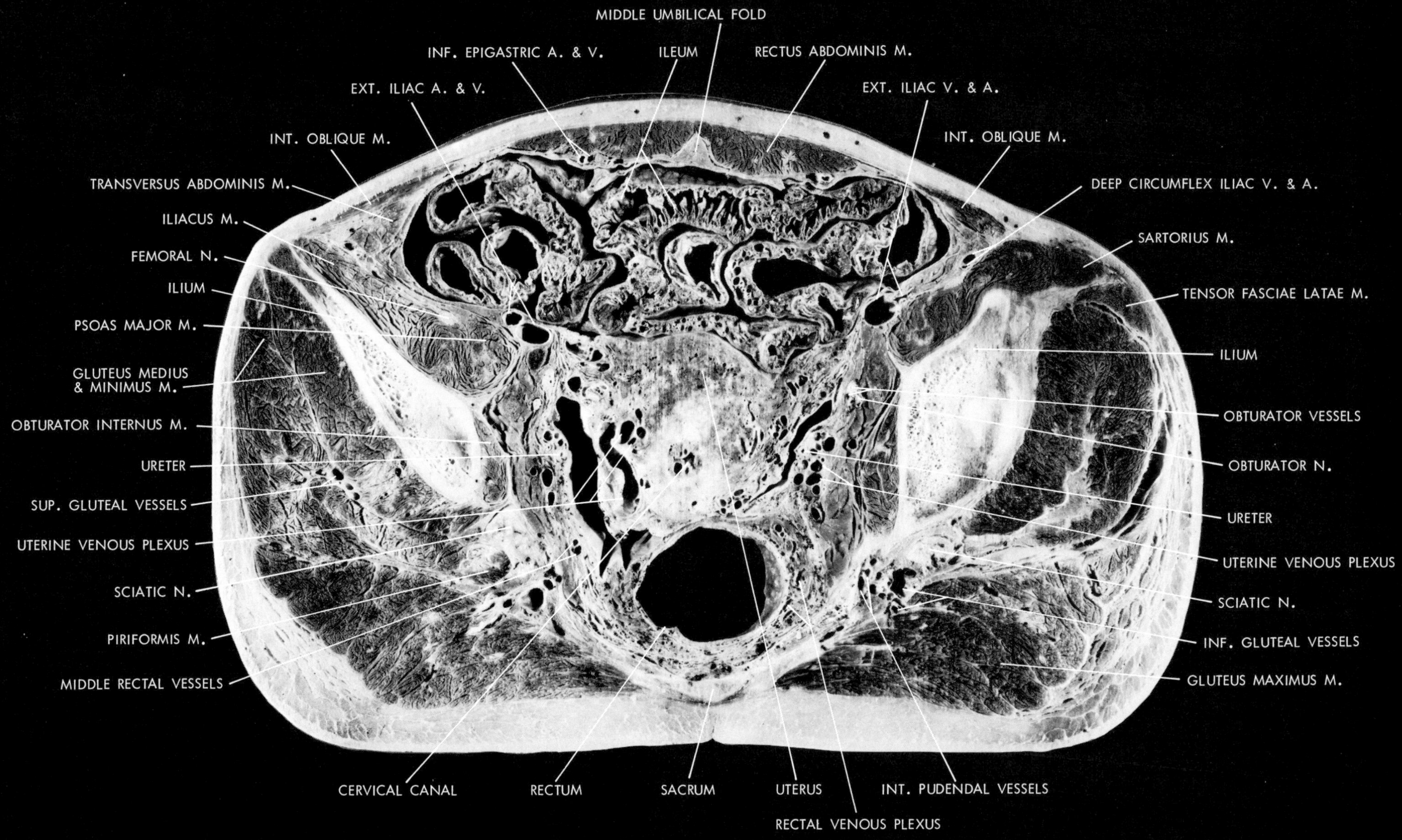

MIDDLE UMBILICAL FOLD

INF. EPIGASTRIC A. & V.   ILEUM   RECTUS ABDOMINIS M.

EXT. ILIAC A. & V.   EXT. ILIAC V. & A.

INT. OBLIQUE M.   INT. OBLIQUE M.

TRANSVERSUS ABDOMINIS M.   DEEP CIRCUMFLEX ILIAC V. & A.

ILIACUS M.   SARTORIUS M.

FEMORAL N.

ILIUM   TENSOR FASCIAE LATAE M.

PSOAS MAJOR M.   ILIUM

GLUTEUS MEDIUS
& MINIMUS M.   OBTURATOR VESSELS

OBTURATOR INTERNUS M.   OBTURATOR N.

URETER   URETER

SUP. GLUTEAL VESSELS   UTERINE VENOUS PLEXUS

UTERINE VENOUS PLEXUS   SCIATIC N.

SCIATIC N.   INF. GLUTEAL VESSELS

PIRIFORMIS M.   GLUTEUS MAXIMUS M.

MIDDLE RECTAL VESSELS

CERVICAL CANAL   RECTUM   SACRUM   UTERUS   INT. PUDENDAL VESSELS

RECTAL VENOUS PLEXUS

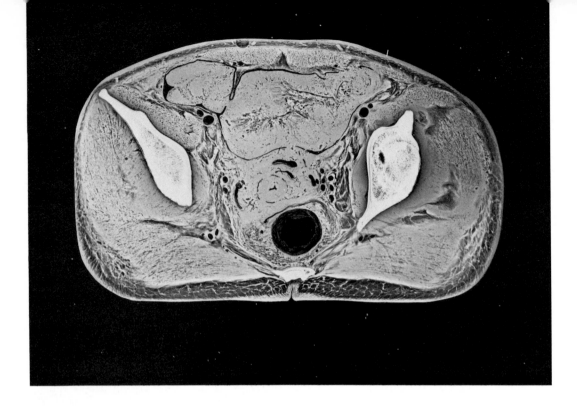

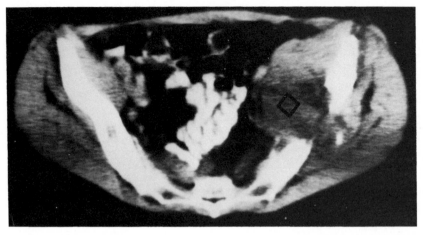

This cadaveric section clearly demonstrates, as do the preceding three illustrations, that the female pelvis has three horizontally distinct parts: (1) an anterior sector consisting of the ileal loops; (2) a middle sector containing the uterus, uterine cervix, and contiguous venous plexuses, as well as the obturator internus muscle more laterally; and (3) a posterior sector containing the rectum and tip of the sacrum.

The identification of the obturator internus muscle is important in the event that an abnormality such as an enlarged lymph node occurs and requires documentation. In patients with carcinoma of the cervix, for example, an enlargement of an obturator lymph node immediately establishes this malignancy as a Stage 3, irrespective of other involvement. This is a relatively far advanced malignancy and of considerable importance clinically.

SECTION 5–6

Through the uterus, 1 cm below the preceding section

Anatomic Considerations

In this section, the uterine artery can be observed directly anterior to the ureter. As the ureter approaches the urinary bladder in the female, it passes through the base of the broad ligament and crosses the uterine artery in an oblique fashion approximately 1 to 3 cm lateral to the uterine cervix.

The uterine artery is the chief blood supply to the uterus, although the ovarian artery can help supply it through the anastomosis between the ovarian artery and ovarian branch of the uterine artery. The uterine artery arises from the internal iliac and passes across the pelvis in the lateral cervical ligament to the cervix, where it divides into a larger ascending branch along the side of the uterus and a smaller descending branch to the vagina.

Clinical Considerations

This representative CT scan of the female pelvis demonstrates a recurrent mass from carcinoma of the cervix that has invaded and partially destroyed the iliac bone (diamond) (Stage 4).

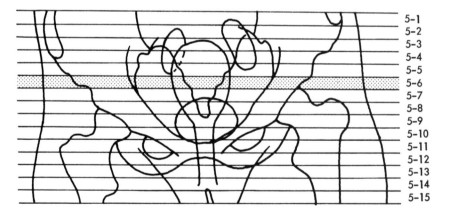

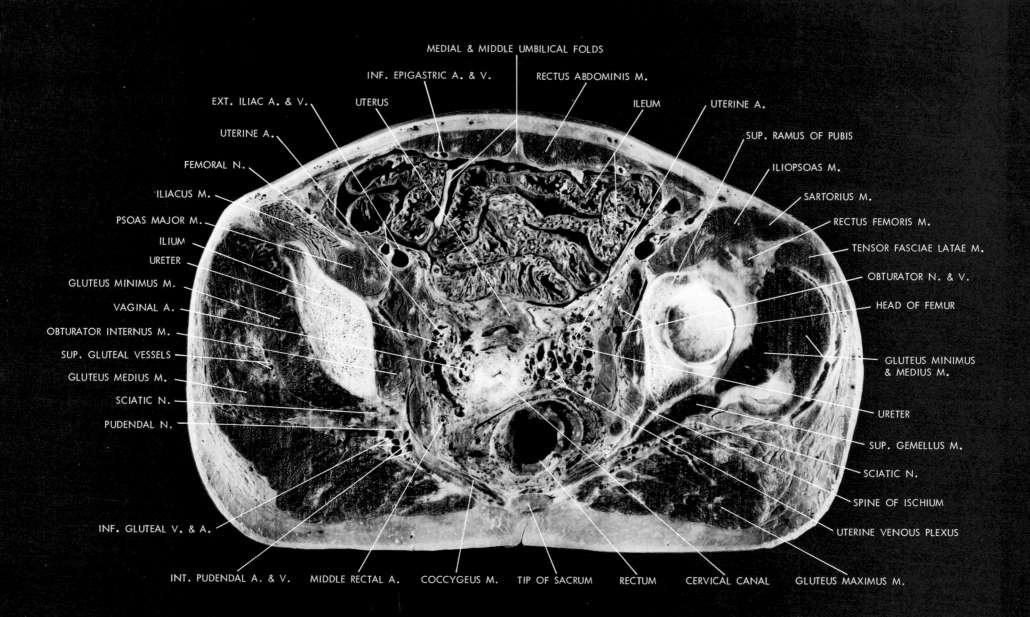

MEDIAL & MIDDLE UMBILICAL FOLDS

INF. EPIGASTRIC A. & V.

RECTUS ABDOMINIS M.

EXT. ILIAC A. & V.

UTERUS

ILEUM

UTERINE A.

UTERINE A.

SUP. RAMUS OF PUBIS

FEMORAL N.

ILIOPSOAS M.

ILIACUS M.

SARTORIUS M.

PSOAS MAJOR M.

RECTUS FEMORIS M.

ILIUM

TENSOR FASCIAE LATAE M.

URETER

OBTURATOR N. & V.

GLUTEUS MINIMUS M.

HEAD OF FEMUR

VAGINAL A.

OBTURATOR INTERNUS M.

GLUTEUS MINIMUS & MEDIUS M.

SUP. GLUTEAL VESSELS

GLUTEUS MEDIUS M.

URETER

SCIATIC N.

PUDENDAL N.

SUP. GEMELLUS M.

SCIATIC N.

SPINE OF ISCHIUM

INF. GLUTEAL V. & A.

UTERINE VENOUS PLEXUS

INT. PUDENDAL A. & V.   MIDDLE RECTAL A.   COCCYGEUS M.   TIP OF SACRUM   RECTUM   CERVICAL CANAL   GLUTEUS MAXIMUS M.

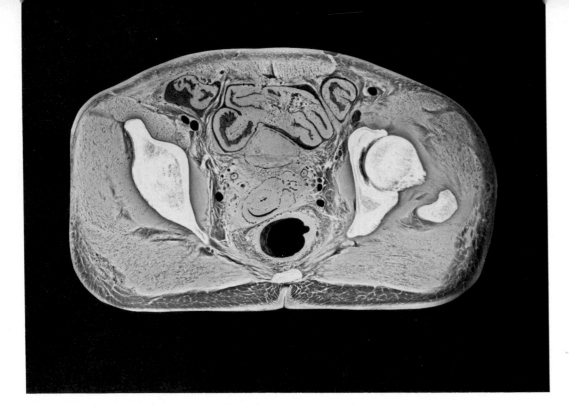

This close proximity of the urinary bladder anteriorly, and the rectum posteriorly, is important clinically relative to the spread of tumors from the uterine cervix; involvement of the urinary bladder or the rectum immediately establishes the lesion as a Stage 4 lesion.

The medial umbilical folds visualized in this section are of some importance in the event of a pneumoperitoneum in a newborn infant. They may be visualized in the midline, with somewhat similar folds being situated lateral to the midline, giving rise to a so-called "football sign." Also notable is the ligamentum teres, which becomes accentuated in its appearance in the presence of a pneumoperitoneum in the infant.

The exact position of the obturator internus muscle is of some importance in routine radiography in that the so-called obturator line is a landmark along the lateral border of the pelvis near the iliopectineal line on an antero-posterior view of the pelvis. Inflammatory lesions involving the hip or its bursae or inflammatory lesions descending from the region of the iliopsoas may push the obturator line medially and thus can establish their presence radiologically.

Occasionally, in conditions such as rheumatoid arthritis of the hips, bursal structures may extend inward into the pelvis through the fovea centralis of the acetabulum and present clinically as masses that are palpable in the pelvis, often so tense that they give the clinical impression of solid masses. With computed tomography, these can be distinguished by their different absorption coefficients.

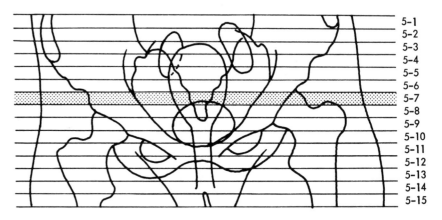

5–1
5–2
5–3
5–4
5–5
5–6
5–7
5–8
5–9
5–10
5–11
5–12
5–13
5–14
5–15

SECTION
5–7

Through the superior portion of the urinary bladder

Anatomic Considerations

The vagina joins the cervix above the caudal extension of the cervix and divides it into a supravaginal and a vaginal portion. A circular fissure, the vaginal fornices, is formed between the wall of the vagina and the vaginal portion of the cervix. The fornices are divided into anterior, posterior, and lateral portions. The posterior fornix is closely related to the pouch of Douglas.

In this section the prominent middle and medial umbilical folds can be observed. The former is formed by the remnant of the urachus and the latter by the obliterated umbilical artery.

Clinical Considerations

In this section, the urinary bladder, in close proximity to the cervical canal, becomes part of the middle compartment of the female pelvis just posterior to the ileal loops.

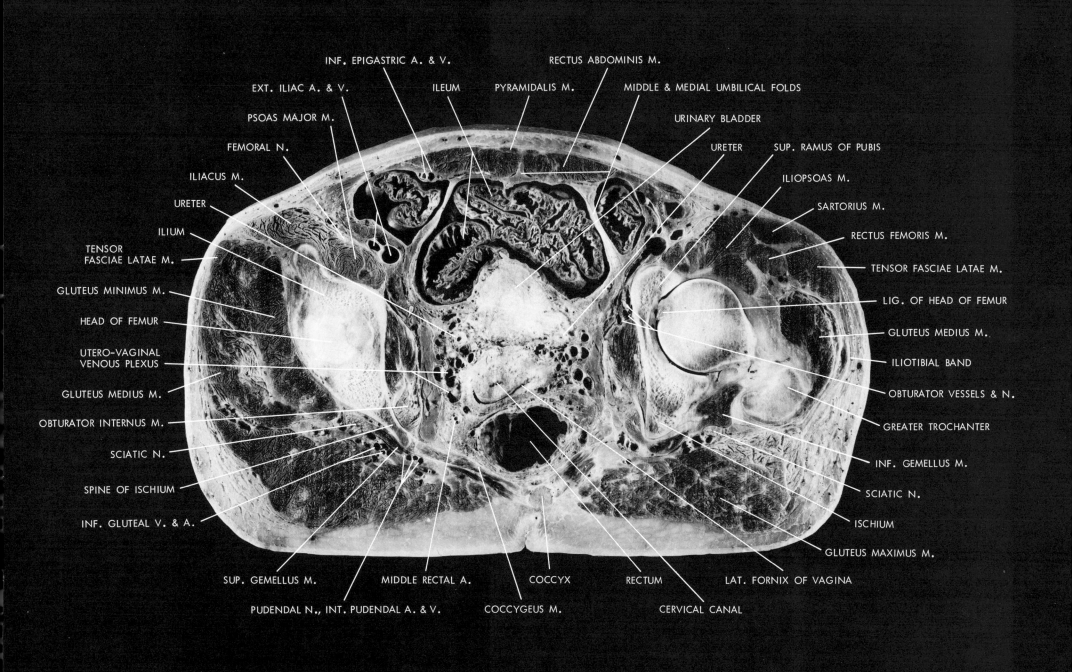

INF. EPIGASTRIC A. & V.

RECTUS ABDOMINIS M.

EXT. ILIAC A. & V.

ILEUM

PYRAMIDALIS M.

MIDDLE & MEDIAL UMBILICAL FOLDS

PSOAS MAJOR M.

URINARY BLADDER

FEMORAL N.

URETER

SUP. RAMUS OF PUBIS

ILIACUS M.

ILIOPSOAS M.

URETER

SARTORIUS M.

ILIUM

RECTUS FEMORIS M.

TENSOR
FASCIAE LATAE M.

TENSOR FASCIAE LATAE M.

GLUTEUS MINIMUS M.

LIG. OF HEAD OF FEMUR

HEAD OF FEMUR

GLUTEUS MEDIUS M.

UTERO-VAGINAL
VENOUS PLEXUS

ILIOTIBIAL BAND

GLUTEUS MEDIUS M.

OBTURATOR VESSELS & N.

OBTURATOR INTERNUS M.

GREATER TROCHANTER

SCIATIC N.

INF. GEMELLUS M.

SPINE OF ISCHIUM

SCIATIC N.

INF. GLUTEAL V. & A.

ISCHIUM

GLUTEUS MAXIMUS M.

SUP. GEMELLUS M.

MIDDLE RECTAL A.

COCCYX

RECTUM

LAT. FORNIX OF VAGINA

PUDENDAL N., INT. PUDENDAL A. & V.

COCCYGEUS M.

CERVICAL CANAL

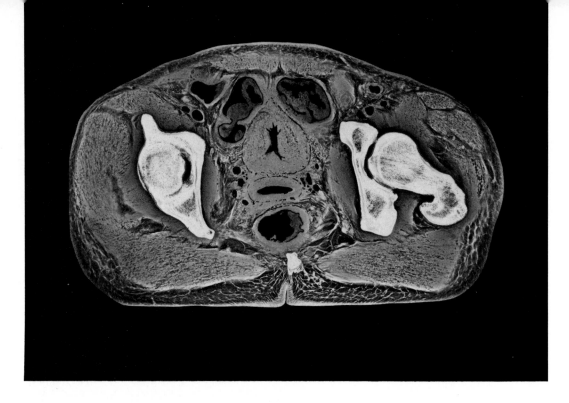

connected to the adjacent muscular coat and therefore appears folded or convoluted. However, in the area of the trigone, a small triangular area bounded by the urethra and two ureteric openings, the mucous membrane is firmly attached to the muscle and appears smooth.

Clinical Considerations

In this section, the close relationship between the vault of the vagina and the urinary bladder is evident. This is of some significance in malignancies that involve the vagina and invade the urinary bladder secondarily, creating fistulous communication between these two structures. Likewise, the close contiguity of the vagina and rectum becomes readily apparent.

In this section the ischiorectal fossa is in evidence. This contains a great deal of fat and allows easy dissection of a gaseous medium that may be introduced into this area and that may ascend to other portions of the abdomen and even into the mediastinum. Prior to the advent of computed tomography, the injection of air into the ischiorectal fossa ascended to the perirenal space as well as around the suprarenal glands and allowed one to visualize the structural boundaries with greater clarity. With computed tomography, visualization of the suprarenal gland can be accomplished so accurately with this modality that perirenal insufflation of gas is very seldom if ever necessary.

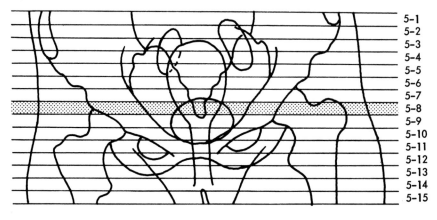

	5–1
	5–2
	5–3
	5–4
	5–5
	5–6
	5–7
	5–8
	5–9
	5–10
	5–11
	5–12
	5–13
	5–14
	5–15

SECTION 5–8

Through the urinary bladder

Anatomic Considerations

The peritoneum covers the pelvic viscera to a variable extent. It is reflected from the rectum onto the uterus to form the rectouterine pouch (pouch of Douglas), which is the most inferior portion of the peritoneal cavity in the female. The peritoneum reflects from the uterus onto the urinary bladder to form the uterovesical pouch and continues across the bladder to the anterior abdominal wall.

The urachus is the fibrous obliterated connection between the apex of the urinary bladder and umbilicus. During *in utero* development, the bladder communicated with the allantois by the urachus.

The mucous lining of a great portion of the urinary bladder is loosely

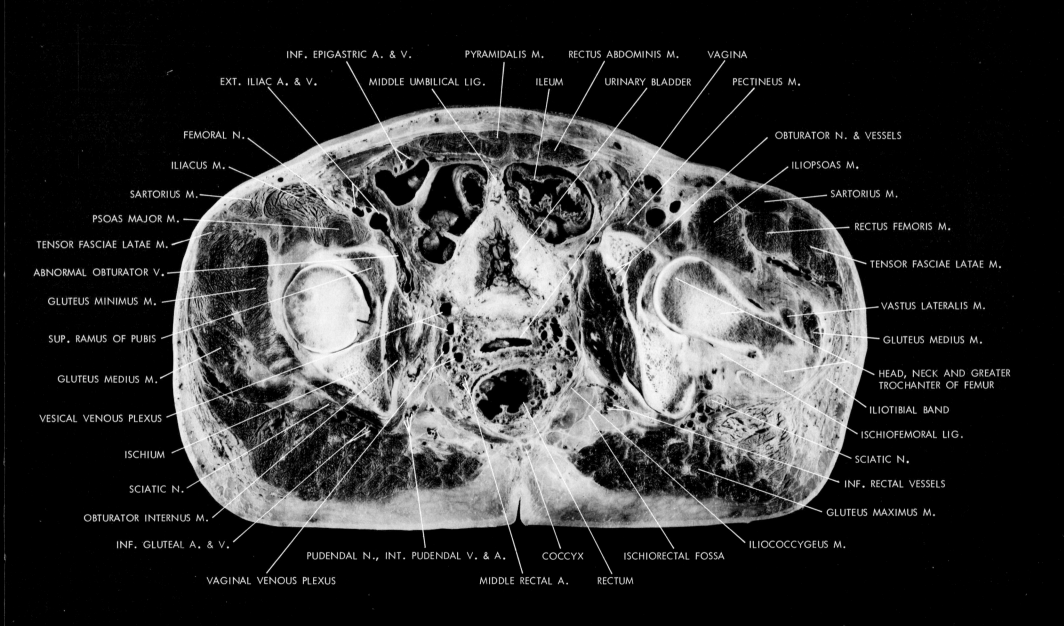

INF. EPIGASTRIC A. & V. PYRAMIDALIS M. RECTUS ABDOMINIS M. VAGINA

EXT. ILIAC A. & V. MIDDLE UMBILICAL LIG. ILEUM URINARY BLADDER PECTINEUS M.

FEMORAL N. OBTURATOR N. & VESSELS

ILIACUS M. ILIOPSOAS M.

SARTORIUS M. SARTORIUS M.

PSOAS MAJOR M. RECTUS FEMORIS M.

TENSOR FASCIAE LATAE M. TENSOR FASCIAE LATAE M.

ABNORMAL OBTURATOR V. VASTUS LATERALIS M.

GLUTEUS MINIMUS M. GLUTEUS MEDIUS M.

SUP. RAMUS OF PUBIS HEAD, NECK AND GREATER TROCHANTER OF FEMUR

GLUTEUS MEDIUS M. ILIOTIBIAL BAND

VESICAL VENOUS PLEXUS ISCHIOFEMORAL LIG.

ISCHIUM SCIATIC N.

SCIATIC N. INF. RECTAL VESSELS

OBTURATOR INTERNUS M. GLUTEUS MAXIMUS M.

INF. GLUTEAL A. & V. ILIOCOCCYGEUS M.

PUDENDAL N., INT. PUDENDAL V. & A. COCCYX ISCHIORECTAL FOSSA

VAGINAL VENOUS PLEXUS MIDDLE RECTAL A. RECTUM

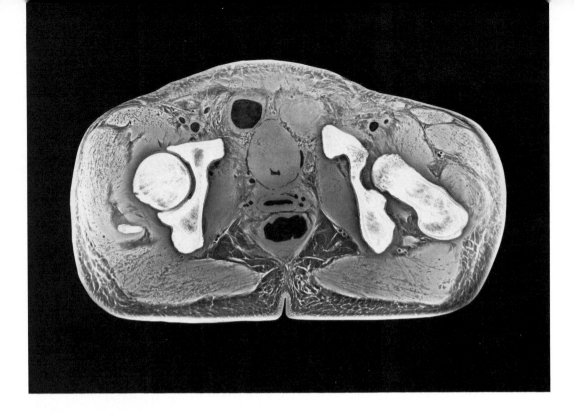

the anal canal. Laterally, the vagina is related to the levator ani, the pelvic fascia, and the ureters, which lie close to the lateral fornices.

Clinical Considerations

In this section, not only the urinary bladder but also the urethra, vagina, and rectum may all be visualized, and their relationship becomes of considerable importance clinically. The urethra in the female is in essence equivalent to the posterior urethra of the male; its relationship to the urinary bladder and the base of the urinary bladder is virtually identical.

Note the prominence of the vesical and vaginal venous plexuses, which may be visualized when diatrazoates are used intravenously in conjunction with computed tomography.

Note also in this section the relationships of the femoral artery, vein, nerve, and iliopsoas muscle. These structures are in close contiguity with one another at this level. The artery and vein (the latter particularly) may be distinguished with contrast enhancement during computed tomography. The nerve is always lateral to the artery and the iliopsoas muscle lateral to the nerve.

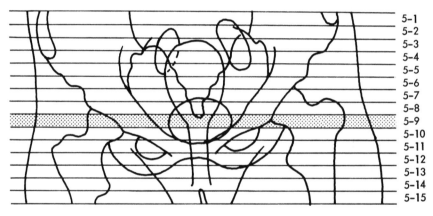

5–1
5–2
5–3
5–4
5–5
5–6
5–7
5–8
5–9
5–10
5–11
5–12
5–13
5–14
5–15

SECTION
5–9

Through the urinary bladder, 1 cm below the preceding section

Anatomic Considerations

The vagina extends from the uterus to the vestibule of the external genitalia. It passes through the pelvic fascia, between the two levator ani muscles, and through the sphincter urethrae muscle and pierces the perineal membrane. It therefore lies partly in the pelvis and partly in the perineum.

The long axis of the vagina meets the cervix approximately at a right angle. Anteriorly, the vagina is related to the posterior wall of the bladder and urethra. Posteriorly, from superior to inferior, the vagina is related to the pouch of Douglas, the rectum, and the perineal body, which separates it from

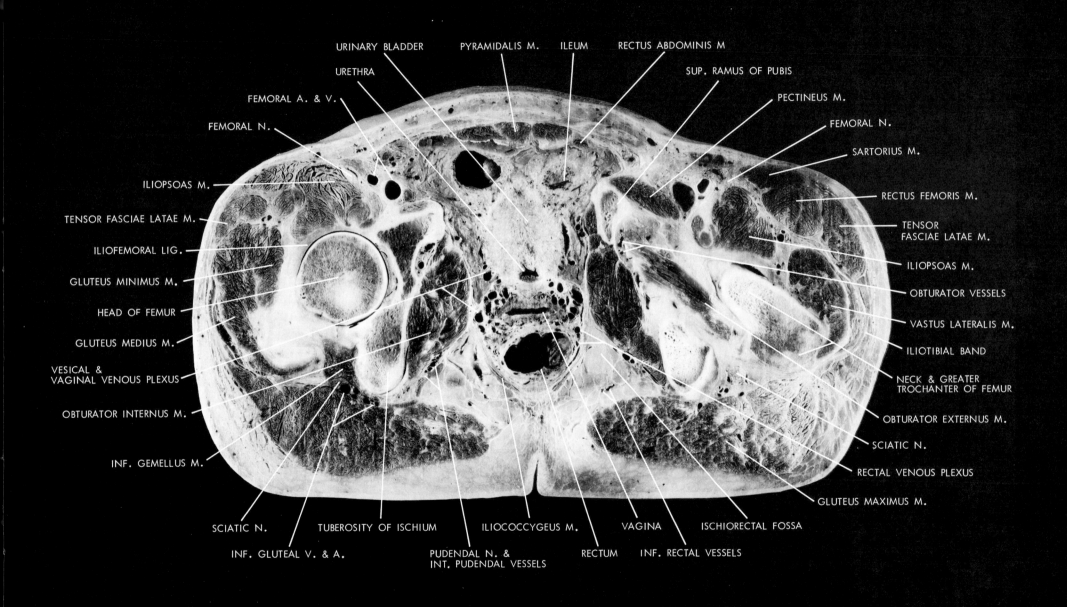

URINARY BLADDER   PYRAMIDALIS M.   ILEUM   RECTUS ABDOMINIS M

URETHRA   SUP. RAMUS OF PUBIS

FEMORAL A. & V.   PECTINEUS M.

FEMORAL N.   FEMORAL N.

                                                      SARTORIUS M.

ILIOPSOAS M.   RECTUS FEMORIS M.

TENSOR FASCIAE LATAE M.   TENSOR
                                                      FASCIAE LATAE M.

ILIOFEMORAL LIG.   ILIOPSOAS M.

GLUTEUS MINIMUS M.   OBTURATOR VESSELS

HEAD OF FEMUR   VASTUS LATERALIS M.

GLUTEUS MEDIUS M.   ILIOTIBIAL BAND

VESICAL &   NECK & GREATER
VAGINAL VENOUS PLEXUS   TROCHANTER OF FEMUR

OBTURATOR INTERNUS M.   OBTURATOR EXTERNUS M.

INF. GEMELLUS M.   SCIATIC N.

                                                      RECTAL VENOUS PLEXUS

                                                      GLUTEUS MAXIMUS M.

SCIATIC N.   TUBEROSITY OF ISCHIUM   ILIOCOCCYGEUS M.   VAGINA   ISCHIORECTAL FOSSA

INF. GLUTEAL V. & A.   PUDENDAL N. &   RECTUM   INF. RECTAL VESSELS
                         INT. PUDENDAL VESSELS

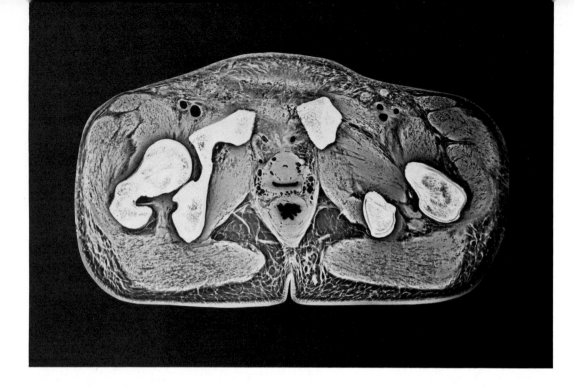

vessels and pudendal nerve. The pudendal nerve and internal pudendal artery are the chief innervation and blood supply to the urogenital triangle.

Clinical Considerations

In this section the supportive relationship of the iliococcygeus muscle in respect to the vagina and anal canal is clearly identified. Injuries to the muscle during parturition give rise to a lack of perineal support in the female; it can thus be readily understood why at times urinary problems are encountered in such female patients. Reconstructive surgery is sometimes required as a result of such tears and injuries during the parturition process.

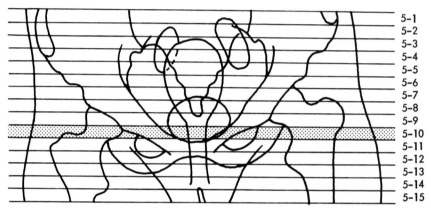

5-1
5-2
5-3
5-4
5-5
5-6
5-7
5-8
5-9
5-10
5-11
5-12
5-13
5-14
5-15

SECTION
5–10

Through the superior aspect of the anal canal

Anatomic Considerations

Alcock's (pudendal) canal is formed by a splitting of the fascia of the obturator internus muscle. This canal is found in the lateral wall of the ischiorectal fossa; it extends from the lesser sciatic foramen to the posterior margin of the urogenital diaphragm of the perineum and conveys the internal pudendal

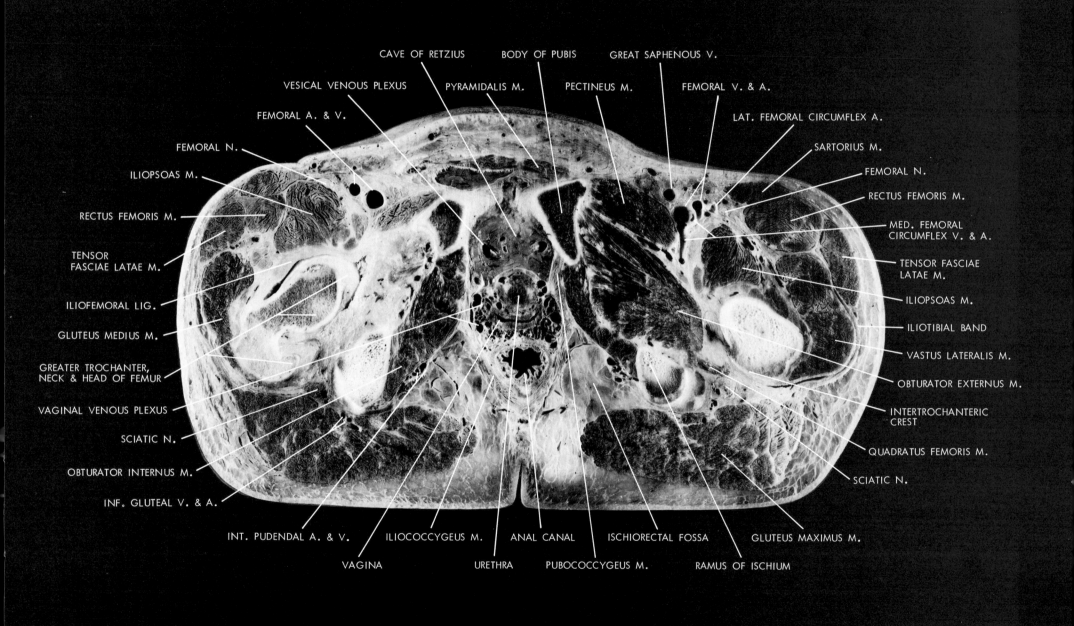

CAVE OF RETZIUS   BODY OF PUBIS   GREAT SAPHENOUS V.

VESICAL VENOUS PLEXUS   PYRAMIDALIS M.   PECTINEUS M.   FEMORAL V. & A.

FEMORAL A. & V.   LAT. FEMORAL CIRCUMFLEX A.

FEMORAL N.   SARTORIUS M.

ILIOPSOAS M.   FEMORAL N.

RECTUS FEMORIS M.   RECTUS FEMORIS M.

MED. FEMORAL
CIRCUMFLEX V. & A.

TENSOR
FASCIAE LATAE M.   TENSOR FASCIAE
LATAE M.

ILIOFEMORAL LIG.   ILIOPSOAS M.

ILIOTIBIAL BAND

GLUTEUS MEDIUS M.   VASTUS LATERALIS M.

GREATER TROCHANTER,
NECK & HEAD OF FEMUR   OBTURATOR EXTERNUS M.

VAGINAL VENOUS PLEXUS   INTERTROCHANTERIC
CREST

SCIATIC N.

OBTURATOR INTERNUS M.   QUADRATUS FEMORIS M.

SCIATIC N.

INF. GLUTEAL V. & A.

INT. PUDENDAL A. & V.   ILIOCOCCYGEUS M.   ANAL CANAL   ISCHIORECTAL FOSSA   GLUTEUS MAXIMUS M.

VAGINA   URETHRA   PUBOCOCCYGEUS M.   RAMUS OF ISCHIUM

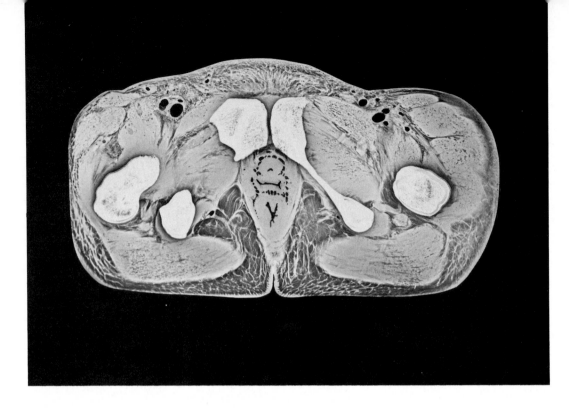

The vaginal venous plexus can be seen in this illustration. This plexus communicates with the uterine, vesical, and rectal plexuses and drains into the internal iliac veins.

Clinical Considerations

In this section the close relationship of the urethra to the pubococcygeus as well as to the vagina and anal canal is emphasized. Also, the fatty content of the ischiorectal fossa is once again identified. This rather large fossa, it will be recalled, acts as a conduit for the injection of gases that may rise in the abdominal fascial planes to surround the kidney and suprarenal gland as well as the region of the mediastinum for more conventional methods of radiography. On the other hand, the ischiorectal fossa may become the pathway for descent of infectious processes from the lumbar or even thoracic regions to give rise to perirectal as well as perianal abscesses. Tuberculosis is a frequent offender along these lines; often it is presumed that a perianal infectious sinus making its appearance because of this descent is tuberculous in origin.

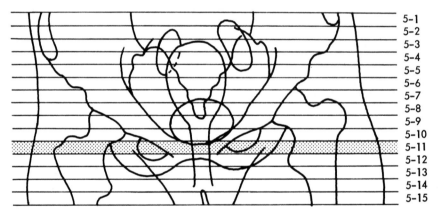

5-1
5-2
5-3
5-4
5-5
5-6
5-7
5-8
5-9
5-10
5-11
5-12
5-13
5-14
5-15

SECTION
5-11

Through the anal canal

Anatomic Considerations

The pelvic diaphragm, composed of the levator ani and coccygeus muscles and their investing fasciae, stretches across the floor of the pelvis like a hammock and separates the pelvis from the perineum. In the female, the diaphragm is pierced by the urethra, vagina, and anal canal. The pelvic diaphragm closes off the pelvic inlet and serves to support the pelvic viscera.

The levator ani muscle is further subdivided according to its attachments. The pubococcygeus and iliococcygeus muscles are attached to the coccyx; the pubovaginalis and puborectalis muscles form slings around the vagina and rectum, respectively.

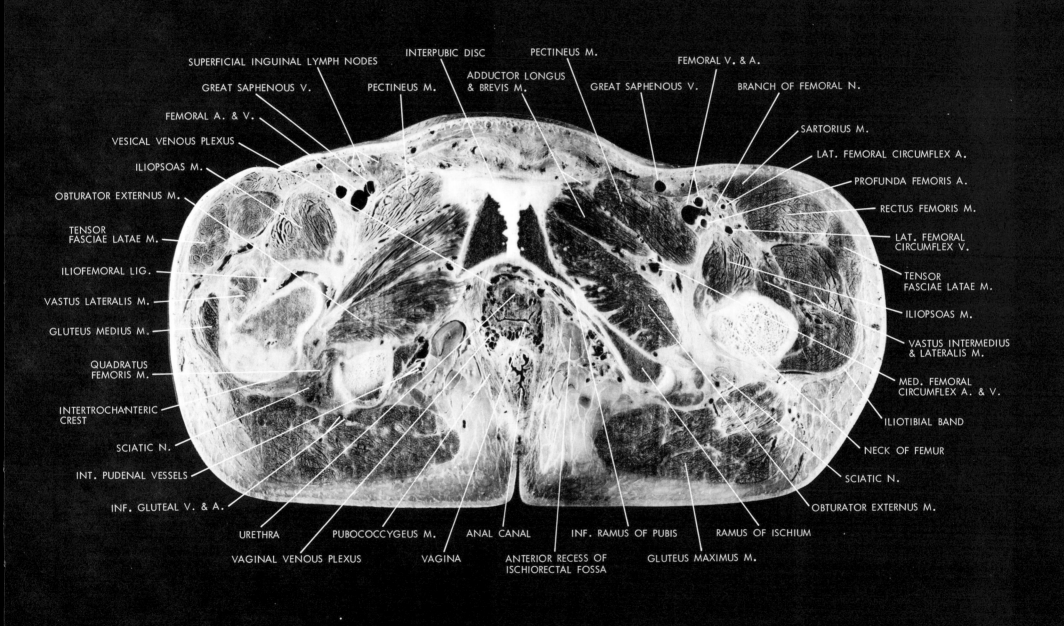

SUPERFICIAL INGUINAL LYMPH NODES

INTERPUBIC DISC

PECTINEUS M.

FEMORAL V. & A.

GREAT SAPHENOUS V.

PECTINEUS M.

ADDUCTOR LONGUS & BREVIS M.

GREAT SAPHENOUS V.

BRANCH OF FEMORAL N.

FEMORAL A. & V.

SARTORIUS M.

VESICAL VENOUS PLEXUS

LAT. FEMORAL CIRCUMFLEX A.

ILIOPSOAS M.

PROFUNDA FEMORIS A.

OBTURATOR EXTERNUS M.

RECTUS FEMORIS M.

TENSOR FASCIAE LATAE M.

LAT. FEMORAL CIRCUMFLEX V.

ILIOFEMORAL LIG.

TENSOR FASCIAE LATAE M.

VASTUS LATERALIS M.

ILIOPSOAS M.

GLUTEUS MEDIUS M.

VASTUS INTERMEDIUS & LATERALIS M.

QUADRATUS FEMORIS M.

MED. FEMORAL CIRCUMFLEX A. & V.

INTERTROCHANTERIC CREST

ILIOTIBIAL BAND

SCIATIC N.

NECK OF FEMUR

INT. PUDENAL VESSELS

SCIATIC N.

INF. GLUTEAL V. & A.

OBTURATOR EXTERNUS M.

URETHRA

PUBOCOCCYGEUS M.

ANAL CANAL

INF. RAMUS OF PUBIS

RAMUS OF ISCHIUM

VAGINAL VENOUS PLEXUS

VAGINA

ANTERIOR RECESS OF ISCHIORECTAL FOSSA

GLUTEUS MAXIMUS M.

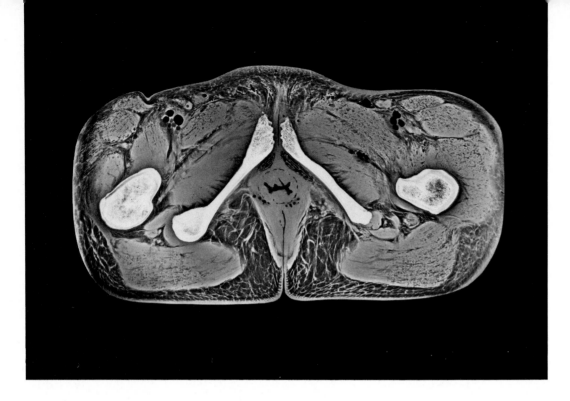

located in the deep pouch of the perineum. In the female, however, the homologous structures (greater vestibular glands) are found in the superficial pouch of the perineum.

Clinical Consideration

In this section the anal canal, with the vagina just anterior to it, can readily be identified. Anterior to this are the urethra and the crura of the clitoris.

The parametrial relationship of these structures, particularly in association with the perineal vessels, is readily apparent and is of particular significance in computed tomography of this area. This provides a contrast to the three horizontal zones described in Section 5–6.

Just anterior and lateral to the wall of this "pyramid" are the obturator externus muscle, and pectineus muscle, and the various major blood vessels, such as the femoral artery and vein. The iliopsoas muscle is even more lateral to this wall. The "pyramid" is an important landmark in computed tomography and cross-sectional anatomy.

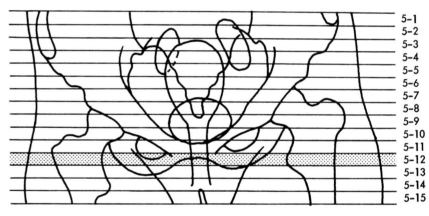

5–1
5–2
5–3
5–4
5–5
5–6
5–7
5–8
5–9
5–10
5–11
5–12
5–13
5–14
5–15

SECTION
5–12

Through the anal canal, 1 cm below the preceding section

Anatomic Considerations

After passing through the pelvic diaphragm, the vagina and urethra pass through the urogenital diaphragm. The urogenital diaphragm extends from the rami of the pubis and ischium (conjoint rami) on one side to the conjoint rami of the other side. The diaphragm consists of two layers of fascia, superior and inferior (perineal membrane), which enclose the deep pouch of the perineum. Within the pouch are found the vagina, the urethra, the sphincter urethrae, deep transverse perineii muscles, and branches of the pudendal nerve and internal pudendal vessels. In the male, the bulbourethral glands are

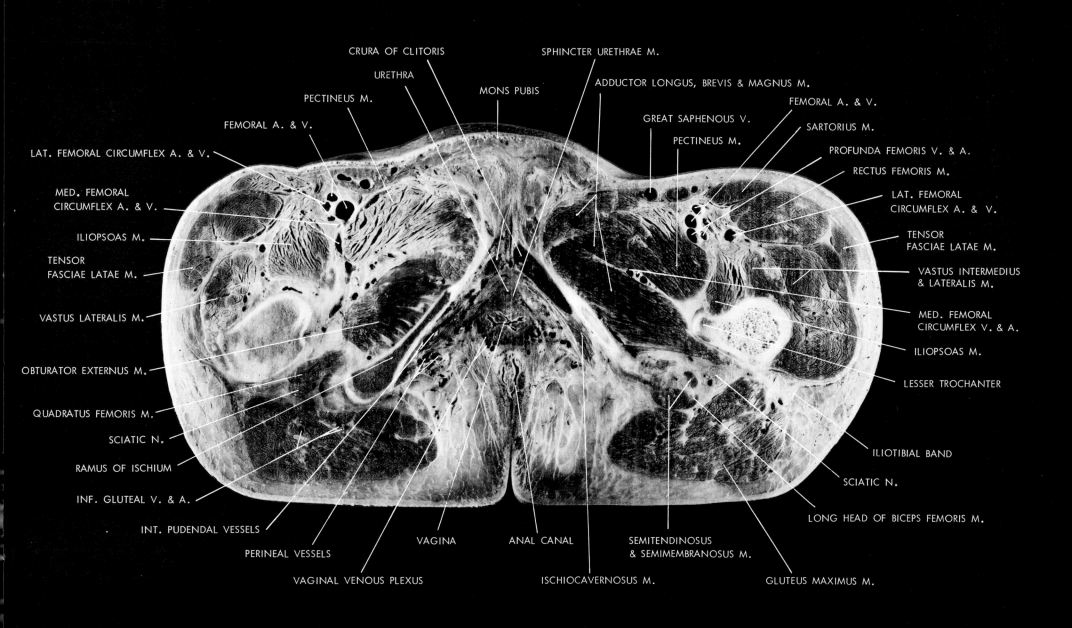

CRURA OF CLITORIS

SPHINCTER URETHRAE M.

URETHRA

ADDUCTOR LONGUS, BREVIS & MAGNUS M.

PECTINEUS M.

MONS PUBIS

FEMORAL A. & V.

GREAT SAPHENOUS V.

SARTORIUS M.

FEMORAL A. & V.

PECTINEUS M.

PROFUNDA FEMORIS V. & A.

LAT. FEMORAL CIRCUMFLEX A. & V.

RECTUS FEMORIS M.

MED. FEMORAL
CIRCUMFLEX A. & V.

LAT. FEMORAL
CIRCUMFLEX A. & V.

ILIOPSOAS M.

TENSOR
FASCIAE LATAE M.

TENSOR
FASCIAE LATAE M.

VASTUS INTERMEDIUS
& LATERALIS M.

VASTUS LATERALIS M.

MED. FEMORAL
CIRCUMFLEX V. & A.

OBTURATOR EXTERNUS M.

ILIOPSOAS M.

QUADRATUS FEMORIS M.

LESSER TROCHANTER

SCIATIC N.

RAMUS OF ISCHIUM

ILIOTIBIAL BAND

INF. GLUTEAL V. & A.

SCIATIC N.

LONG HEAD OF BICEPS FEMORIS M.

INT. PUDENDAL VESSELS

VAGINA

ANAL CANAL

SEMITENDINOSUS
& SEMIMEMBRANOSUS M.

PERINEAL VESSELS

GLUTEUS MAXIMUS M.

VAGINAL VENOUS PLEXUS

ISCHIOCAVERNOSUS M.

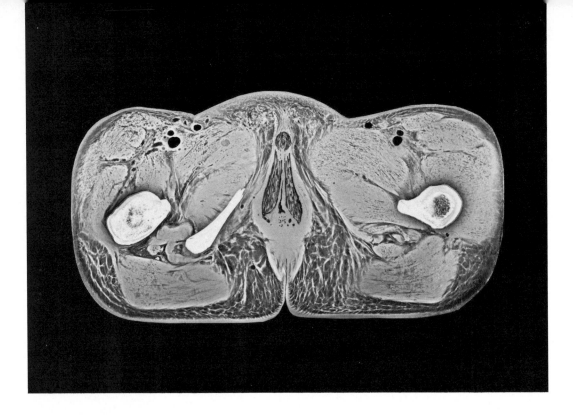

The vestibular bulbs are loosely encapsulated masses of erectile tissue. The convex surface of each bulb is lateral and covered by the bulbospongiosus muscle, whereas the concave surface is medial and covered by the perineal membrane. As can be seen in the illustration, the greater vestibular glands (Bartholin's glands) lie posterior to the vestibular bulbs.

Clinical Considerations

In this section, the middle segment from anterior to posterior is more readily separable from the rest of the pelvis, and the triangular relationship of this section is apparent. The clitoris forms the apex anteriorly of this "pyramid," whereas the wall of the "pyramid" is provided by the bulb of the vestibule and the vagina is situated rather centrally to this. If a tampon is inserted into the vagina at the time of computed tomography, it can readily be discerned from the bulb of the vestibule laterally and the anal sphincter posteriorly. The urethra is seen as a very small slit-like structure just anterior to the vagina but posterior to the clitoris near the apex created by the oblique bulb of the vestibule.

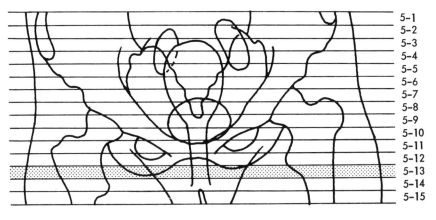

5–1
5–2
5–3
5–4
5–5
5–6
5–7
5–8
5–9
5–10
5–11
5–12
5–13
5–14
5–15

SECTION
5–13

Through the superficial pouch of the perineum

Anatomic Considerations

This section shows some of the contents of the superficial pouch of the perineum. The pouch is located between the perineal membrane and Colles' fascia. The latter is attached laterally to the rami of the pubis and ischium and posteriorly to the posterior boundary of the urogenital diaphragm. In the female, the pouch contains the crura of the clitoris; the vestibular bulbs; the ischiocavernosus, bulbospongiosus, and superficial transverse perineii muscles; the greater vestibular gland; and the posterior labial nerves and arteries.

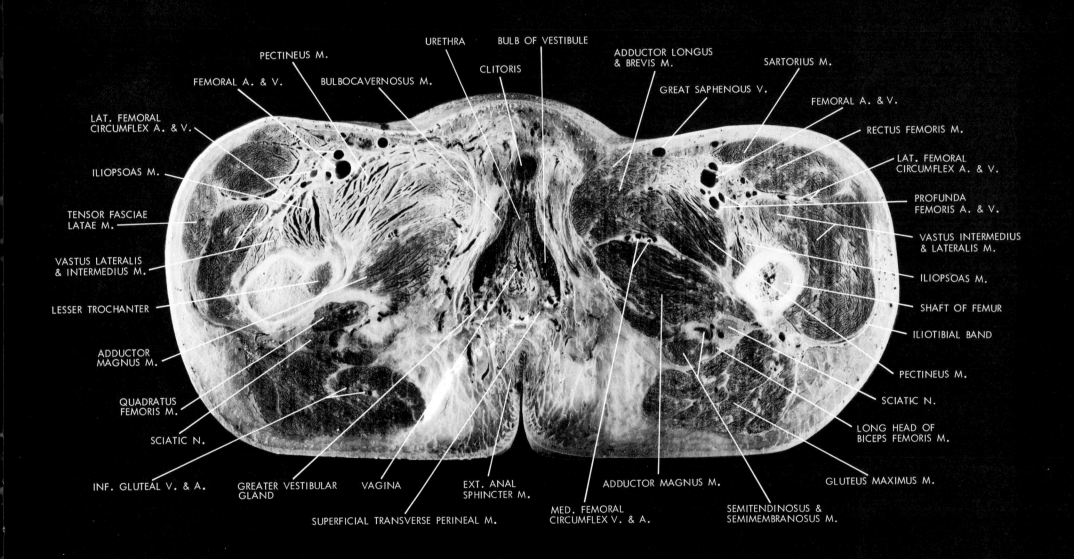

URETHRA

BULB OF VESTIBULE

PECTINEUS M.

ADDUCTOR LONGUS
& BREVIS M.

SARTORIUS M.

CLITORIS

FEMORAL A. & V.

BULBOCAVERNOSUS M.

GREAT SAPHENOUS V.

FEMORAL A. & V.

LAT. FEMORAL
CIRCUMFLEX A. & V.

RECTUS FEMORIS M.

LAT. FEMORAL
CIRCUMFLEX A. & V.

ILIOPSOAS M.

PROFUNDA
FEMORIS A. & V.

TENSOR FASCIAE
LATAE M.

VASTUS INTERMEDIUS
& LATERALIS M.

VASTUS LATERALIS
& INTERMEDIUS M.

ILIOPSOAS M.

LESSER TROCHANTER

SHAFT OF FEMUR

ILIOTIBIAL BAND

ADDUCTOR
MAGNUS M.

PECTINEUS M.

QUADRATUS
FEMORIS M.

SCIATIC N.

SCIATIC N.

LONG HEAD OF
BICEPS FEMORIS M.

INF. GLUTEAL V. & A.

GREATER VESTIBULAR
GLAND

VAGINA

EXT. ANAL
SPHINCTER M.

ADDUCTOR MAGNUS M.

GLUTEUS MAXIMUS M.

MED. FEMORAL
CIRCUMFLEX V. & A.

SEMITENDINOSUS &
SEMIMEMBRANOSUS M.

SUPERFICIAL TRANSVERSE PERINEAL M.

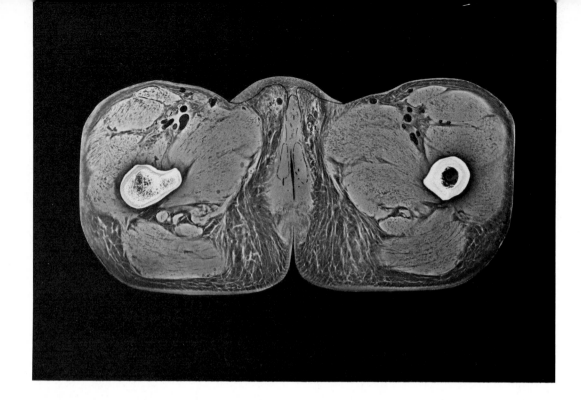

The inner portions of this section extending from the anterior surface to the posterior are most readily available to external examination, so the clitoris and the vestibule of the vagina become important landmarks. The other structures visualized herein are largely vascular, muscular, and nervous in origin.

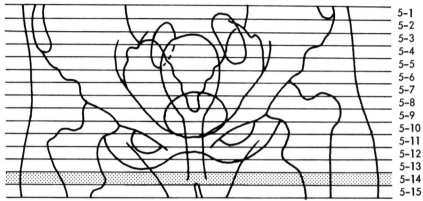

5-1
5-2
5-3
5-4
5-5
5-6
5-7
5-8
5-9
5-10
5-11
5-12
5-13
5-14
5-15

SECTION

5-14

Through the external genital organs

Anatomic Considerations

The external genital organs of the female consist of the mons pubis, vestibule, clitoris, labia majora, labia minora, vestibular bulbs and greater vestibular glands. The vestibule is the cleft between the labia minora. Opening into the vestibule are the vagina, urethra, greater and lesser vestibular glands, and paraurethral glands.

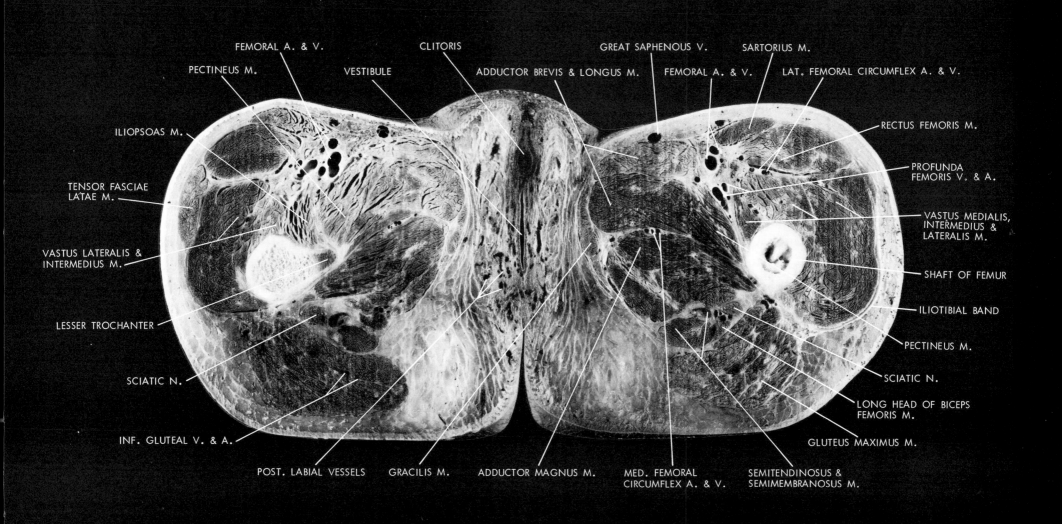

FEMORAL A. & V. CLITORIS GREAT SAPHENOUS V. SARTORIUS M.

PECTINEUS M. VESTIBULE ADDUCTOR BREVIS & LONGUS M. FEMORAL A. & V. LAT. FEMORAL CIRCUMFLEX A. & V.

ILIOPSOAS M. RECTUS FEMORIS M.

TENSOR FASCIAE LATAE M. PROFUNDA FEMORIS V. & A.

VASTUS MEDIALIS, INTERMEDIUS & LATERALIS M.

VASTUS LATERALIS & INTERMEDIUS M. SHAFT OF FEMUR

LESSER TROCHANTER ILIOTIBIAL BAND

PECTINEUS M.

SCIATIC N. SCIATIC N.

LONG HEAD OF BICEPS FEMORIS M.

INF. GLUTEAL V. & A. GLUTEUS MAXIMUS M.

POST. LABIAL VESSELS GRACILIS M. ADDUCTOR MAGNUS M. MED. FEMORAL CIRCUMFLEX A. & V. SEMITENDINOSUS & SEMIMEMBRANOSUS M.

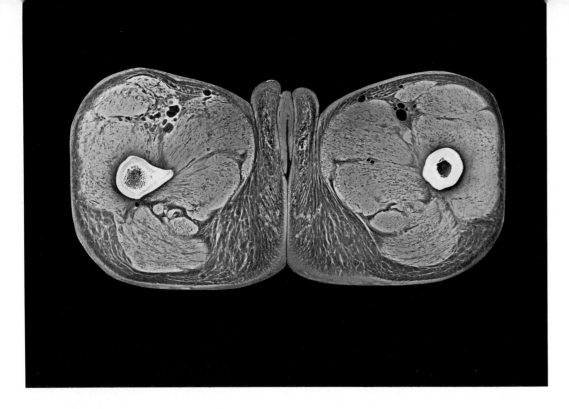

and veins, and the perineal branch of the posterior femoral cutaneous nerve. The labia majora are homologous to the scrotum in the male.

The labia minora are small cutaneous folds located between the labia majora that extend posteriorly, inferiorly, and laterally from the clitoris. The labia minora are homologous to the penile urethra of the male.

Clinical Considerations

At this level, the labia minora become separately identifiable from the labia majora. These compose the major structures in the inner zone from front to back; otherwise, the greatest consideration is to the mass of musculature separable by fascial planes on either side. The vessels, such as the femoral artery and vein, can still be visualized by contrast enhancement during computed tomography. The shafts of the femurs are clearly evident and begin to compose the structures of the thighs.

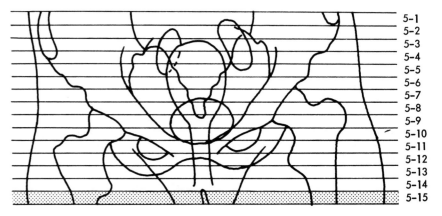

SECTION
5–15

Through the external genital organs, 1 cm below the preceding section

Anatomic Considerations

The labia majora are two longitudinal folds that extend posteriorly and inferiorly from the mons pubis. The external pudendal artery and vein and a branch of the ilioinguinal nerve enter each labium from the front. Entering each labium from behind are the lateral and medial labial nerves, the arteries

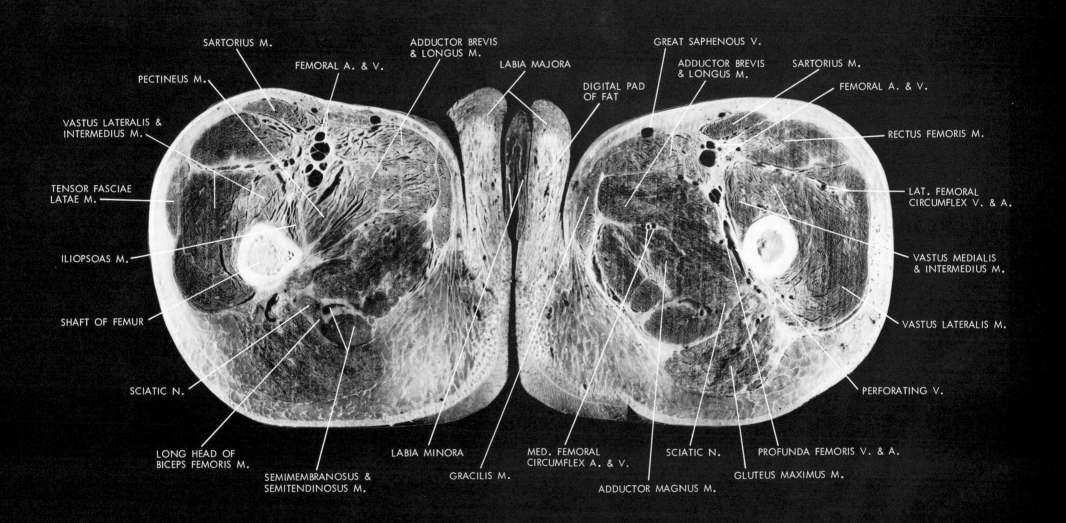

SARTORIUS M.

ADDUCTOR BREVIS
& LONGUS M.

GREAT SAPHENOUS V.

PECTINEUS M.

FEMORAL A. & V.

LABIA MAJORA

ADDUCTOR BREVIS
& LONGUS M.

SARTORIUS M.

DIGITAL PAD
OF FAT

FEMORAL A. & V.

VASTUS LATERALIS &
INTERMEDIUS M.

RECTUS FEMORIS M.

TENSOR FASCIAE
LATAE M.

LAT. FEMORAL
CIRCUMFLEX V. & A.

ILIOPSOAS M.

VASTUS MEDIALIS
& INTERMEDIUS M.

SHAFT OF FEMUR

VASTUS LATERALIS M.

SCIATIC N.

PERFORATING V.

LONG HEAD OF
BICEPS FEMORIS M.

LABIA MINORA

MED. FEMORAL
CIRCUMFLEX A. & V.

SCIATIC N.

PROFUNDA FEMORIS V. & A.

SEMIMEMBRANOSUS &
SEMITENDINOSUS M.

GRACILIS M.

GLUTEUS MAXIMUS M.

ADDUCTOR MAGNUS M.

6

Lower Extremity

INTRODUCTION

Although 1 cm–thick sections of the entire lower extremity were prepared, only 27 illustrations of the unattached lower extremity are presented in this chapter, as indicated in the drawing. We selected sections that did not excessively duplicate the structures shown in a preceding section yet allowed for a continuity in following the various structures of the lower extremity. The sections of the upper portion of the thigh, which are attached to the torso, are presented in Chapters 4 and 5. The illustrations of the lower extremity in this chapter are from a male specimen different from the one shown in Chapter 4.

Our consideration in the clinical applications of the cross-sectional anatomy has largely represented applied computed tomography with occasional reference to ultrasound. Since the utilization of computed tomography in the evaluation of the living cross-sectional anatomy of the extremities is still in its preliminary phase, the clinical considerations will be presented in a general way instead by individual illustration, as was done in the preceding chapters.

The evaluation of computed tomography in respect to the lower extremities evolves from the following:

1. An evaluation of sarcomatous tumors of the thigh (Weinberger and Levinsohn, 1978; de Santos et al., 1979).
2. A distinction between various types of tissue that might occupy the lower extremities different from the normal, such as myositis ossificans or primary bone tumors, as indicated previously.
3. The differentiation of a discrete versus an infiltrating mass occupying the lower extremity (Forrester and Becker, 1977).
4. The determination of accurate cross-sectional areas of various muscles to differentiate normal from abnormal (Hiaggmark et al., 1978).
5. The establishment of the relationship of certain muscle bundles and fascial planes with respect to one another prior to surgery. This involves the determination of both the size and the extent of a lesion and of vital structures that may be involved to achieve a tumor-free margin at surgery. The computed tomograph of the cross-section also may help plan subsequent reconstruction. Of particular importance is the determination of the relationship of lesion to bone, such as might occur with a synovial sarcoma of the thigh, a liposarcoma, or osteogenic sarcoma (Weis et al., 1978).
6. The accurate location of the sciatic nerve and the femoral artery in the event radical surgery is contemplated (Pritchard et al., 1977). Pritchard and his coworkers also use whole-lung tomography routinely with computed tomography to determine small foci of metastases, which may not be revealed by routine radiography.
7. The determination of the presence of denervation, reinnervation, or hypertrophic fibers in the event that a painless enlargement of a weak muscle such as a gastrocnemius occurs (Bernat and Ochor, 1978).

Other individuals who have presented preliminary investigations in respect to computed tomography in diagnosis and management of lesions of the musculoskeletal system are Schumacher and associates (1978). They have presented illustrative cases, including a lipoma of the thigh, osteochondroma of a simple cyst of the ilium, recurrent liposarcoma, desmoid tumor in the gluteal region, and applications in respect to the postoperative spine, particularly in the determination of interspace infections.

O'Doherty and coworkers (1977) have presented special computed tomographic patterns of pseudohypertrophic muscular dystrophy and showed how these scans may differ from the normal, polymyositis, and sarcoid myopathy. The two most frequent computed tomographic patterns in this pathologic condition consist of diminished tissue density of the affected muscles, contrasting these with the muscle fasciae that have normal density characteristics, and the representation of residual islands of normal muscle among the abnormal. A decreased muscle density has been represented in their cases. At times, symmetric patchy fatty degeneration has also been presented, particularly in the case of the leg involving the soleus and gastrocnemius muscles.

An effort has been made to devise ways and means of using computed tomography in the demonstration of internal structures of the knee (Archer and Yeager, 1978; Pavlov et al., 1978). In general, this application has been disappointing. It is true that the internal structure of specimens of the knee can be visualized by computed tomography, but this is dependent directly on very thin (3 mm) scans in the coronal or sagittal planes with a contrast enhancement with air particularly, or occasionally with a combination of air and an opaque medium. These visualizations can hardly compare with arthrography of the knee by conventional radiographic techniques, and it is not envisioned at this time that computed tomography will play a significant role along these lines when the accurate means available to us by arthrography of the knee can be employed. Without air as a contrast agent, none of the soft tissues within the joint space could be distinguished from one another. After the injection of air into the joint space, however, the cruciate ligaments and the menisci were visualized in both the coronal and the sagittal planes. Portions of the central areas of the cruciate ligaments could also be detected. The attenuation values of the identifiable portions of the cruciate ligaments were considerably lower than those of the isolated muscle samples. This may be due in part to partial volume effect and in part to the fact that samples were not scanned with a bone simulating ring, as suggested by Zatz and Alvarez (1977).

SUMMARY. In utilizing computed tomography, one may detect muscle size, presence and extent of disease, and invasiveness; one also may predict accurately the anatomic location of a lesion for its subsequent surgical removal, so that an appropriate plan of action may be formed prior to surgery, both for the surgery itself and for postoperative repair. At times one may want to determine the distinction between different types of tissue, especially those that contain fat, as in atrophy or in pseudomuscular hypertrophy; or to discriminate discrete from infiltrating masses. Calcific masses, as in myositis ossificans, may be detected. Muscle size and extremity size can be accurately measured in cross section. Finally, one may determine accurately the vital structures that are involved by a lesion in anticipation of surgery, so that a lesion might be removed to its entire free margin.

In all of these no mention has been made of ultrasound, although one particular reference (Lawson and Mitter, 1978) has pointed out that there is some value in the ultrasonic evaluation of extremity soft-tissue lesions with arthrographic correlation. They used diagnostic ultrasound to detect soft-tissue lesions, such as Baker's cysts, abscesses, rupture of suprapatellar bursae, peripheral artery aneurysms, and soft-tissue tumors.

Thus, a careful knowledge of cross-sectional anatomy is actually vital for ultimate diagnosis in these various and sundry applications.

Archer CR and Yeager V: Internal structures of the knee visualized by computed tomography. J Computer Assisted Tomography 2:181–183, 1978.

Bernat JL and Ochor JL: Muscle hypertrophy after partial denervation: a human case. J Neurol Neurosurg Psychiatry 41:719–725, 1978.

de Santos LA, Bernardino ME, and Murray JA: CT in the evaluation of osteosarcoma: experience with 25 cases. AJR 132:535–540, 1979.

Forrester DM and Becker TS: The radiology of bone and soft tissue sarcomas. Orthop Clin North Am 8:986, 1977.

Hiaggmark T, Jansson E, and Svane B: Cross-sectional area of the thigh muscle in man measured by computed tomography. Scan J Clin Lab Invest 38:355–360, 1978.

Lawson TL and Mitter S: Ultrasonic evaluation of extremity soft tissue lesions with arthrographic correlation. J Can Assoc Radiol 29:58–61, 1978.

O'Doherty DS, Dieter Schellinger D, and Raptopoulos V: Computed tomographic patterns of pseudohypertrophic muscular dystrophy: preliminary results. J Computer Assisted Tomography 1:482–486, 1977.

Pavlov H, Freiberger RH, Deck MF, Marshall JL, and Morrissey JK: Computer-assisted tomography of the knee. Invest Radiol 13:57–62, 1978.

Pritchard DJ, Sim FH, Ivins JC, Soule EH, and Dahlin DC: Fibrosarcoma of bone and soft tissues of the trunk and extremities. Orthop Clin North Am 8:869–881, 1977.

Schumacher TM, Genant HK, Korobkin M, and Bovill EF Jr: Computed tomography. Its use in space-occupying lesions of the musculoskeletal system. J Bone Joint Surg (Am) 60:600–607, 1978.

Weinberger G and Levinsohn EM: Computed tomography in the evaluation of sarcomatous tumors of the thigh. AJR 130:115–118, 1978.

Weis L, Heelan RT and Watson RC: Computed tomography of orthopedic tumors of the pelvis and lower extremities. Clin Orthop 130:254–259, 1978.

Zatz LM and Alvarez RE: An inaccuracy in computed tomography: the energy dependence of CT values. Radiology 124:91–97, 1977.

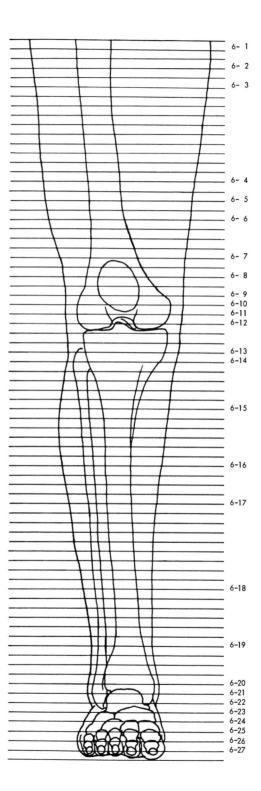

6- 1
6- 2
6- 3
6- 4
6- 5
6- 6
6- 7
6- 8
6- 9
6-10
6-11
6-12
6-13
6-14
6-15
6-16
6-17
6-18
6-19
6-20
6-21
6-22
6-23
6-24
6-25
6-26
6-27

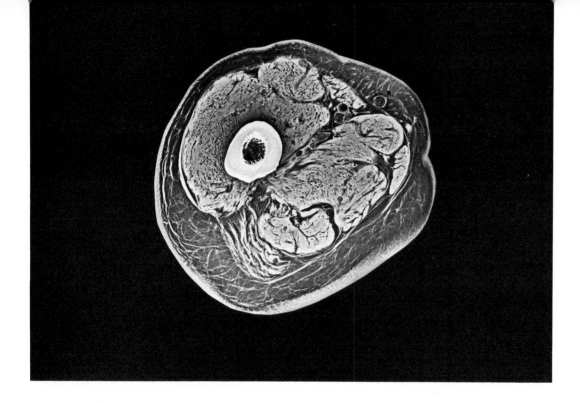

forms a posterior wall at the upper part of the canal (as is shown in this section); the adductor magnus forms the posterior wall at the lower end of the canal. The femoral artery, femoral vein, and saphenous nerve are found throughout the entire extent of the subsartorial canal. Additionally, the nerve to the vastus medialis is found within the upper portion of the canal (shown in this illustration), and the descending genicular artery, with its saphenous branch, is present in the lower part of the canal.

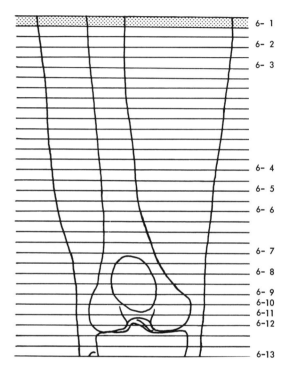

SECTION
6–1

Through the upper half of the shaft of the femur, 9 cm below the lesser trochanter

Anatomic Considerations

The adductor (subsartorial) canal is an intermuscular cleft located in the medial aspect of the middle third of the thigh. It extends from the apex of the femoral triangle to the hiatus of the adductor magnus. As can be seen in this and subsequent illustrations, the canal is triangular in shape, possessing anteromedial, lateral, and posterior walls. The adductor canal lies deep to the sartorius and is bounded laterally by the vastus medialis. The adductor longus

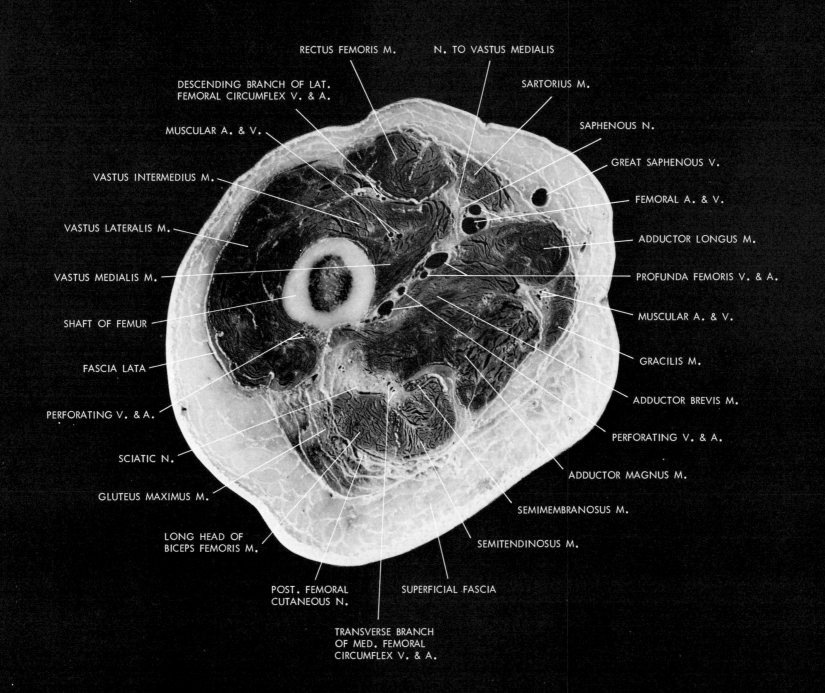

RECTUS FEMORIS M.

N. TO VASTUS MEDIALIS

DESCENDING BRANCH OF LAT.
FEMORAL CIRCUMFLEX V. & A.

SARTORIUS M.

MUSCULAR A. & V.

SAPHENOUS N.

VASTUS INTERMEDIUS M.

GREAT SAPHENOUS V.

FEMORAL A. & V.

VASTUS LATERALIS M.

ADDUCTOR LONGUS M.

VASTUS MEDIALIS M.

PROFUNDA FEMORIS V. & A.

SHAFT OF FEMUR

MUSCULAR A. & V.

FASCIA LATA

GRACILIS M.

PERFORATING V. & A.

ADDUCTOR BREVIS M.

SCIATIC N.

PERFORATING V. & A.

GLUTEUS MAXIMUS M.

ADDUCTOR MAGNUS M.

LONG HEAD OF
BICEPS FEMORIS M.

SEMIMEMBRANOSUS M.

SEMITENDINOSUS M.

POST. FEMORAL
CUTANEOUS N.

SUPERFICIAL FASCIA

TRANSVERSE BRANCH
OF MED. FEMORAL
CIRCUMFLEX V. & A.

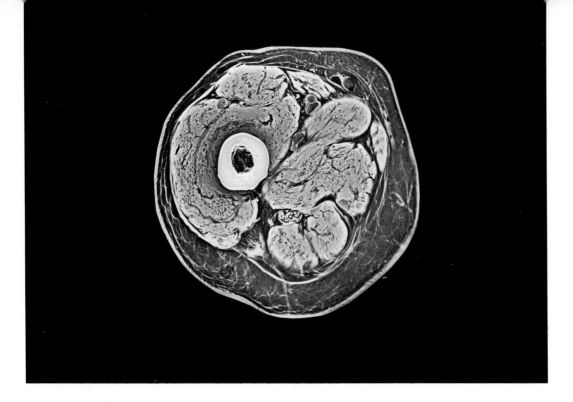

artery. As the femoral artery exits the adductor canal at the hiatus of the adductor magnus, it becomes the popliteal artery.

The course of the femoral artery from the inguinal ligament to the adductor hiatus can be followed in the illustrations. As the artery descends, it undergoes a change in position in regard to the femur from anterior to posterior. This positional change in the femoral artery is due, in part, to the 90° medial rotation of the lower limb during development *in utero*. A key feature of the femoral artery being anterior at its upper end and posterior at the lower end is that it passes on the flexor sides of the hip and knee joints.

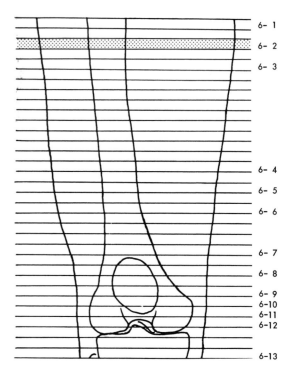

SECTION
6–2

Through the shaft of the femur, 2 cm below the preceding section

Anatomic Considerations

The femoral artery is the continuation of the external iliac artery as the latter passes posterior to the inguinal ligament, which is the base of the femoral triangle. In the femoral triangle, the femoral artery gives rise to the profunda femoris and unnamed muscular branches. The femoral artery also often gives rise to the medial femoral circumflex artery and, more rarely, to the lateral femoral circumflex artery. The femoral artery exits the femoral triangle at its apex and continues into the adductor (subsartorial) canal. In this canal, the femoral artery gives rise to muscular arteries and the descending genicular

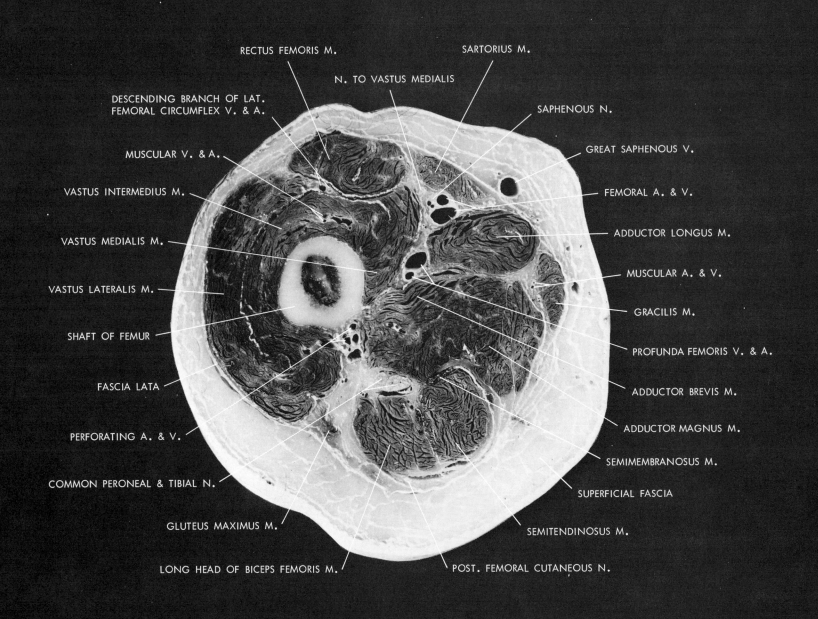

RECTUS FEMORIS M.

SARTORIUS M.

N. TO VASTUS MEDIALIS

DESCENDING BRANCH OF LAT.
FEMORAL CIRCUMFLEX V. & A.

SAPHENOUS N.

MUSCULAR V. & A.

GREAT SAPHENOUS V.

VASTUS INTERMEDIUS M.

FEMORAL A. & V.

VASTUS MEDIALIS M.

ADDUCTOR LONGUS M.

MUSCULAR A. & V.

VASTUS LATERALIS M.

GRACILIS M.

SHAFT OF FEMUR

PROFUNDA FEMORIS V. & A.

FASCIA LATA

ADDUCTOR BREVIS M.

PERFORATING A. & V.

ADDUCTOR MAGNUS M.

COMMON PERONEAL & TIBIAL N.

SEMIMEMBRANOSUS M.

SUPERFICIAL FASCIA

GLUTEUS MAXIMUS M.

SEMITENDINOSUS M.

LONG HEAD OF BICEPS FEMORIS M.

POST. FEMORAL CUTANEOUS N.

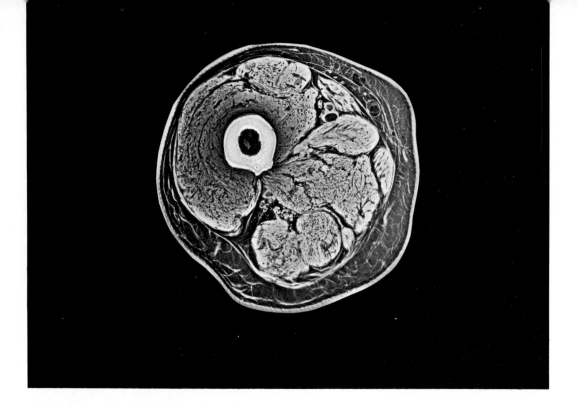

As described elsewhere, the profunda femoris artery may give rise to the medial and lateral femoral circumflex arteries. The profunda femoris artery invariably gives rise to three perforating arteries (the fourth perforating is the termination of the profunda femoris) and a variable number of muscular arteries. These cross sections are especially helpful in distinguishing between the perforating and muscular arteries. The perforating arteries penetrate the adductor magnus to reach the back of the thigh, as shown in this section. In this course to the back of the thigh, the perforating arteries lie very close to the femur under the cover of tendinous arches in the adductor magnus, as can be seen in the preceding illustration.

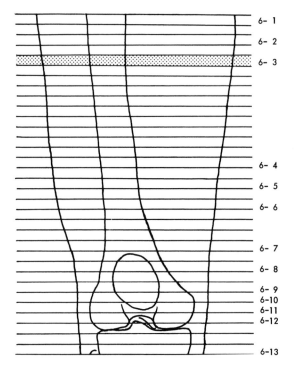

SECTION
6–3

Through the shaft of the femur, 2 cm below the preceding section

Anatomic Considerations

The profunda femoris (deep femoral) artery is the largest branch of the femoral artery. The profunda femoris artery can be observed in this and the preceding sections of the thigh, including those shown with the lower portion of the pelvis. As can be seen in this illustration, the adductor longus muscle lies anterior to the profunda femoris and separates this artery from the femoral artery. The pectineus and adductor brevis muscles lie posterior to the profunda femoris artery at a higher level; the adductor magnus lies posterior to the lower portion of the artery, as shown in this illustration.

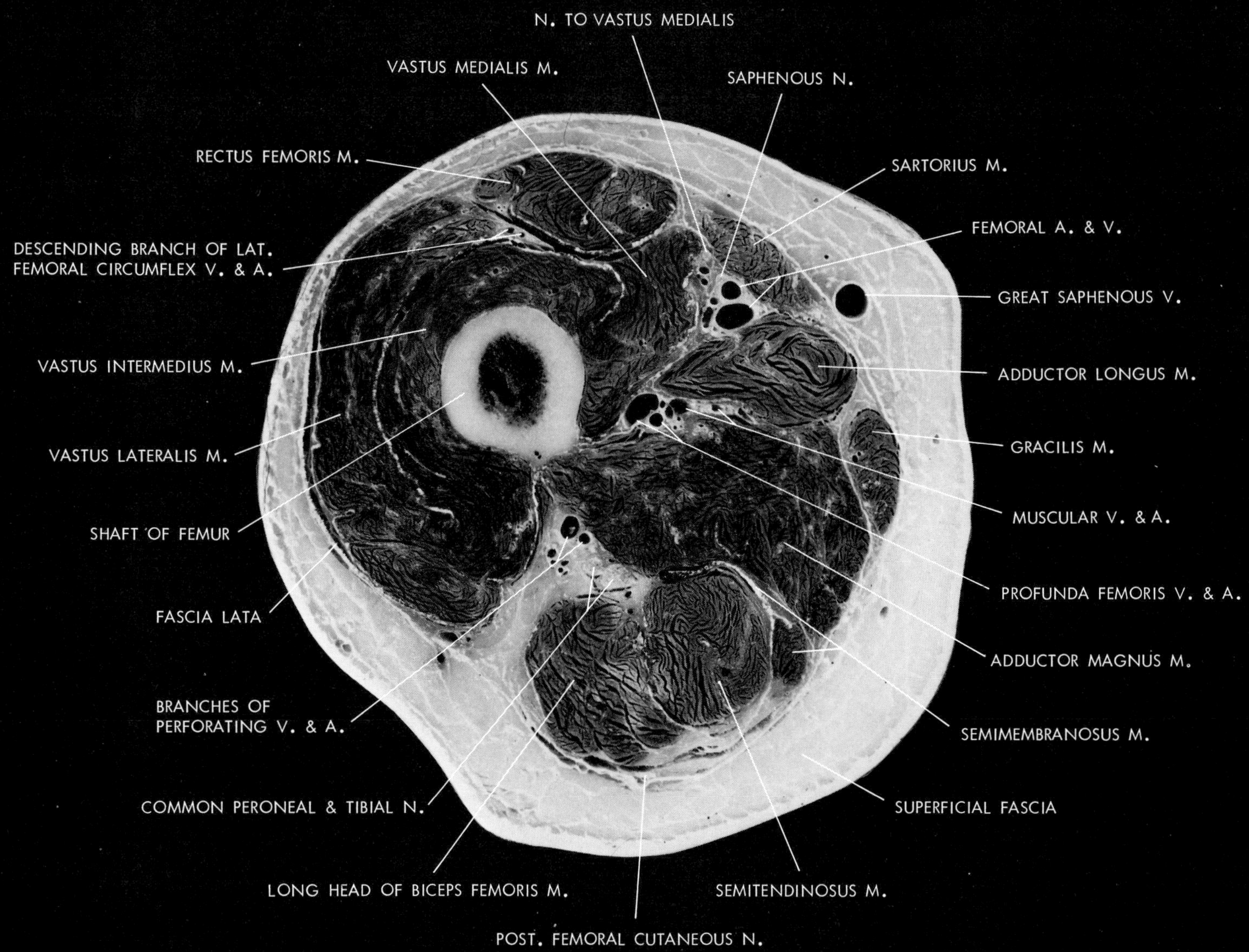

N. TO VASTUS MEDIALIS

VASTUS MEDIALIS M.

SAPHENOUS N.

RECTUS FEMORIS M.

SARTORIUS M.

DESCENDING BRANCH OF LAT.
FEMORAL CIRCUMFLEX V. & A.

FEMORAL A. & V.

GREAT SAPHENOUS V.

VASTUS INTERMEDIUS M.

ADDUCTOR LONGUS M.

VASTUS LATERALIS M.

GRACILIS M.

SHAFT OF FEMUR

MUSCULAR V. & A.

FASCIA LATA

PROFUNDA FEMORIS V. & A.

BRANCHES OF
PERFORATING V. & A.

ADDUCTOR MAGNUS M.

SEMIMEMBRANOSUS M.

COMMON PERONEAL & TIBIAL N.

SUPERFICIAL FASCIA

LONG HEAD OF BICEPS FEMORIS M.

SEMITENDINOSUS M.

POST. FEMORAL CUTANEOUS N.

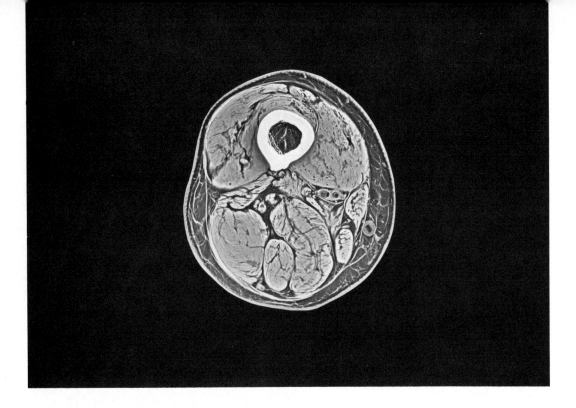

lateral side it is very dense and thickened, forming a long, strong band called the iliotibial tract, which stretches from the iliac crest to the lateral condyle of the tibia.

Proximally, the fascia lata is attached to the anterior part of the iliac crest, inguinal ligament, body of the pubis, margin of the pubic arch, ischial tuberosity, and gluteal fascia, through which it is attached to the sacro-tuberous ligament, coccyx, sacrum, and iliac crest. Distally, it is attached to the capsule of the knee joint, patella, tuberosity of the tibia, condyles of the tibia and femur, and head of the fibula; it is continuous posteriorly as the popliteal fascia.

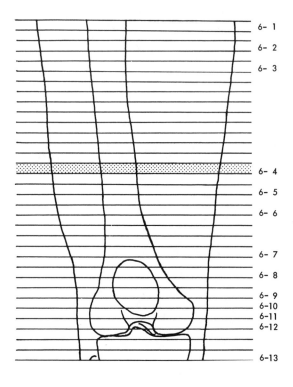

SECTION
6–4

Approximately through the lower half of the shaft of the femur, 10 cm below the preceding section

Anatomic Considerations

The superficial fascia forms a distinct layer over the entire thigh and is usually abundant on the medial side of the thigh. At times it is possible to distinguish two layers — a superficial fatty layer and a deep membranous layer. The two layers are separated from each other by the superficial vessels and nerves, the superficial inguinal lymph nodes, and the great saphenous vein. The superficial fascia is continuous with that of the abdomen, leg, and gluteal region.

The deep fascia of the thigh is called the fascia lata; because of its different morphology, there is a marked difference in strength between it and the superficial fascia. On the medial side the fascia is very thin, whereas on the

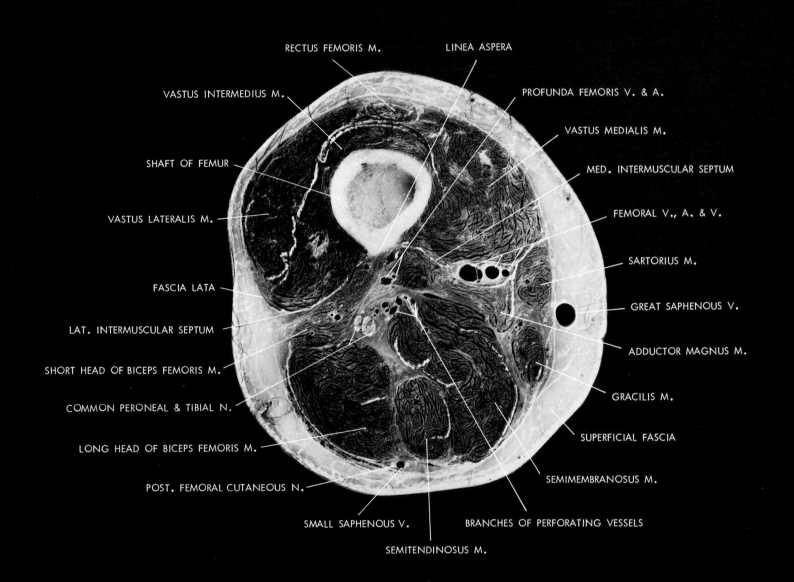

RECTUS FEMORIS M.

LINEA ASPERA

VASTUS INTERMEDIUS M.

PROFUNDA FEMORIS V. & A.

VASTUS MEDIALIS M.

SHAFT OF FEMUR

MED. INTERMUSCULAR SEPTUM

VASTUS LATERALIS M.

FEMORAL V., A. & V.

SARTORIUS M.

FASCIA LATA

GREAT SAPHENOUS V.

LAT. INTERMUSCULAR SEPTUM

ADDUCTOR MAGNUS M.

SHORT HEAD OF BICEPS FEMORIS M.

GRACILIS M.

COMMON PERONEAL & TIBIAL N.

LONG HEAD OF BICEPS FEMORIS M.

SUPERFICIAL FASCIA

SEMIMEMBRANOSUS M.

POST. FEMORAL CUTANEOUS N.

SMALL SAPHENOUS V.

BRANCHES OF PERFORATING VESSELS

SEMITENDINOSUS M.

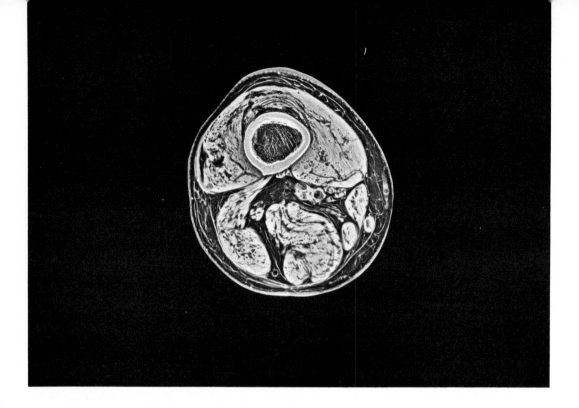

is composed of four large muscles that are collectively called the quadriceps femoris muscle. The femoral nerve also is associated with this compartment. The medial compartment is found between the medial and posterior intermuscular septa and contains the adductor muscles, which are innervated by the obturator nerve. The posterior or flexor compartment is found between the posterior and lateral intermuscular septa. The sciatic nerve innervates the hamstring muscles of this compartment.

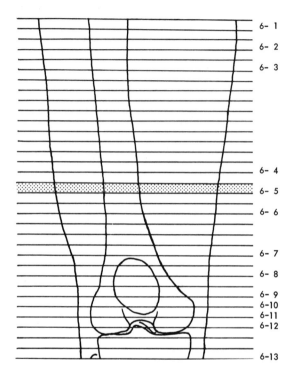

SECTION
6–5

Through the shaft of the femur, 2 cm below the preceding section

Anatomic Considerations

There are septa that pass from the deep surface of the fascia lata to the linea aspera of the femur. The two most prominent are the lateral and medial intermuscular septa. The posterior intermuscular septum is thin and difficult to demonstrate. The septa divide the thigh in three osteofascial compartments for the three great groups of muscles of the thigh. The extensor or anterior compartment is found between the medial and lateral intermuscular septa. It

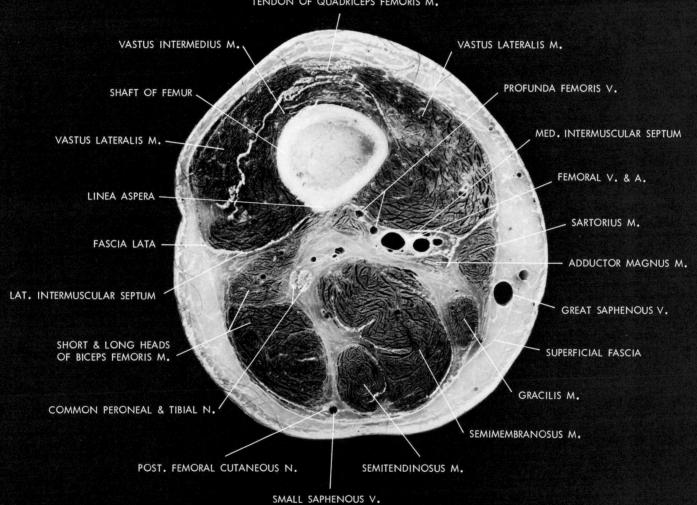

TENDON OF QUADRICEPS FEMORIS M.

VASTUS INTERMEDIUS M.

VASTUS LATERALIS M.

SHAFT OF FEMUR

PROFUNDA FEMORIS V.

VASTUS LATERALIS M.

MED. INTERMUSCULAR SEPTUM

LINEA ASPERA

FEMORAL V. & A.

SARTORIUS M.

FASCIA LATA

ADDUCTOR MAGNUS M.

LAT. INTERMUSCULAR SEPTUM

GREAT SAPHENOUS V.

SHORT & LONG HEADS
OF BICEPS FEMORIS M.

SUPERFICIAL FASCIA

COMMON PERONEAL & TIBIAL N.

GRACILIS M.

SEMIMEMBRANOSUS M.

POST. FEMORAL CUTANEOUS N.

SEMITENDINOSUS M.

SMALL SAPHENOUS V.

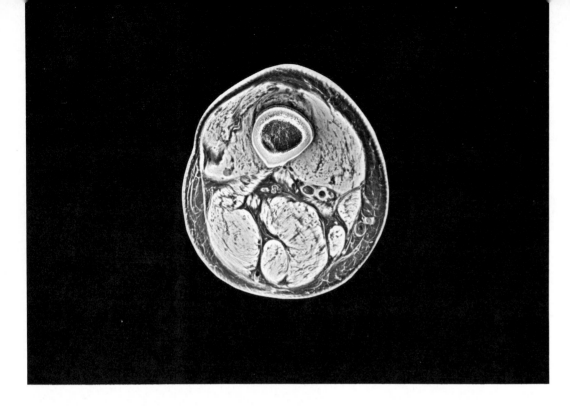

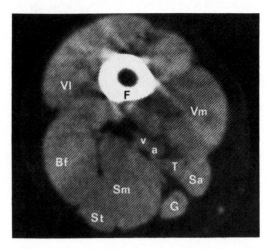

membranosus muscle (Sm), and gracilis muscle (G). F = femur, v = femoral vein, St = semitendinosus muscle, Bf = biceps femoris muscle, Vl = vastus lateralis muscle (courtesy Drs. Weinberger and Levinsohn and the publishers of the AJR).

SECTION
6–6

Through the shaft of the femur, 2 cm below the preceding section

Anatomic Considerations

Within the thickness of this section the femoral artery and vein exit the adductor canal and then become the popliteal artery and vein. The popliteal vessels can be followed in the next eight sections. At a higher level (as is shown here), the popliteal artery lies medial to the popliteal vein. At a lower level (Section 6–11), the popliteal artery lies anterior to the popliteal vein. In addition to muscular branches, the popliteal artery gives rise to two superior, one middle, and two inferior genicular arteries that participate in the arterial anastomosis around the knee joint. The popliteal artery terminates at the inferior margin of the popliteus muscle by dividing into the anterior and posterior tibial arteries.

Clinical Considerations

The CT scan of the distal thigh demonstrates a soft-tissue mass (T) obliterating the deep border of the sartorius muscle (SA). The mass occupies space between the sartorius muscle, vastus medialis muscle (Vm), femoral artery (a), semi-

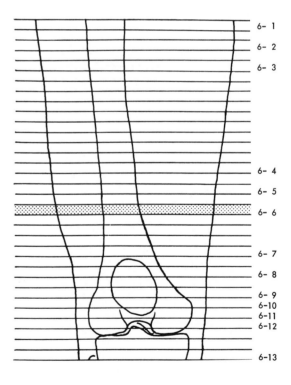

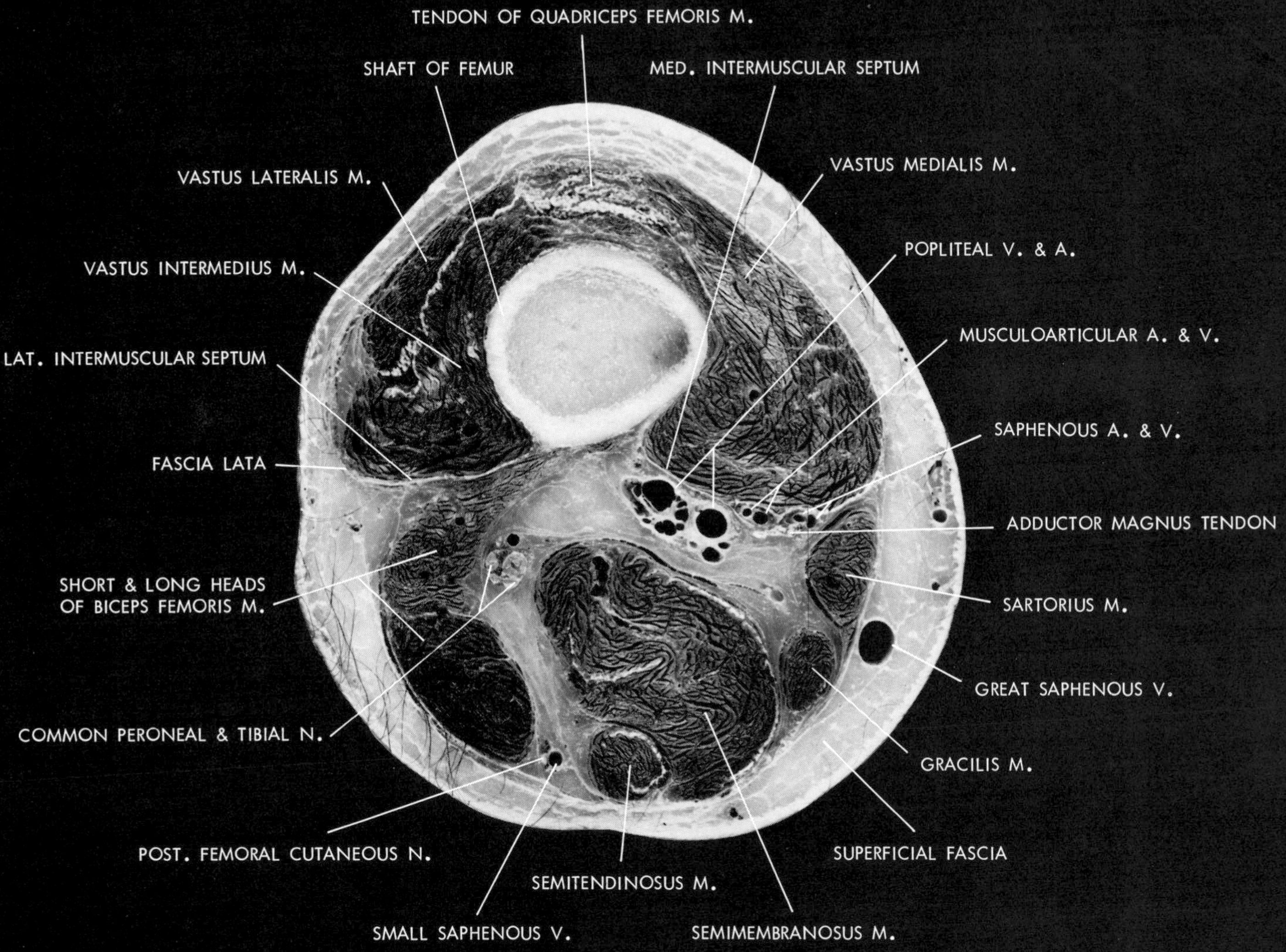

TENDON OF QUADRICEPS FEMORIS M.

SHAFT OF FEMUR

MED. INTERMUSCULAR SEPTUM

VASTUS LATERALIS M.

VASTUS MEDIALIS M.

VASTUS INTERMEDIUS M.

POPLITEAL V. & A.

LAT. INTERMUSCULAR SEPTUM

MUSCULOARTICULAR A. & V.

SAPHENOUS A. & V.

FASCIA LATA

ADDUCTOR MAGNUS TENDON

SHORT & LONG HEADS
OF BICEPS FEMORIS M.

SARTORIUS M.

GREAT SAPHENOUS V.

COMMON PERONEAL & TIBIAL N.

GRACILIS M.

POST. FEMORAL CUTANEOUS N.

SUPERFICIAL FASCIA

SMALL SAPHENOUS V.

SEMITENDINOSUS M.

SEMIMEMBRANOSUS M.

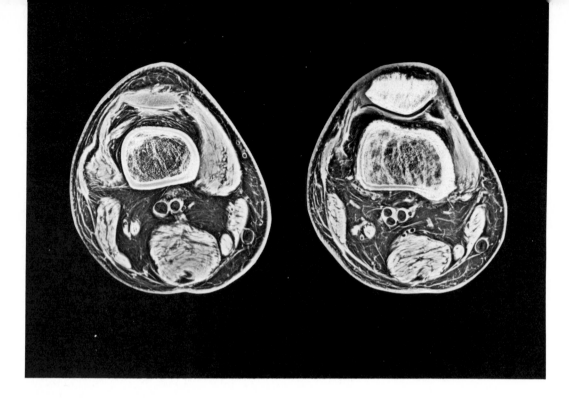

All four heads are the chief extensors of the leg; the last 15° of extension is chiefly due to the vasti muscles. Branches of the femoral nerve innervate each head of the muscle.

The patella, known as the kneecap, is a sesamoid bone set in the tendon of the quadriceps femoris muscle. Posteriorly, it articulates with the patellar surface of the femur. The anterior surface is covered by the expansion of the quadriceps tendon. The medial and lateral borders give attachment to the vasti medialis and lateralis. The patellar ligament (Sections 6–10 through 6–14), a continuation of the quadriceps femoris tendon, is attached to the apex of the patella and continues to the tuberosity of the tibia.

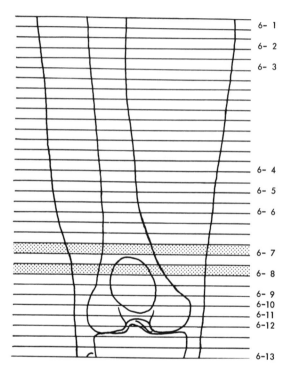

SECTION
6–7

Through the shaft of the femur, 4 cm below the preceding section

SECTION
6–8

Through the proximal portion of the patella, 2 cm below the preceding section

Anatomic Considerations

The quadriceps femoris muscle covers the anterior, medial, and lateral aspects of the thigh. It consists of the rectus femoris, vastus medialis, vastus intermedius, and vastus lateralis. All of these have been observed in the preceding sections.

The rectus femoris is the most anterior and arises by two tendons. It is the only component of the quadriceps muscle that passes across the hip joint and is a flexor of the joint.

The other three heads of the quadriceps are difficult to separate from each other. All three vasti muscles unite with the rectus femoris to form the tendon of the quadriceps and insert on the patella; through the patellar ligament the muscles attach to the tibial tuberosity.

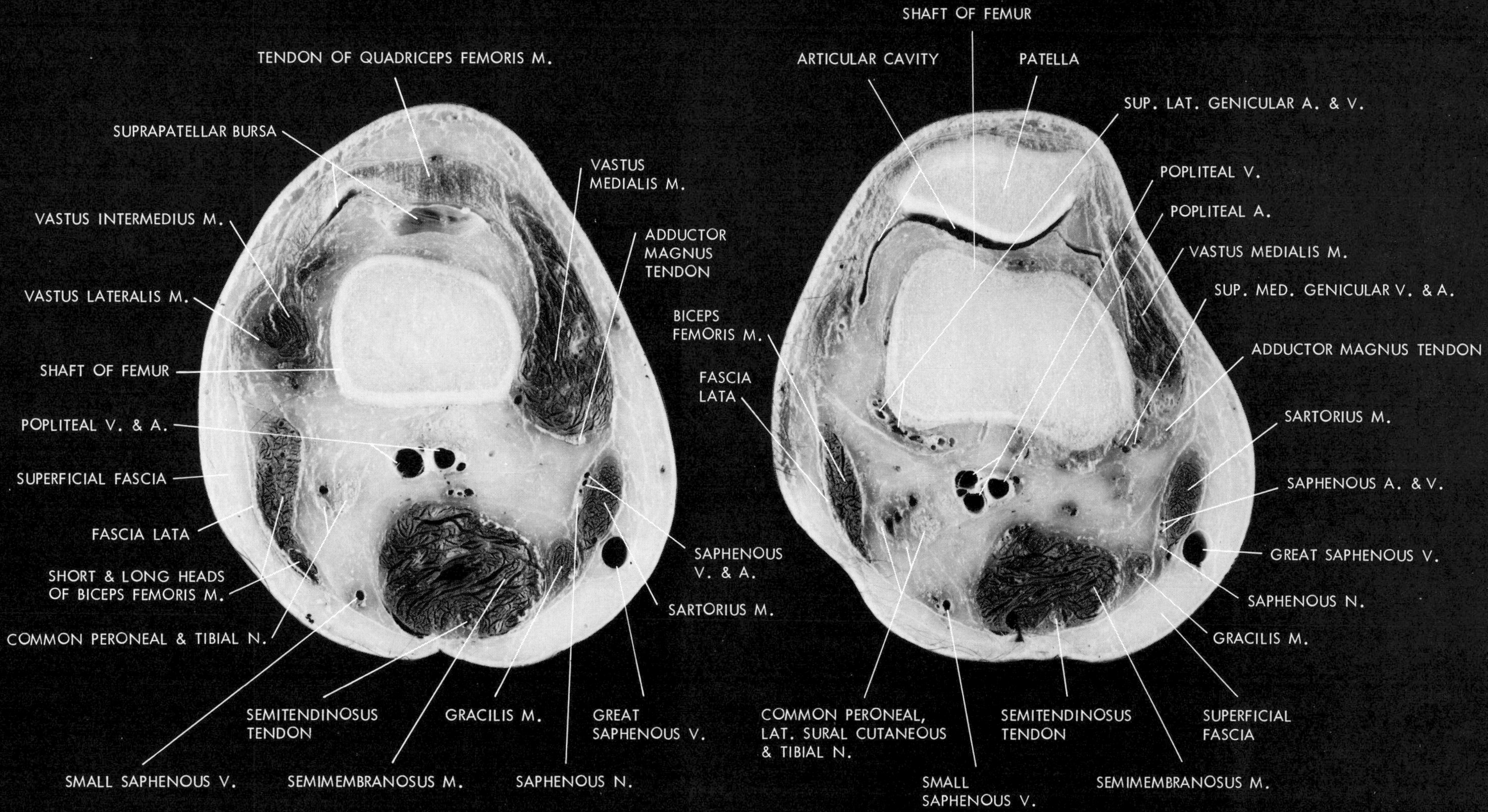

TENDON OF QUADRICEPS FEMORIS M.

SUPRAPATELLAR BURSA

VASTUS INTERMEDIUS M.

VASTUS LATERALIS M.

SHAFT OF FEMUR

POPLITEAL V. & A.

SUPERFICIAL FASCIA

FASCIA LATA

SHORT & LONG HEADS OF BICEPS FEMORIS M.

COMMON PERONEAL & TIBIAL N.

VASTUS MEDIALIS M.

ADDUCTOR MAGNUS TENDON

BICEPS FEMORIS M.

FASCIA LATA

SAPHENOUS V. & A.

SARTORIUS M.

SMALL SAPHENOUS V.

SEMITENDINOSUS TENDON

SEMIMEMBRANOSUS M.

GRACILIS M.

GREAT SAPHENOUS V.

SAPHENOUS N.

SHAFT OF FEMUR

ARTICULAR CAVITY

PATELLA

SUP. LAT. GENICULAR A. & V.

POPLITEAL V.

POPLITEAL A.

VASTUS MEDIALIS M.

SUP. MED. GENICULAR V. & A.

ADDUCTOR MAGNUS TENDON

SARTORIUS M.

SAPHENOUS A. & V.

GREAT SAPHENOUS V.

SAPHENOUS N.

GRACILIS M.

COMMON PERONEAL, LAT. SURAL CUTANEOUS & TIBIAL N.

SMALL SAPHENOUS V.

SEMITENDINOSUS TENDON

SEMIMEMBRANOSUS M.

SUPERFICIAL FASCIA

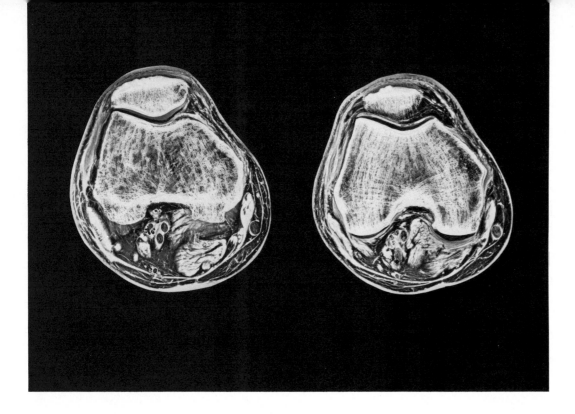

ligaments of the knee joint are extracapsular or intracapsular (the latter are considered in Section 6–11). In addition to the patellar ligament, the extracapsular ligaments include the medial and lateral collateral, the arcuate, and the oblique popliteal ligaments. The medial (tibial) collateral ligament, which is shown in several of the following illustrations, is a broad flat band extending from the medial femoral condyle to the medial aspect of the shaft of the tibia. The innermost portion of this ligament is attached to the edge of the medial meniscus. The lateral (fibular) collateral ligament is a cord-like structure extending from the lateral femoral condyle to the head of the fibula. The arcuate ligament arches over the popliteus, and the oblique ligament is a tendinous reflection derived from the semimembranosus.

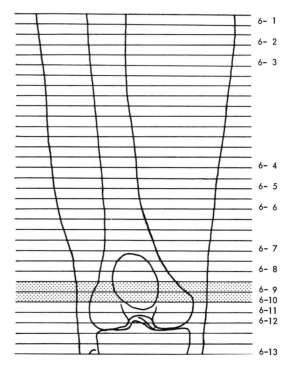

SECTION
6–9

Through the knee joint, 2 cm below the preceding section

SECTION
6–10

Through the knee joint, 1 cm below the preceding section

Anatomic Considerations

The knee joint is a synovial one and may be considered as three articulations: one between the femur and patella and two between the condyles of the femur and tibia. As with other synovial joints, the articulating surfaces of the bones are covered with hyaline cartilage and the joint is surrounded by an articular capsule. Anteriorly, the capsule is deficient and is replaced by the tendon of the quadriceps femoris, the patella, and the patellar ligament. The capsule is strengthened by expansions from the tendons of the vastus medialis and lateralis on each side of the patella. Posteriorly, there is an opening in the capsule behind the lateral tibial condyle for the tendon of the popliteus. The

LOWER EXTREMITY
260

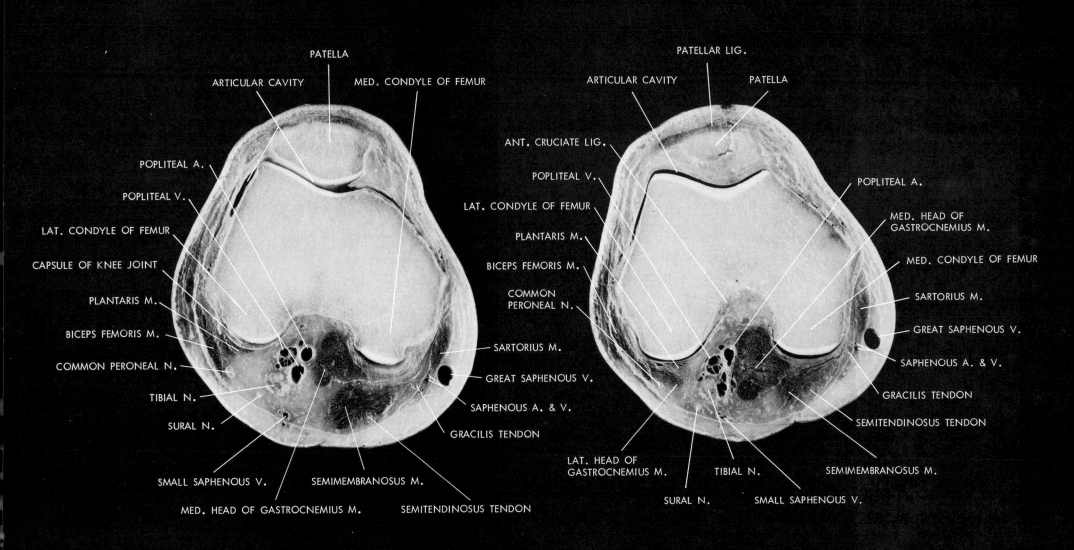

PATELLA

ARTICULAR CAVITY   MED. CONDYLE OF FEMUR

POPLITEAL A.

POPLITEAL V.

LAT. CONDYLE OF FEMUR

CAPSULE OF KNEE JOINT

PLANTARIS M.

BICEPS FEMORIS M.

COMMON PERONEAL N.

TIBIAL N.

SURAL N.

SMALL SAPHENOUS V.

SEMIMEMBRANOSUS M.

MED. HEAD OF GASTROCNEMIUS M.

SEMITENDINOSUS TENDON

SARTORIUS M.

GREAT SAPHENOUS V.

SAPHENOUS A. & V.

GRACILIS TENDON

PATELLAR LIG.

ARTICULAR CAVITY   PATELLA

ANT. CRUCIATE LIG.

POPLITEAL V.

LAT. CONDYLE OF FEMUR

PLANTARIS M.

BICEPS FEMORIS M.

COMMON PERONEAL N.

POPLITEAL A.

MED. HEAD OF GASTROCNEMIUS M.

MED. CONDYLE OF FEMUR

SARTORIUS M.

GREAT SAPHENOUS V.

SAPHENOUS A. & V.

GRACILIS TENDON

SEMITENDINOSUS TENDON

SEMIMEMBRANOSUS M.

LAT. HEAD OF GASTROCNEMIUS M.

TIBIAL N.

SURAL N.

SMALL SAPHENOUS V.

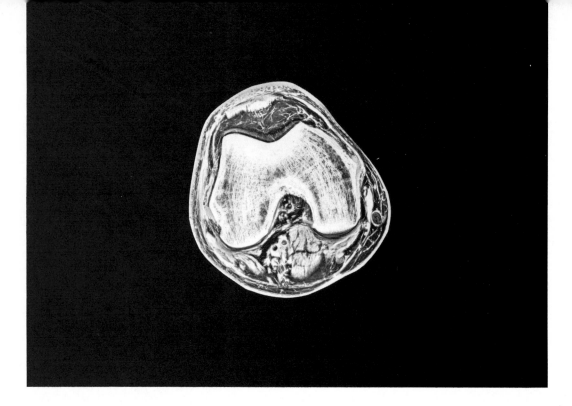

SECTION
6–11

Through the knee joint, 1 cm below the preceding section

Anatomic Considerations

The two cruciate ligaments (shown in this section) are strong intracapsular ligaments that cross each other within the joint cavity. While these ligaments are intracapsular they are also extrasynovial; this occurs because during the development of the knee joint three separate articulations are formed: two between the tibia and femur and the third between the femur and patella.

The anterior cruciate ligament extends from the anterior part of the intercondylar region of the tibia to the posterior part of the medial surface of the lateral condyle of the femur. The posterior cruciate ligament passes from the posterior part of the intracondylar fossa of the tibia to the anterior part of the lateral surface of the medial condyle of the femur.

The medial and lateral menisci are semilunar cartilages that deepen the cavities on the surfaces of the tibial condyles and act as shock absorbers. The medial meniscus is semicircular, whereas the lateral one is circular in form. These fibrocartilaginous structures have thick peripheral margins that attach to the capsule and to the head of the tibia and thin inner margins that are free. The transverse ligament connects the anterior portion of the two menisci. Like the cruciate ligaments, the transverse ligament is intracapsular.

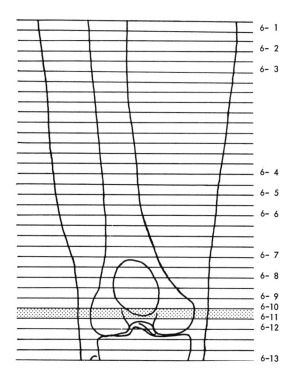

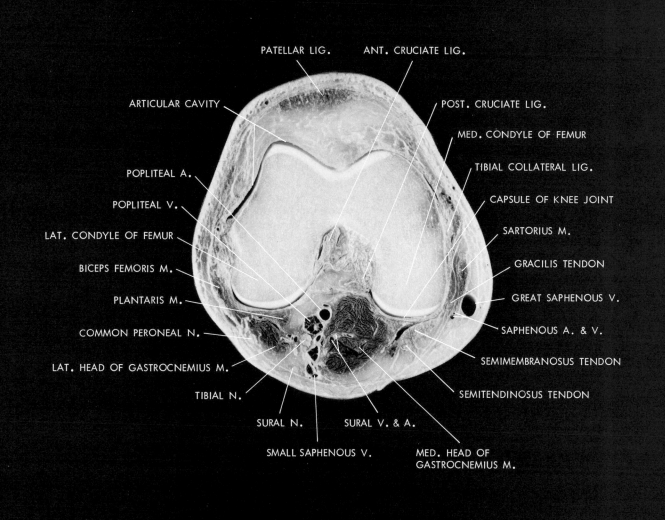

PATELLAR LIG.   ANT. CRUCIATE LIG.

ARTICULAR CAVITY   POST. CRUCIATE LIG.

MED. CONDYLE OF FEMUR

TIBIAL COLLATERAL LIG.

POPLITEAL A.   CAPSULE OF KNEE JOINT

POPLITEAL V.   SARTORIUS M.

LAT. CONDYLE OF FEMUR   GRACILIS TENDON

BICEPS FEMORIS M.   GREAT SAPHENOUS V.

PLANTARIS M.

COMMON PERONEAL N.   SAPHENOUS A. & V.

LAT. HEAD OF GASTROCNEMIUS M.   SEMIMEMBRANOSUS TENDON

TIBIAL N.   SEMITENDINOSUS TENDON

SURAL N.   SURAL V. & A.

SMALL SAPHENOUS V.   MED. HEAD OF
GASTROCNEMIUS M.

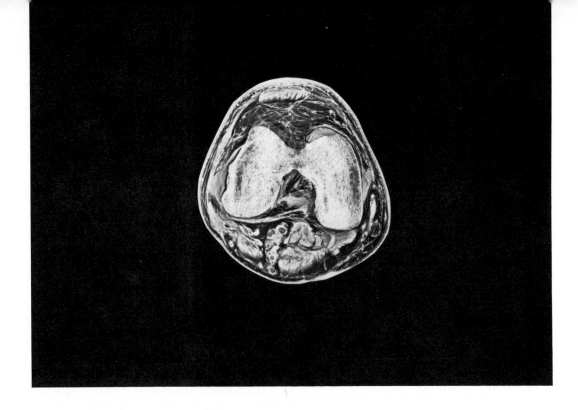

femoris, semitendinosus, and semimembranosus muscles). Extension is performed by the quadriceps femoris. Medial rotation is performed mainly by the sartorius, gracilis, and semitendinosus muscles, and lateral rotation is by the biceps femoris. The relationships of the knee joint to surrounding structures can be seen in this and adjacent illustrations. Certain relationships, especially those posterior to the knee, are important to consider; these posterior structures include the popliteal artery and vein, the tibial and common peroneal nerves, and the gastrocnemius and hamstring muscles.

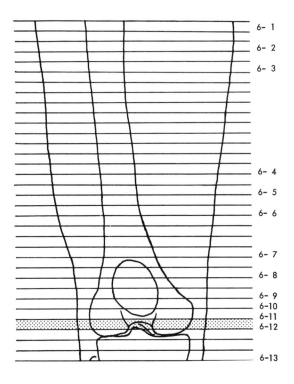

SECTION 6–12

Through the knee joint, 1 cm below the preceding section

Anatomic Considerations

The chief movements that occur at the knee joint are flexion and extension. Additional movements of gliding, rolling, and rotation also occur, because the shapes and curvatures of the articulating surfaces differ. Since the lateral condyle of the femur is shorter and more curved than the medial femoral condyle, it completes its forward roll on the tibia before the medial condyle during extension of the knee joint.

Flexion of the knee joint is produced mainly by the hamstrings (biceps

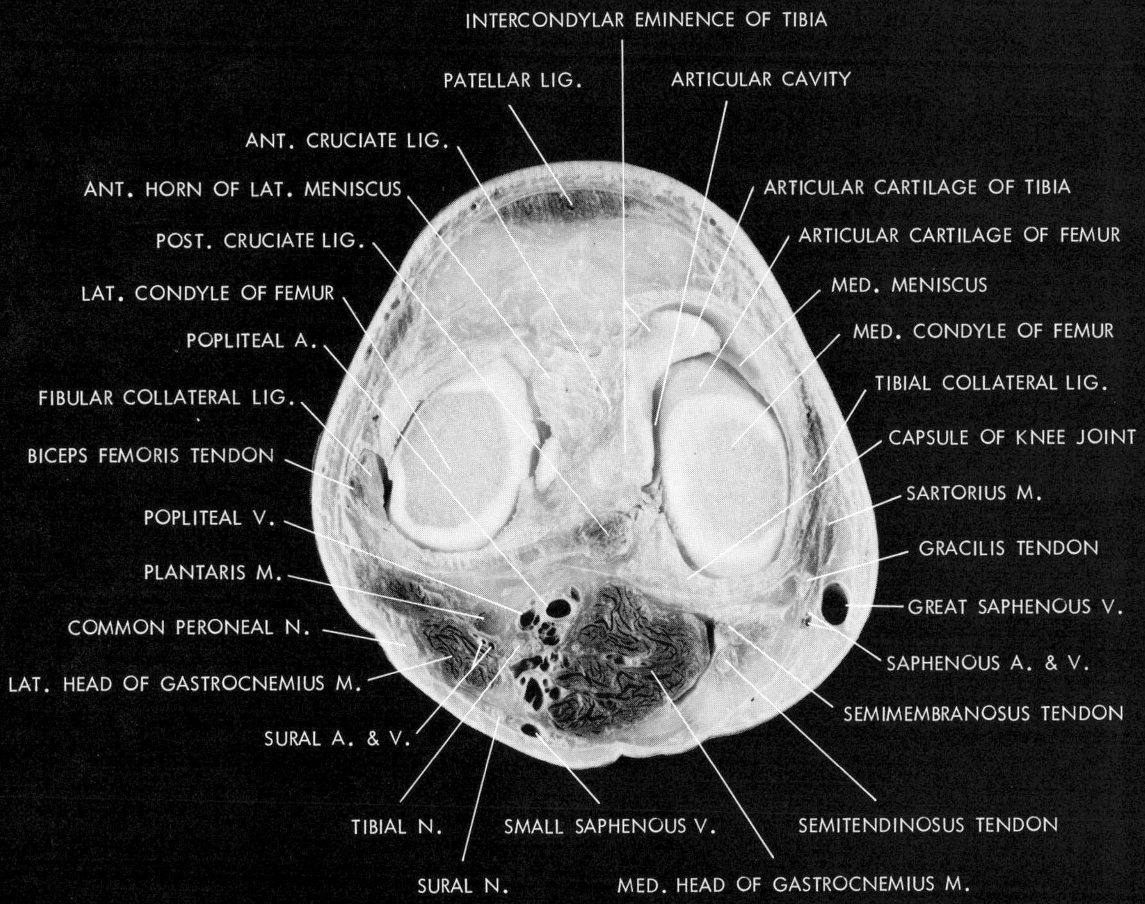

INTERCONDYLAR EMINENCE OF TIBIA

PATELLAR LIG. ARTICULAR CAVITY

ANT. CRUCIATE LIG.

ANT. HORN OF LAT. MENISCUS ARTICULAR CARTILAGE OF TIBIA

POST. CRUCIATE LIG. ARTICULAR CARTILAGE OF FEMUR

LAT. CONDYLE OF FEMUR MED. MENISCUS

POPLITEAL A. MED. CONDYLE OF FEMUR

FIBULAR COLLATERAL LIG. TIBIAL COLLATERAL LIG.

BICEPS FEMORIS TENDON CAPSULE OF KNEE JOINT

POPLITEAL V. SARTORIUS M.

PLANTARIS M. GRACILIS TENDON

COMMON PERONEAL N. GREAT SAPHENOUS V.

LAT. HEAD OF GASTROCNEMIUS M. SAPHENOUS A. & V.

SURAL A. & V. SEMIMEMBRANOSUS TENDON

TIBIAL N. SMALL SAPHENOUS V. SEMITENDINOSUS TENDON

SURAL N. MED. HEAD OF GASTROCNEMIUS M.

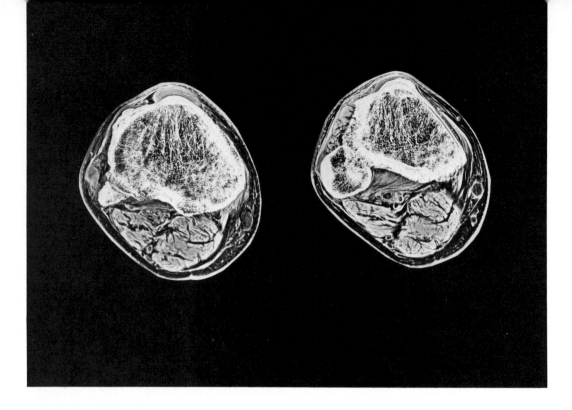

and the fibular notch of the distal end of the tibia. The bones are not in contact with each other but are separated by the interosseous ligament that binds them together. The joint is strengthened by anterior and posterior tibiofibular ligaments.

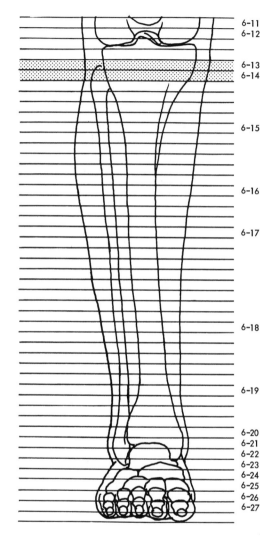

SECTION 6–13

Through the superior tibiofibular joint, 3 cm below the preceding section

SECTION 6–14

Through the head of the fibula, 1 cm below the preceding section

Anatomic Considerations

The tibia and fibula are connected by the superior and inferior tibiofibular joints and the interosseous membrane. These illustrations demonstrate the superior tibiofibular joint. It is a synovial joint between the head of the fibula and the lateral condyle of the tibia. The bones are united by a fibrous capsule and strengthened by anterior and posterior ligaments.

The interosseous membrane can be observed in Sections 6–15 to 6–19. It stretches across the interval between the interosseous borders of the two bones and separates the muscles on the anterior from those on the posterior aspect of the leg. In the proximal part there is an oval opening for the passage of the anterior tibial vessels, and distally, just superior to the ankle joint, there is a small opening for the perforating branch of the peroneal artery.

The inferior tibiofibular joint can be seen in Section 6–20. It is a syndesmosis type of joint between the medial side of the distal end of the fibula

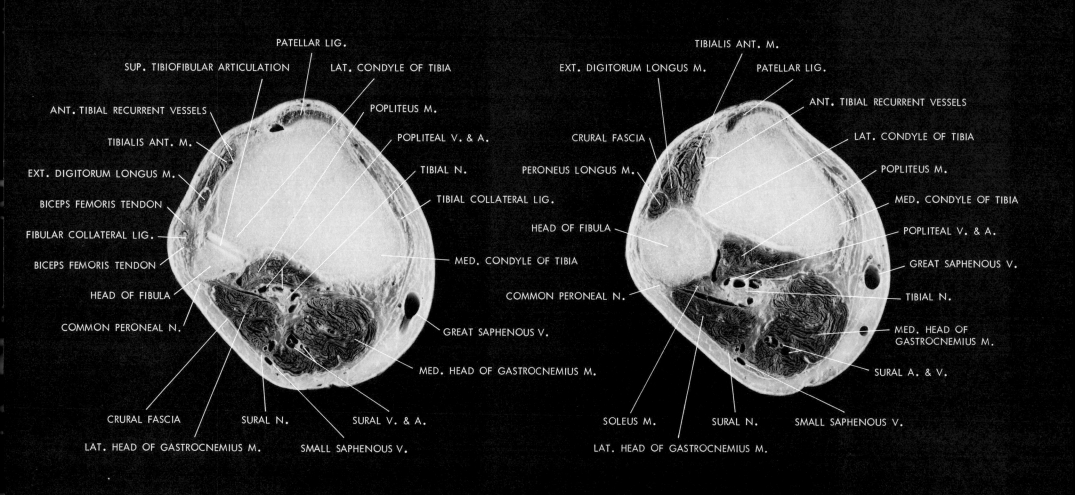

PATELLAR LIG.

SUP. TIBIOFIBULAR ARTICULATION

LAT. CONDYLE OF TIBIA

ANT. TIBIAL RECURRENT VESSELS

POPLITEUS M.

TIBIALIS ANT. M.

POPLITEAL V. & A.

EXT. DIGITORUM LONGUS M.

TIBIAL N.

BICEPS FEMORIS TENDON

TIBIAL COLLATERAL LIG.

FIBULAR COLLATERAL LIG.

BICEPS FEMORIS TENDON

MED. CONDYLE OF TIBIA

HEAD OF FIBULA

COMMON PERONEAL N.

GREAT SAPHENOUS V.

MED. HEAD OF GASTROCNEMIUS M.

CRURAL FASCIA

SURAL N.

SURAL V. & A.

LAT. HEAD OF GASTROCNEMIUS M.

SMALL SAPHENOUS V.

TIBIALIS ANT. M.

EXT. DIGITORUM LONGUS M.

PATELLAR LIG.

ANT. TIBIAL RECURRENT VESSELS

CRURAL FASCIA

LAT. CONDYLE OF TIBIA

PERONEUS LONGUS M.

POPLITEUS M.

MED. CONDYLE OF TIBIA

HEAD OF FIBULA

POPLITEAL V. & A.

GREAT SAPHENOUS V.

COMMON PERONEAL N.

TIBIAL N.

MED. HEAD OF
GASTROCNEMIUS M.

SURAL A. & V.

SOLEUS M.

SURAL N.

SMALL SAPHENOUS V.

LAT. HEAD OF GASTROCNEMIUS M.

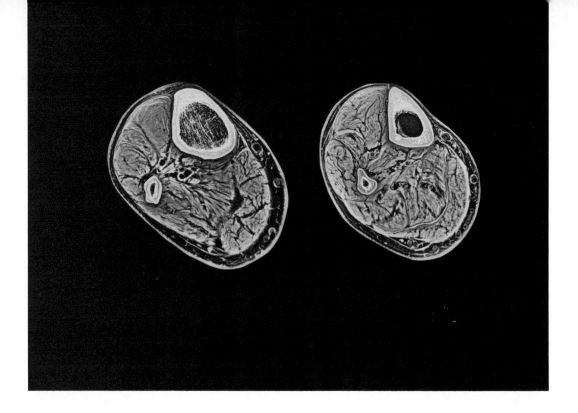

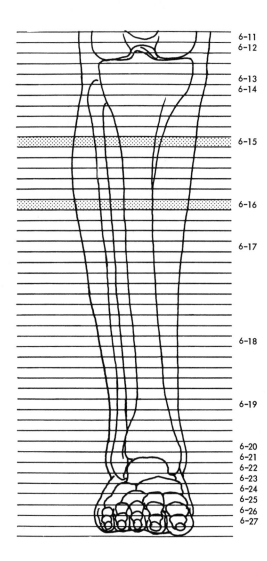

6-11
6-12

6-13
6-14

6-15

6-16

6-17

6-18

6-19

6-20
6-21
6-22
6-23
6-24
6-25
6-26
6-27

SECTION
6–15

*Through the
upper half of the
shafts of the
tibia and fibula,
5 cm below the
preceding section*

SECTION
6–16

*Through the
shafts of the
tibia and fibula,
6 cm below the
preceding section*

Anatomic Considerations

Cross sections are especially valuable in helping to understand the compartments of the leg. The structures that form the boundaries of the osteofascial
compartments of the leg are the two bones (tibia, fibula), the interosseous
membrane (which lies between the bones), and the deep (crural) fascia. These
structures divide the leg into three compartments: the small anterior and
lateral ones and the large posterior compartment. The anterior compartment
lies anterior to the interosseous membrane; the posterior one lies posterior to
it. The lateral compartment is delineated by the anterior and posterior
intermuscular septa, which are prolongations of the crural fasciae that attach to
the fibula. Each compartment contains a group of muscles and a nerve that
innervates the muscles. The anterior and posterior compartments have their
own blood supply; the lateral compartment receives its blood supply from the
posterior compartment.

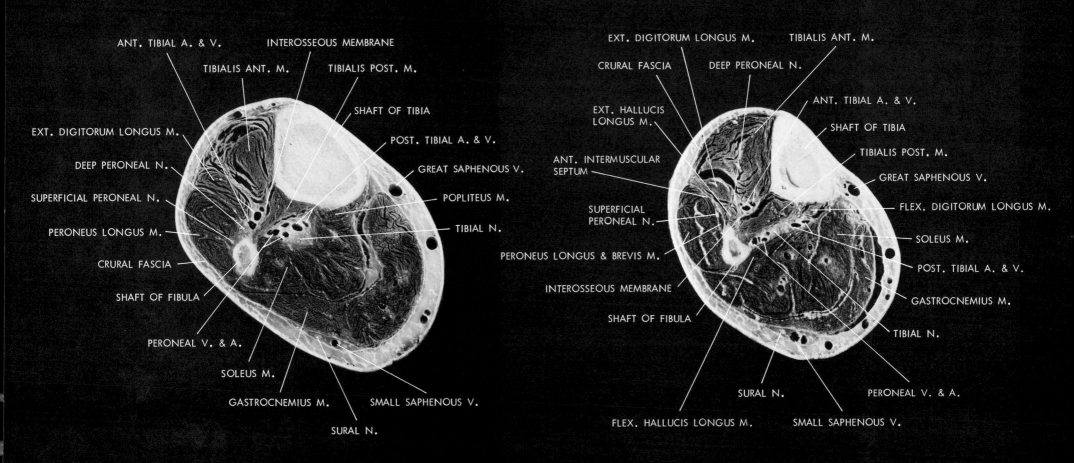

ANT. TIBIAL A. & V.

INTEROSSEOUS MEMBRANE

TIBIALIS ANT. M.

TIBIALIS POST. M.

SHAFT OF TIBIA

EXT. DIGITORUM LONGUS M.

POST. TIBIAL A. & V.

DEEP PERONEAL N.

GREAT SAPHENOUS V.

SUPERFICIAL PERONEAL N.

POPLITEUS M.

PERONEUS LONGUS M.

TIBIAL N.

CRURAL FASCIA

SHAFT OF FIBULA

PERONEAL V. & A.

SOLEUS M.

GASTROCNEMIUS M.

SMALL SAPHENOUS V.

SURAL N.

EXT. DIGITORUM LONGUS M.

TIBIALIS ANT. M.

CRURAL FASCIA

DEEP PERONEAL N.

ANT. TIBIAL A. & V.

EXT. HALLUCIS LONGUS M.

SHAFT OF TIBIA

TIBIALIS POST. M.

ANT. INTERMUSCULAR SEPTUM

GREAT SAPHENOUS V.

FLEX. DIGITORUM LONGUS M.

SUPERFICIAL PERONEAL N.

SOLEUS M.

PERONEUS LONGUS & BREVIS M.

POST. TIBIAL A. & V.

INTEROSSEOUS MEMBRANE

GASTROCNEMIUS M.

SHAFT OF FIBULA

TIBIAL N.

SURAL N.

PERONEAL V. & A.

FLEX. HALLUCIS LONGUS M.

SMALL SAPHENOUS V.

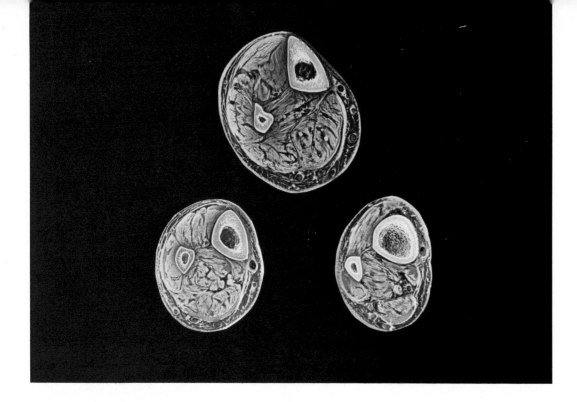

posterior) are located in the deep group. As can be seen in the illustrations, the neurovascular elements are found in the deep group; the peroneal vessels are related posterior to the fibula, and the tibial nerve and posterior tibial vessels are related to the tibia.

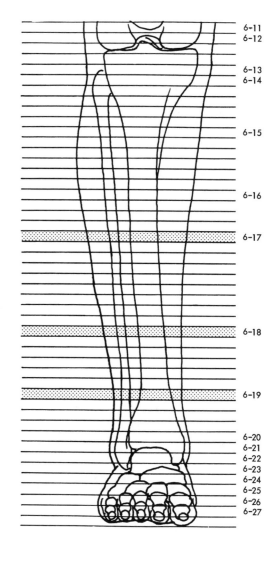

SECTION
6–17

Through the shafts of the tibia and fibula, 4 cm below the preceding section

SECTION
6–18

Through the shafts of the tibia and fibula, 9 cm below the preceding section

SECTION
6–19

Through the shafts of the tibia and fibula, 6 cm below the preceding section

Anatomic Considerations

The anterior compartment of the leg is small and located anterior to the interosseous membrane. This compartment contains a muscle that inverts the foot (tibialis anterior), two muscles that extend the toes (extensor digitorum longus and extensor hallucis longus), and their blood supply and innervation (anterior tibial vessels and deep peroneal nerve).

The lateral compartment contains the muscles that evert the foot, the peroneus longus and brevis, and the nerve that innervates them, the superficial peroneal nerve. There is no major artery located in this compartment. The blood supply to the muscles comes from branches of the peroneal artery that pass through the posterior intermuscular septum from the posterior compartment.

The muscles in the posterior compartment, which is the largest one in the leg, are divided into superficial and deep groups of muscles by a layer of deep fascia. The muscles that act mainly to flex the foot (gastrocnemius, soleus, and plantaris) are found in the superficial group. The muscles that flex the toes (flexor hallucis longus and flexor digitorum longus) and invert the foot (tibialis

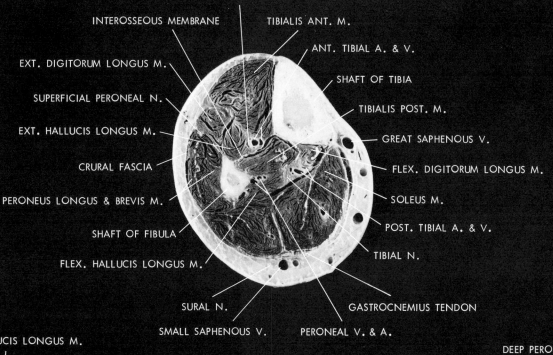

DEEP PERONEAL N.

INTEROSSEOUS MEMBRANE — TIBIALIS ANT. M.

ANT. TIBIAL A. & V.

EXT. DIGITORUM LONGUS M. — SHAFT OF TIBIA

SUPERFICIAL PERONEAL N. — TIBIALIS POST. M.

EXT. HALLUCIS LONGUS M. — GREAT SAPHENOUS V.

CRURAL FASCIA — FLEX. DIGITORUM LONGUS M.

PERONEUS LONGUS & BREVIS M. — SOLEUS M.

SHAFT OF FIBULA — POST. TIBIAL A. & V.

FLEX. HALLUCIS LONGUS M. — TIBIAL N.

SURAL N. — GASTROCNEMIUS TENDON

SMALL SAPHENOUS V. — PERONEAL V. & A.

EXT. HALLUCIS LONGUS M.

CRURAL FASCIA — TIBIALIS ANT. M.

EXT. DIGITORUM LONGUS M. — DEEP PERONEAL N.

SUPERFICIAL PERONEAL N. — ANT. TIBIAL V. & A.

ANT. INTERMUSCULAR SEPTUM — SHAFT OF TIBIA

SHAFT OF FIBULA — INTEROSSEOUS MEMBRANE

TIBIALIS POST. M.

PERONEUS LONGUS & BREVIS M. — GREAT SAPHENOUS V.

PERONEAL A. & V. — FLEX. DIGITORUM LONGUS M.

POST. INTERMUSCULAR SEPTUM — POST. TIBIAL V. & A.

FLEX. HALLUCIS LONGUS M. — TIBIAL N.

SURAL N. — SOLEUS M.

SMALL SAPHENOUS V. — GASTROCNEMIUS TENDON

DEEP PERONEAL N.

EXT. HALLUCIS LONGUS M. — TIBIALIS ANT. M.

PERONEAL A. & V. — ANT. TIBIAL A. & V.

EXT. DIGITORUM LONGUS M. — SHAFT OF TIBIA

CRURAL FASCIA — FLEX. HALLUCIS LONGUS M.

INTEROSSEOUS MEMBRANE — GREAT SAPHENOUS V.

SHAFT OF FIBULA — TIBIALIS POST. M. & TENDON

PERONEUS LONGUS TENDON — FLEX. DIGITORUM LONGUS M. & TENDON

POST. INTERMUSCULAR SEPTUM — POST. TIBIAL V. & A.

PERONEUS BREVIS M. — SOLEUS M.

SURAL N. — TIBIAL N.

SMALL SAPHENOUS V. — TENDO CALCANEUS

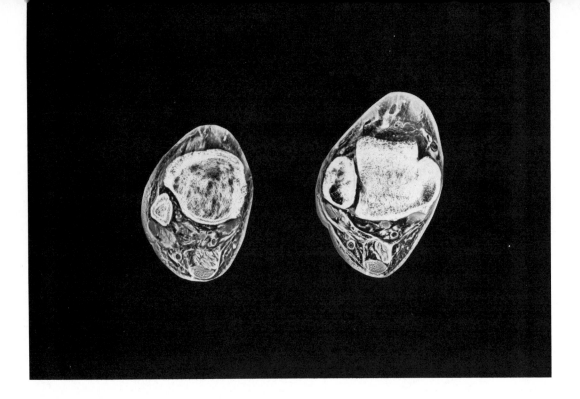

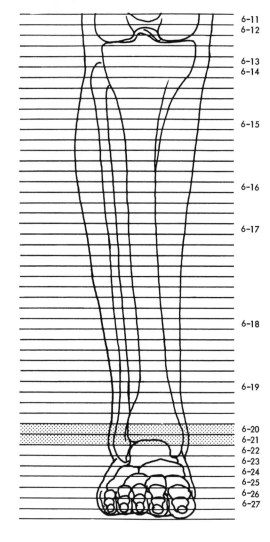

SECTION
6–20

Through the inferior tibiofibular joint, 4 cm below the preceding section

SECTION
6–21

Through the ankle joint, 1 cm below the preceding section

Anatomic Considerations

The ankle joint is a synovial joint of the hinge type. The bony structures involved are the distal end of the tibia and its malleolus, the lateral malleolus of the fibula, and the trochlea of the talus. It is a joint of great strength because of the powerful ligaments and tendons around it and the interlocking of the articulating surfaces.

The capsule of the joint is thin anteriorly and posteriorly but is reinforced by strong ligaments on the medial and lateral sides. The medial, or deltoid, ligament is extremely strong and passes from the lower border of the medial malleolus to the body of the talus, sustentaculum tali, neck of the talus, plantar calcaneonavicular ligament, and tuberosity of the navicular bone. By this extensive attachment, it not only supports the ankle but helps to maintain the medial longitudinal arch of the foot. The lateral ligament consists of three bands: The anterior talofibular and posterior talofibular ligaments are thickenings of the capsule, whereas the third band, the calcaneofibular ligament, is a separate cord.

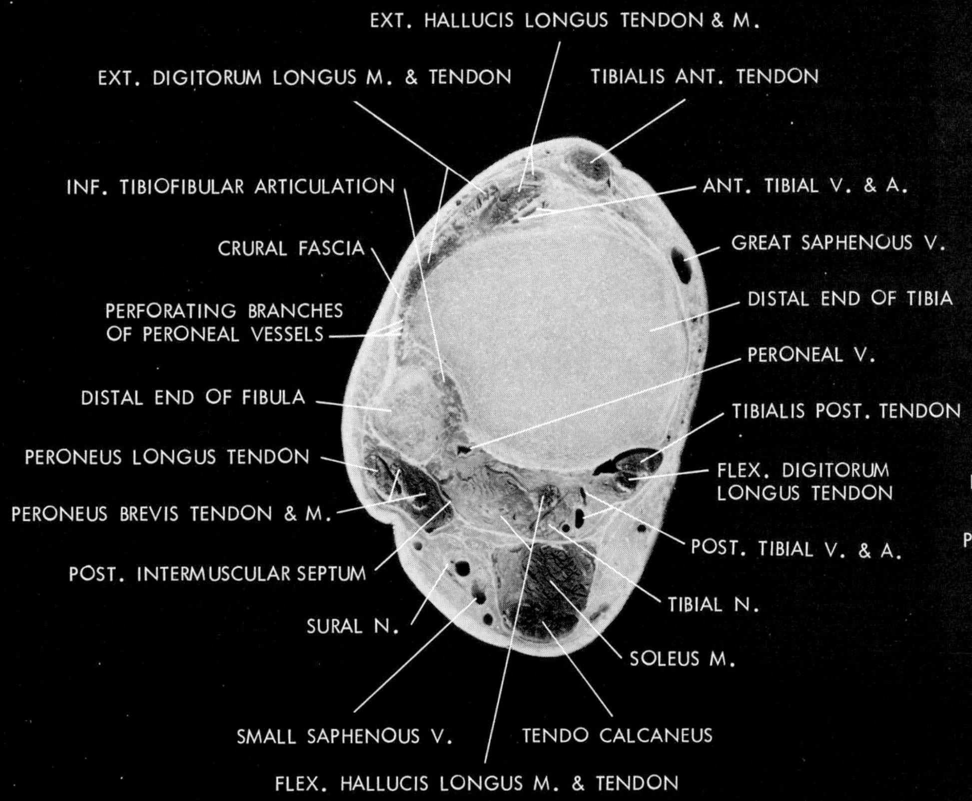

EXT. HALLUCIS LONGUS TENDON & M.

EXT. DIGITORUM LONGUS M. & TENDON

TIBIALIS ANT. TENDON

INF. TIBIOFIBULAR ARTICULATION

ANT. TIBIAL V. & A.

CRURAL FASCIA

GREAT SAPHENOUS V.

PERFORATING BRANCHES
OF PERONEAL VESSELS

DISTAL END OF TIBIA

PERONEAL V.

DISTAL END OF FIBULA

TIBIALIS POST. TENDON

PERONEUS LONGUS TENDON

FLEX. DIGITORUM
LONGUS TENDON

PERONEUS BREVIS TENDON & M.

POST. INTERMUSCULAR SEPTUM

POST. TIBIAL V. & A.

SURAL N.

TIBIAL N.

SOLEUS M.

SMALL SAPHENOUS V.

TENDO CALCANEUS

FLEX. HALLUCIS LONGUS M. & TENDON

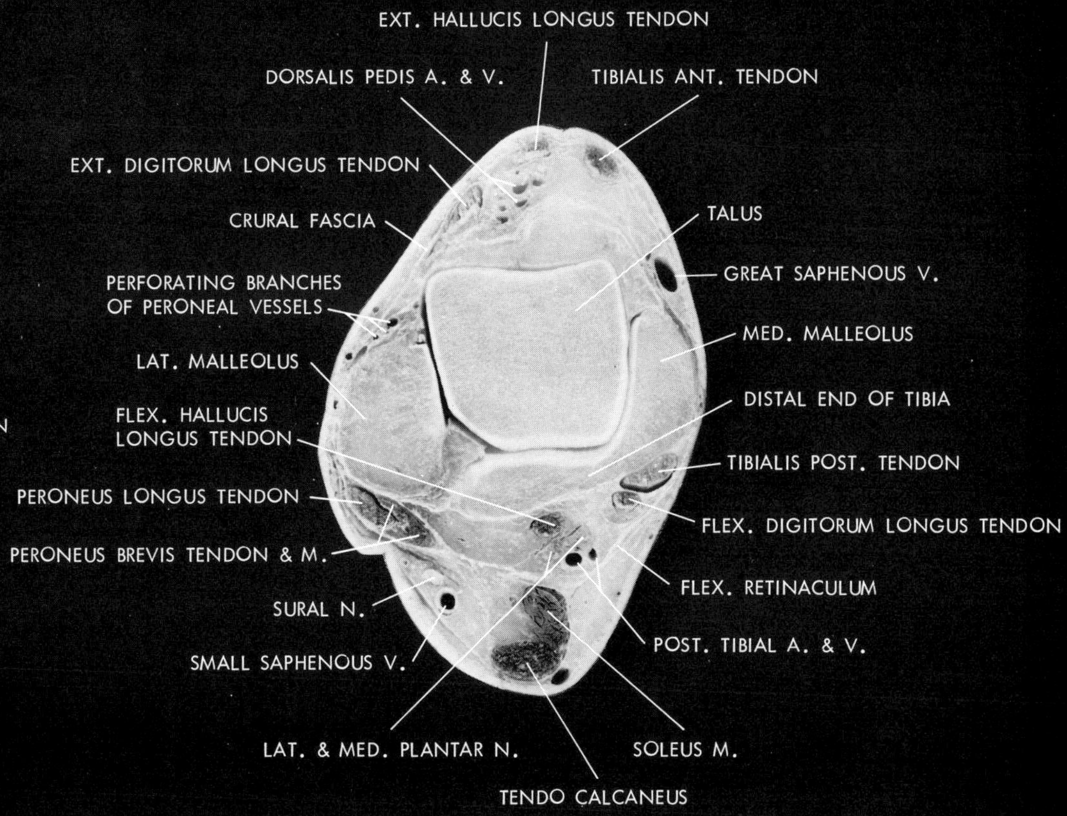

EXT. HALLUCIS LONGUS TENDON

DORSALIS PEDIS A. & V.

TIBIALIS ANT. TENDON

EXT. DIGITORUM LONGUS TENDON

CRURAL FASCIA

TALUS

GREAT SAPHENOUS V.

PERFORATING BRANCHES
OF PERONEAL VESSELS

MED. MALLEOLUS

LAT. MALLEOLUS

DISTAL END OF TIBIA

FLEX. HALLUCIS
LONGUS TENDON

TIBIALIS POST. TENDON

PERONEUS LONGUS TENDON

FLEX. DIGITORUM LONGUS TENDON

PERONEUS BREVIS TENDON & M.

FLEX. RETINACULUM

SURAL N.

POST. TIBIAL A. & V.

SMALL SAPHENOUS V.

LAT. & MED. PLANTAR N.

SOLEUS M.

TENDO CALCANEUS

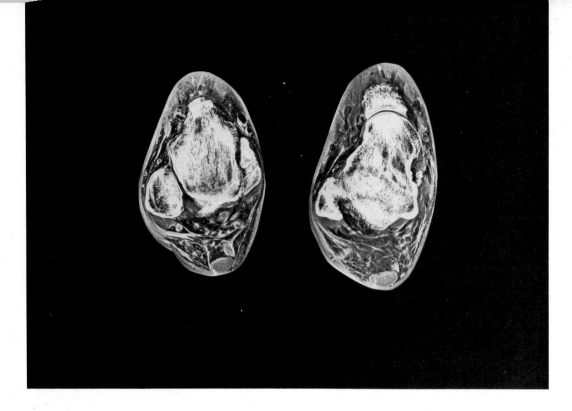

SECTION
6–22

Through a portion of the ankle joint, 1 cm below the preceding section

SECTION
6–23

Through a portion of the tarsal bones, 1 cm below the preceding section

Anatomic Considerations

The flexor retinaculum (laciniate ligament) can be observed in these sections. This is a thickened band of deep fascia that bridges the hollow between the medial tubercle of the calcaneus and the medial malleolus. The relationships of the structures that pass from the leg deep to the flexor retinaculum and enter the sole of the foot can be observed in these two illustrations. From anterior to posterior, these structures are the tendon of the tibialis posterior, the tendon of the flexor digitorum longus, the neurovascular elements, and the tendon of the flexor hallucis longus.

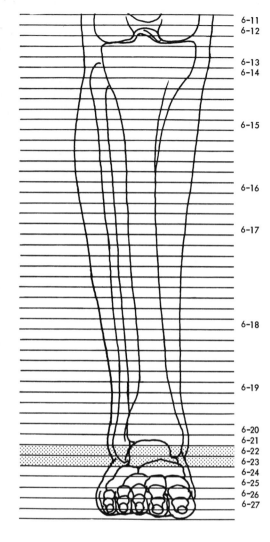

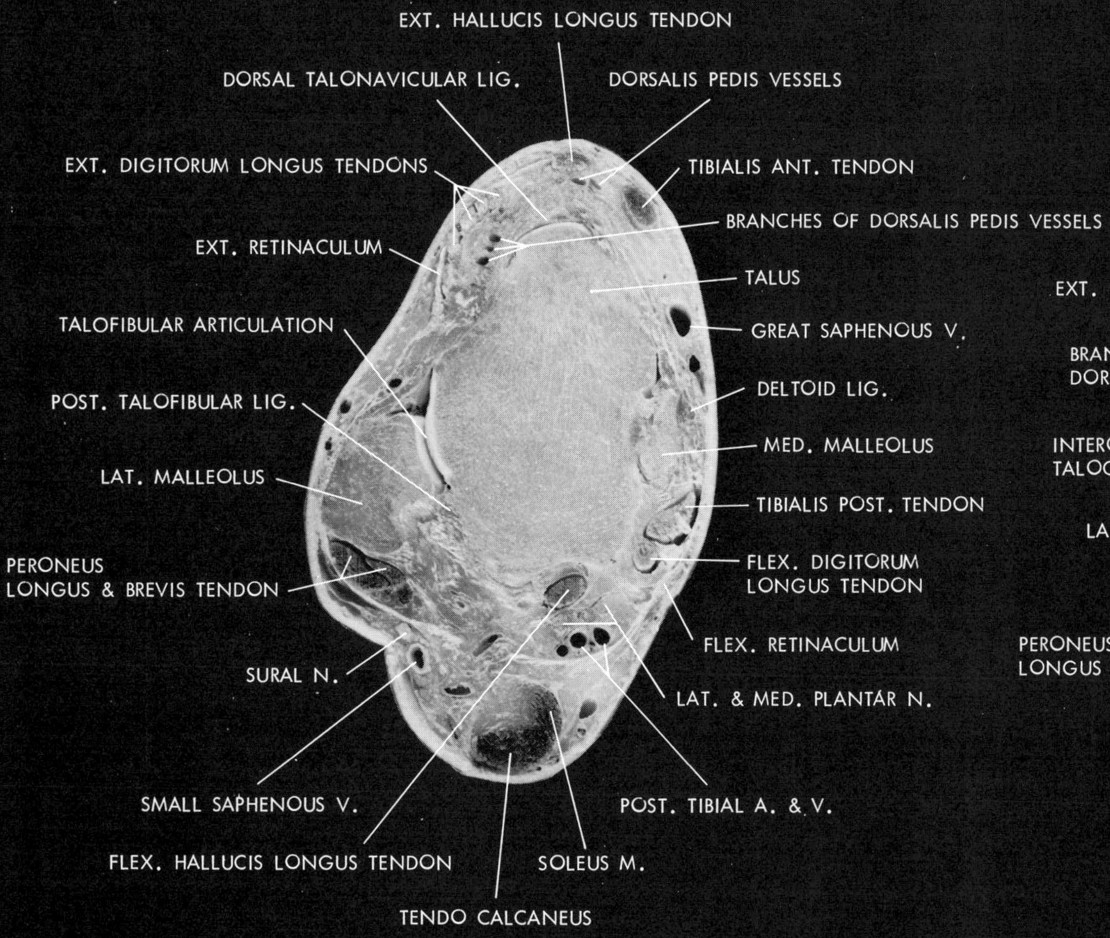

EXT. HALLUCIS LONGUS TENDON

DORSAL TALONAVICULAR LIG.

DORSALIS PEDIS VESSELS

EXT. DIGITORUM LONGUS TENDONS

TIBIALIS ANT. TENDON

EXT. RETINACULUM

BRANCHES OF DORSALIS PEDIS VESSELS

TALOFIBULAR ARTICULATION

TALUS

GREAT SAPHENOUS V.

POST. TALOFIBULAR LIG.

DELTOID LIG.

LAT. MALLEOLUS

MED. MALLEOLUS

TIBIALIS POST. TENDON

PERONEUS
LONGUS & BREVIS TENDON

FLEX. DIGITORUM
LONGUS TENDON

SURAL N.

FLEX. RETINACULUM

LAT. & MED. PLANTAR N.

SMALL SAPHENOUS V.

POST. TIBIAL A. & V.

FLEX. HALLUCIS LONGUS TENDON

SOLEUS M.

TENDO CALCANEUS

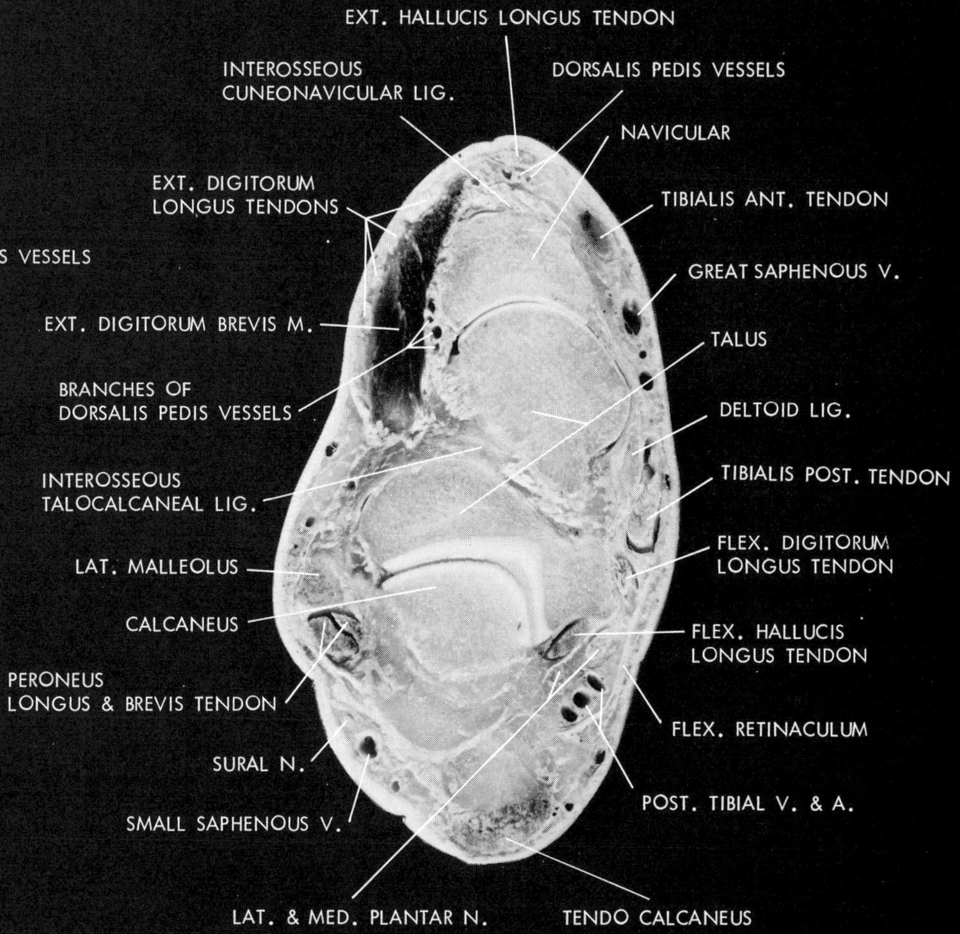

EXT. HALLUCIS LONGUS TENDON

INTEROSSEOUS
CUNEONAVICULAR LIG.

DORSALIS PEDIS VESSELS

NAVICULAR

EXT. DIGITORUM
LONGUS TENDONS

TIBIALIS ANT. TENDON

GREAT SAPHENOUS V.

EXT. DIGITORUM BREVIS M.

TALUS

BRANCHES OF
DORSALIS PEDIS VESSELS

DELTOID LIG.

INTEROSSEOUS
TALOCALCANEAL LIG.

TIBIALIS POST. TENDON

LAT. MALLEOLUS

FLEX. DIGITORUM
LONGUS TENDON

CALCANEUS

FLEX. HALLUCIS
LONGUS TENDON

PERONEUS
LONGUS & BREVIS TENDON

FLEX. RETINACULUM

SURAL N.

POST. TIBIAL V. & A.

SMALL SAPHENOUS V.

LAT. & MED. PLANTAR N.

TENDO CALCANEUS

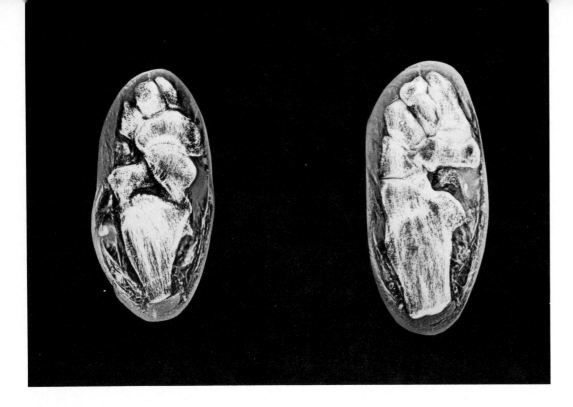

The digits each consist of three phalanges, except the first toe (hallux), which has only two. The base of the proximal phalanx articulates with the metatarsal bone and forms the metatarsophalangeal joint. The phalanges articulate with each other to form the interphalangeal joints.

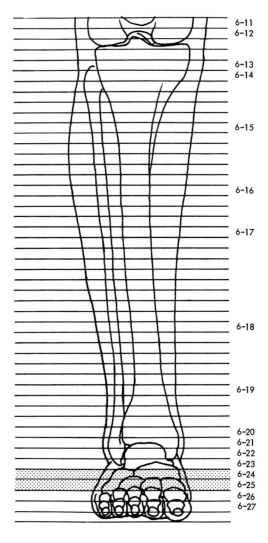

SECTION 6–24

Through a portion of the tarsal bones, 1 cm below the preceding section

SECTION 6–25

Through a portion of the tarsal bones, 1 cm below the preceding section

Anatomic Considerations

The bones of the foot are divided into the tarsus, the metatarsus, and the digits.

The tarsus consists of seven tarsal bones divided essentially into a posterior and an anterior row. The posterior row contains the talus and calcaneus. The talus sits on the calcaneus just distal to the tibia. In the second row there are four bones: From lateral to medial they are the cuboid and three cuneiform bones. The navicular bone separates the cuneiform bones from the talus. The tarsal bones articulate with one another and form the intertarsal joints. The only tarsal bones that have ossification centers at birth are the talus and calcaneus.

The five metatarsal bones articulate at their bases with one another and form the intermetatarsal joints; they articulate with the cuneiforms and cuboid, forming the tarsometatarsal joints.

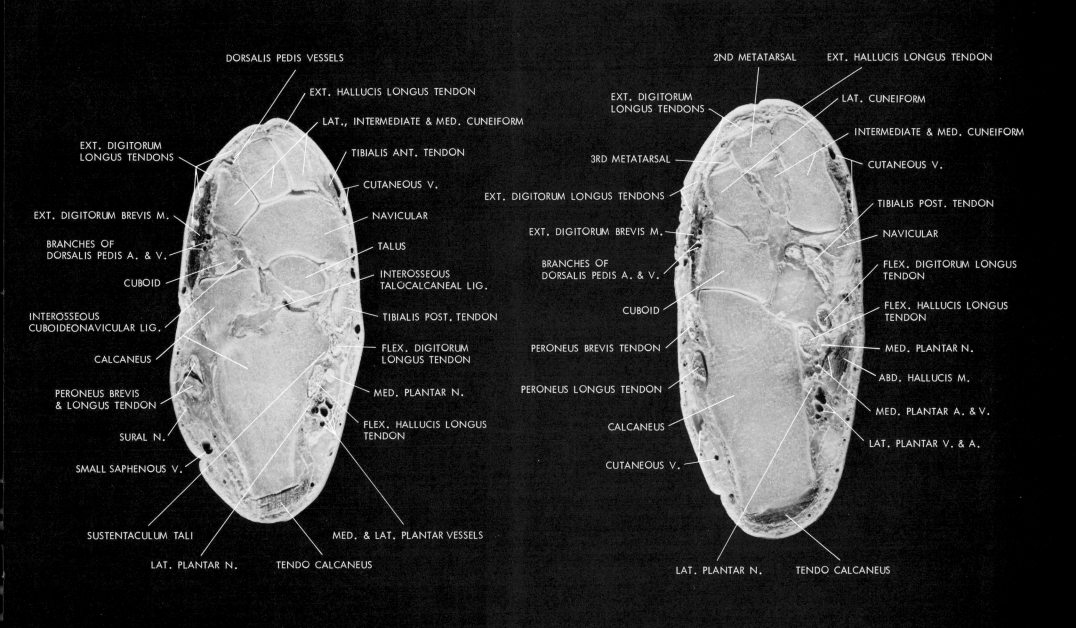

DORSALIS PEDIS VESSELS

EXT. HALLUCIS LONGUS TENDON

LAT., INTERMEDIATE & MED. CUNEIFORM

TIBIALIS ANT. TENDON

CUTANEOUS V.

NAVICULAR

TALUS

INTEROSSEOUS TALOCALCANEAL LIG.

TIBIALIS POST. TENDON

FLEX. DIGITORUM LONGUS TENDON

MED. PLANTAR N.

FLEX. HALLUCIS LONGUS TENDON

MED. & LAT. PLANTAR VESSELS

EXT. DIGITORUM LONGUS TENDONS

EXT. DIGITORUM BREVIS M.

BRANCHES OF DORSALIS PEDIS A. & V.

CUBOID

INTEROSSEOUS CUBOIDEONAVICULAR LIG.

CALCANEUS

PERONEUS BREVIS & LONGUS TENDON

SURAL N.

SMALL SAPHENOUS V.

SUSTENTACULUM TALI

LAT. PLANTAR N.

TENDO CALCANEUS

2ND METATARSAL

EXT. HALLUCIS LONGUS TENDON

LAT. CUNEIFORM

INTERMEDIATE & MED. CUNEIFORM

CUTANEOUS V.

TIBIALIS POST. TENDON

NAVICULAR

FLEX. DIGITORUM LONGUS TENDON

FLEX. HALLUCIS LONGUS TENDON

MED. PLANTAR N.

ABD. HALLUCIS M.

MED. PLANTAR A. & V.

LAT. PLANTAR V. & A.

EXT. DIGITORUM LONGUS TENDONS

3RD METATARSAL

EXT. DIGITORUM LONGUS TENDONS

EXT. DIGITORUM BREVIS M.

BRANCHES OF DORSALIS PEDIS A. & V.

CUBOID

PERONEUS BREVIS TENDON

PERONEUS LONGUS TENDON

CALCANEUS

CUTANEOUS V.

LAT. PLANTAR N.

TENDO CALCANEUS

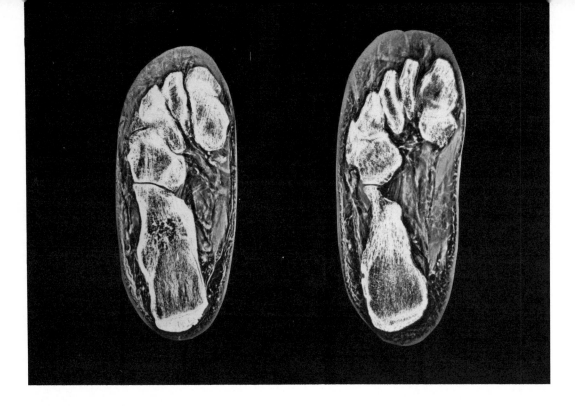

peroneus longus give added support in maintaining the arch, as does the plantar aponeurosis.

The transverse arch is best observed across the line of the tarsometatarsal articulations.

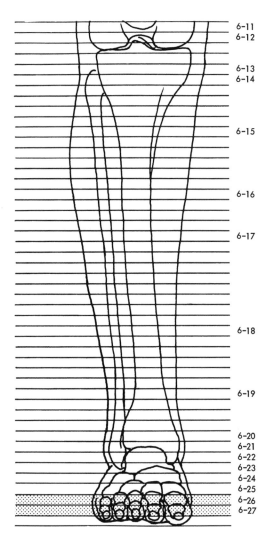

SECTION
6–26

Through the bones of the sole of the foot, 1 cm below the preceding section

SECTION
6–27

Through the bones of the sole of the foot, 1 cm below the preceding section

Anatomic Considerations

The tarsal and metatarsal bones form the longitudinal and transverse arches of the foot. The arches are maintained by the shape of the bones, the tension of the ligaments and plantar aponeurosis, and the action of the long and short muscles of the foot.

The longitudinal arch has its greatest height along the medial side of the foot and the talus is at the summit of the arch. The posterior pillar is formed by the calcaneus. The anterior pillar is formed by the rest of the tarsal and metatarsal bones and is divided into a medial and a lateral column. The medial column is composed of the navicular, three cuneiform, and the medial three metatarsal bones. The lateral column is formed by the cuboid and lateral two metatarsal bones. The ligaments that are most important in preventing flattening of the arch are the plantar calcaneonavicular (spring) ligament and the long and short plantar ligaments. The tendons of the tibialis posterior and

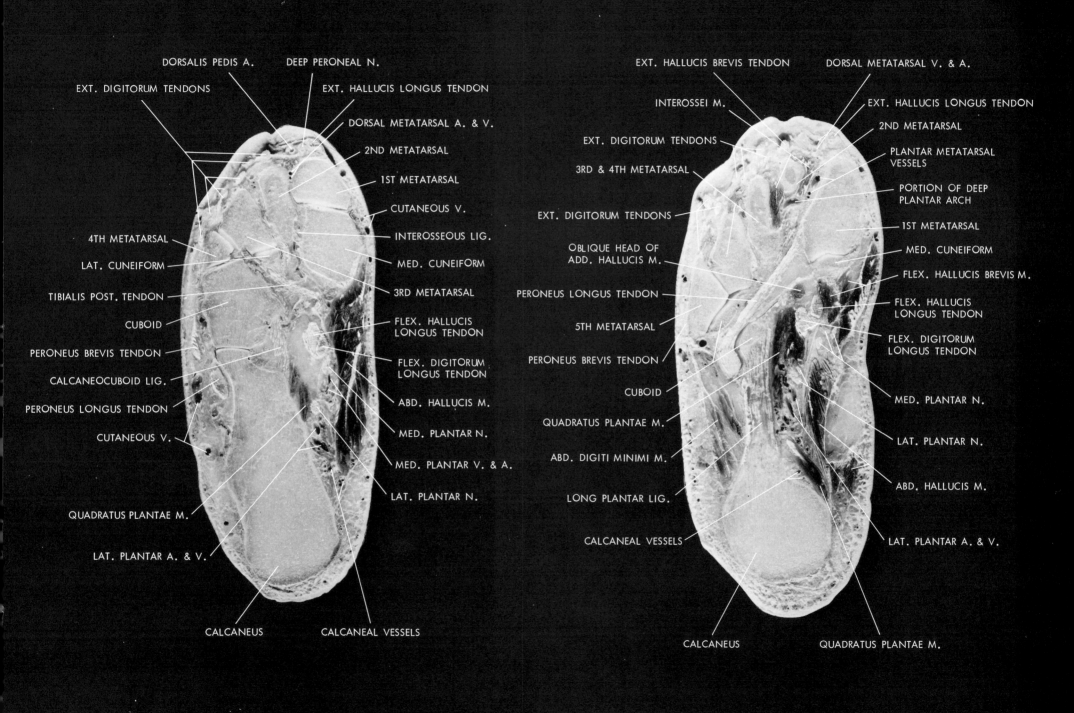

DORSALIS PEDIS A. DEEP PERONEAL N.

EXT. DIGITORUM TENDONS

EXT. HALLUCIS LONGUS TENDON

DORSAL METATARSAL A. & V.

2ND METATARSAL

1ST METATARSAL

CUTANEOUS V.

INTEROSSEOUS LIG.

4TH METATARSAL

MED. CUNEIFORM

LAT. CUNEIFORM

3RD METATARSAL

TIBIALIS POST. TENDON

FLEX. HALLUCIS
LONGUS TENDON

CUBOID

PERONEUS BREVIS TENDON

FLEX. DIGITORUM
LONGUS TENDON

CALCANEOCUBOID LIG.

PERONEUS LONGUS TENDON

ABD. HALLUCIS M.

CUTANEOUS V.

MED. PLANTAR N.

QUADRATUS PLANTAE M.

MED. PLANTAR V. & A.

LAT. PLANTAR A. & V.

LAT. PLANTAR N.

CALCANEUS CALCANEAL VESSELS

EXT. HALLUCIS BREVIS TENDON

DORSAL METATARSAL V. & A.

INTEROSSEI M.

EXT. HALLUCIS LONGUS TENDON

EXT. DIGITORUM TENDONS

2ND METATARSAL

3RD & 4TH METATARSAL

PLANTAR METATARSAL
VESSELS

EXT. DIGITORUM TENDONS

PORTION OF DEEP
PLANTAR ARCH

OBLIQUE HEAD OF
ADD. HALLUCIS M.

1ST METATARSAL

MED. CUNEIFORM

PERONEUS LONGUS TENDON

FLEX. HALLUCIS BREVIS M.

5TH METATARSAL

FLEX. HALLUCIS
LONGUS TENDON

PERONEUS BREVIS TENDON

FLEX. DIGITORUM
LONGUS TENDON

CUBOID

QUADRATUS PLANTAE M.

MED. PLANTAR N.

ABD. DIGITI MINIMI M.

LAT. PLANTAR N.

LONG PLANTAR LIG.

ABD. HALLUCIS M.

CALCANEAL VESSELS

LAT. PLANTAR A. & V.

CALCANEUS QUADRATUS PLANTAE M.

7

Upper Extremity

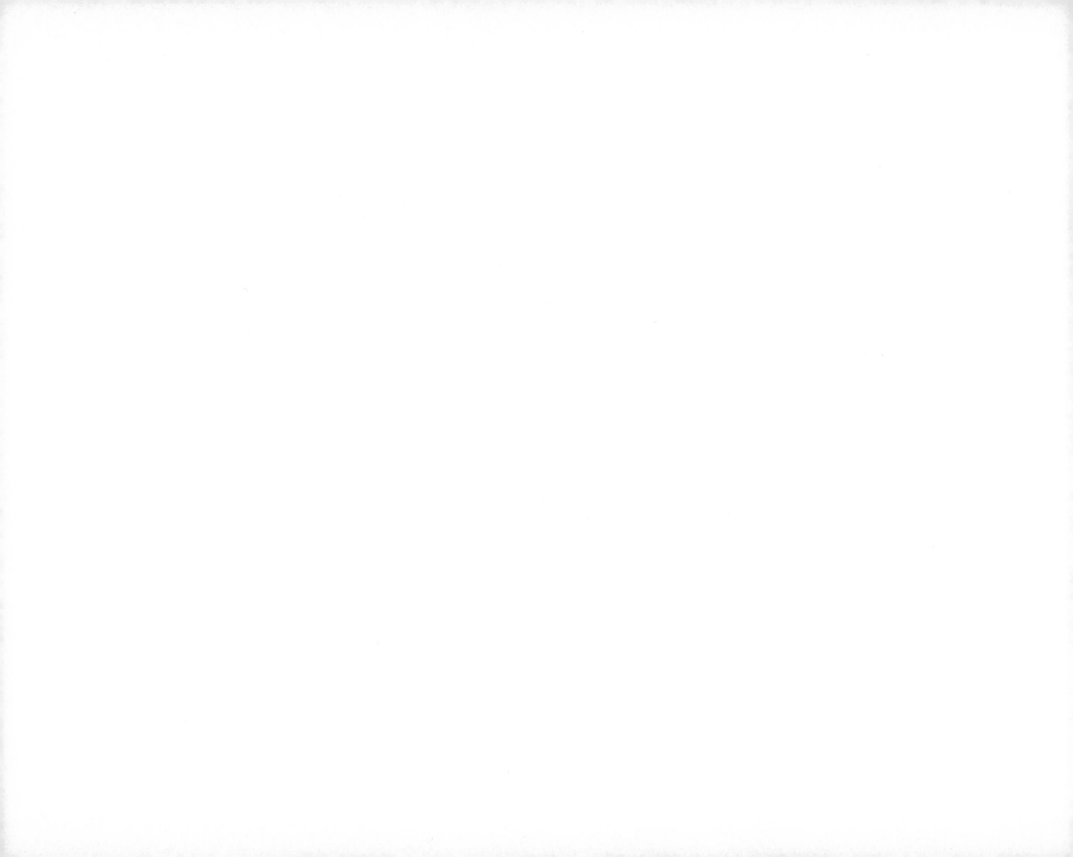

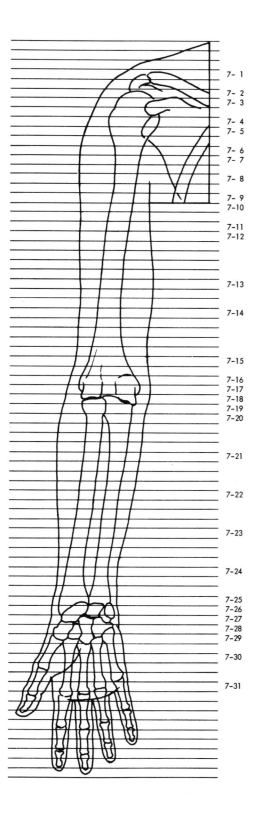

Although we prepared 1 cm-thick sections of the entire upper extremity, only 31 of these are presented. As is indicated in the accompanying sketch, some of the sections are adjacent and others are several cm apart. We selected illustrations that allow for continuity in following the various structures of the upper extremity yet do not excessively duplicate the structures seen in the preceding sections.

Although the magnification was constant for the sections of the upper extremity that are not attached to the torso (Sections 7–10 to 7–31), they were enlarged more than those that are attached (Sections 7–1 to 7–9). Other sections of the upper extremity, which are from a different specimen, can be seen in Chapters 1 and 2.

The clinical applications of the cross-sectional anatomy largely represent an application of computed tomography and it can be anticipated that these concern detailed definition of involvement of contiguous anatomic parts by neoplasia or infectious processes.

The clinical applications of cross-sectional anatomy of the upper extremity are often alluded to in teaching the basic anatomy of this region. It is important to have a "mind's eye concept" of the cross section of the upper extremity in many areas, such as

1. The middle third of the humerus to the radial nerve, since fractures in this area may produce palsies.
2. The relationshp of the integrity of the interosseous membrane to the radius and ulna, since fractures of this area may, when healed, result in a disability to pronate and supinate.
3. Malignant tumors which could conceivably invade critical anatomic areas.

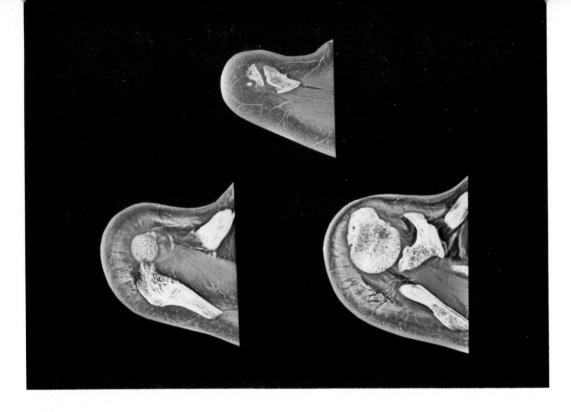

The capsule of the shoulder joint is loose and thin and it forms a sleeve-like structure around the head of the humerus and the glenoid cavity. The capsule is strengthened by the tendons of the supraspinatus, infraspinatus, teres minor, and subscapularis. These muscles form a musculotendinous cuff around the joint capsule; this cuff, often referred to as the rotator cuff, provides major support to the shoulder joint. Sections 7–2 to 7–5 show the relationships of the tendons of the rotator cuff to the shoulder joint. The subscapularis is related anteriorly, the supraspinatus superiorly, and both the infraspinatus and the teres minor posteriorly. The inferior part of the capsule, therefore, is the least supported part. There are usually two and at times three openings in the capsule. One of the constant openings in the fibrous capsule is for the tendon of the long head of the biceps, the other is a communication between the synovial cavity of the shoulder joint and the subscapular bursa. The third opening, which is not always present, is located posteriorly between the joint and a bursal sac under the tendon of the infraspinatus.

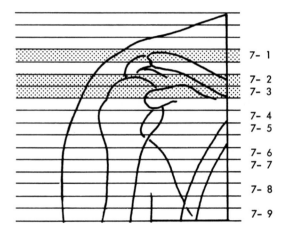

SECTION

7–1

Through the superior portion of the shoulder

SECTION

7–2

Through the shoulder, 2 cm below the preceding section

SECTION

7–3

Through the shoulder joint, 1 cm below the preceding section

Anatomic Considerations

The shoulder joint can be seen here as well as in Sections 7–4 and 7–5. This is a ball and socket type of synovial joint in which the head of the humerus articulates with the glenoid cavity of the scapula. As can be observed in Section 7–3, the glenoid cavity is small in comparison with the humeral head. The shallow glenoid cavity is slightly deepened by the glenoid labrum, which is a fibrocartilaginous ring attached to the margins of the glenoid cavity; the glenoid labrum is shown in Sections 7–4 and 7–5.

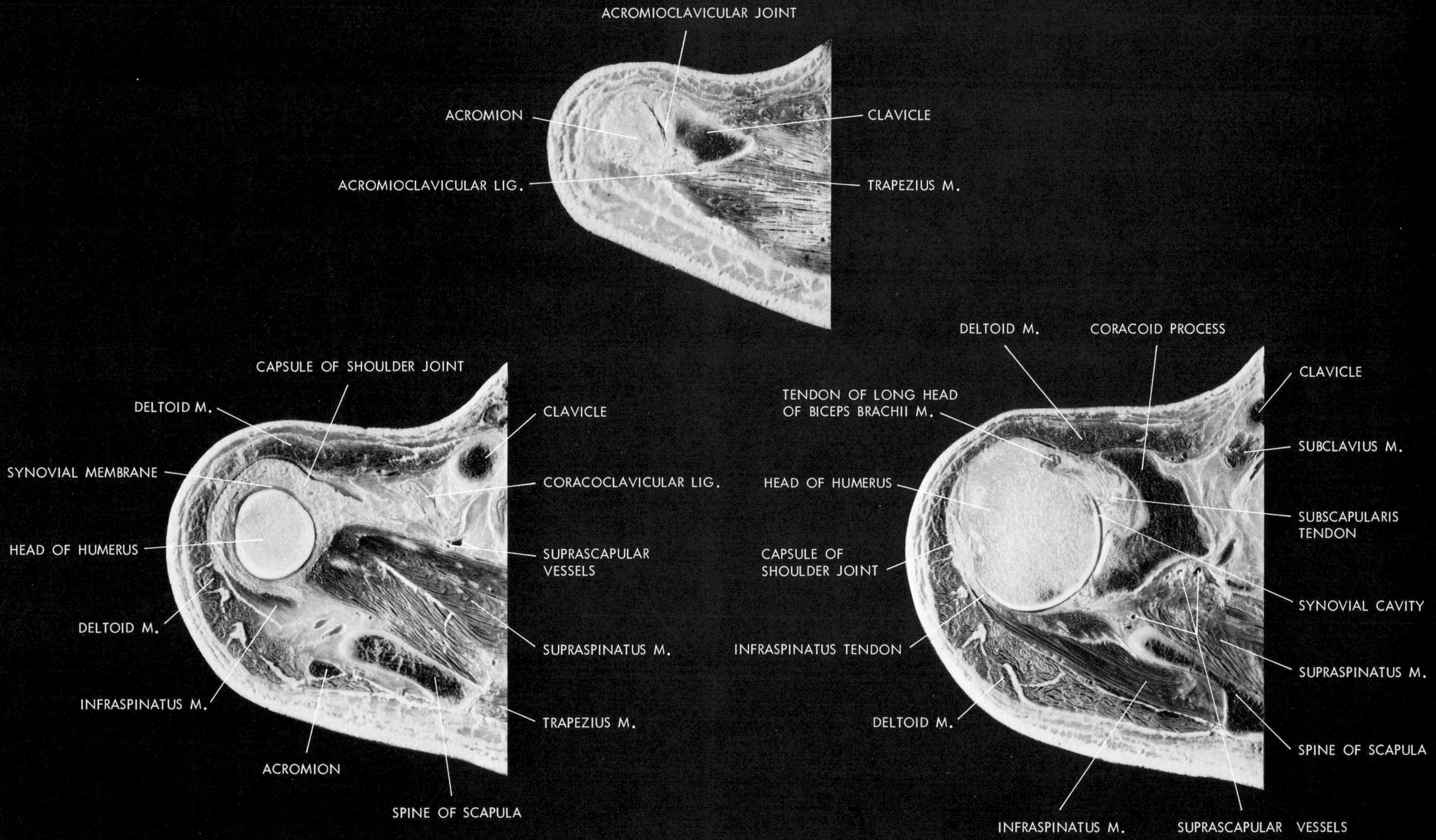

ACROMIOCLAVICULAR JOINT

ACROMION

CLAVICLE

ACROMIOCLAVICULAR LIG.

TRAPEZIUS M.

CAPSULE OF SHOULDER JOINT

DELTOID M.

CLAVICLE

SYNOVIAL MEMBRANE

CORACOCLAVICULAR LIG.

HEAD OF HUMERUS

SUPRASCAPULAR
VESSELS

DELTOID M.

SUPRASPINATUS M.

INFRASPINATUS M.

TRAPEZIUS M.

ACROMION

SPINE OF SCAPULA

DELTOID M.

CORACOID PROCESS

CLAVICLE

TENDON OF LONG HEAD
OF BICEPS BRACHII M.

SUBCLAVIUS M.

HEAD OF HUMERUS

SUBSCAPULARIS
TENDON

CAPSULE OF
SHOULDER JOINT

SYNOVIAL CAVITY

INFRASPINATUS TENDON

SUPRASPINATUS M.

DELTOID M.

SPINE OF SCAPULA

INFRASPINATUS M.

SUPRASCAPULAR VESSELS

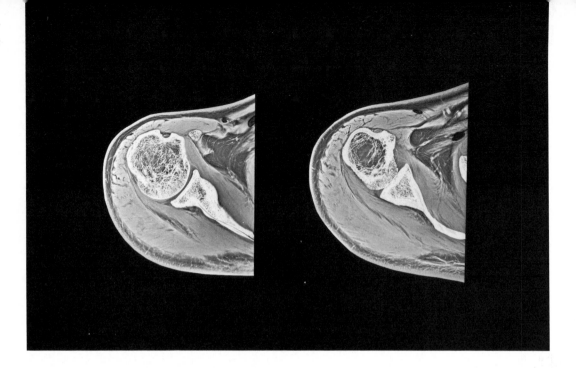

The brachial plexus is formed by the anterior primary rami (roots) of spinal nerves C5 to C8 and T1 and consists of roots, trunks, divisions, cords, and terminal nerves. The trunks, which are superior, middle, and inferior, are formed by the union of the roots. The superior trunk is formed by C5 and C6 spinal nerves, the middle trunk by C7, and the inferior trunk by C8 and T1. The trunks divide into anterior and posterior parts. The anterior divisions of the superior and middle trunks unite and form the lateral cord. The posterior divisions of the superior, middle, and inferior trunks unite to form the posterior cord, and the anterior division of the inferior trunk forms the medial cord. The cords divide into branches that form the terminal nerves.

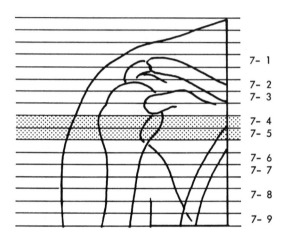

7- 1
7- 2
7- 3
7- 4
7- 5
7- 6
7- 7
7- 8
7- 9

SECTION
7–4

Through the shoulder joint, 2 cm below the preceding section

SECTION
7–5

Through the shoulder joint, 1 cm below the preceding section

Anatomic Considerations

In these sections the three cords (lateral, medial, and posterior) of the brachial plexus can be observed. The relations of the cords to the axillary artery are clearly seen in Section 7–5.

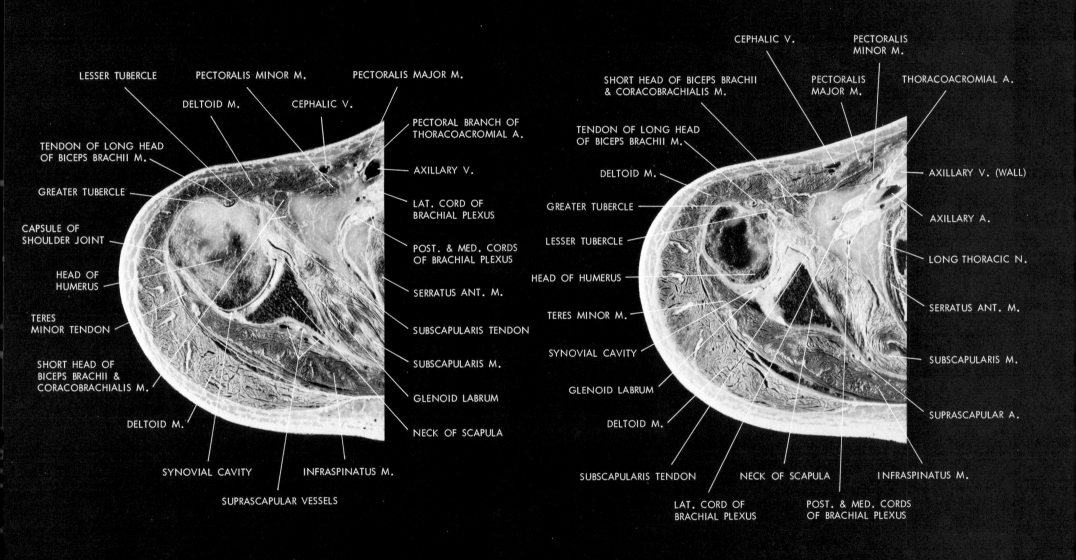

LESSER TUBERCLE

PECTORALIS MINOR M.

PECTORALIS MAJOR M.

DELTOID M.

CEPHALIC V.

PECTORAL BRANCH OF
THORACOACROMIAL A.

TENDON OF LONG HEAD
OF BICEPS BRACHII M.

AXILLARY V.

GREATER TUBERCLE

LAT. CORD OF
BRACHIAL PLEXUS

CAPSULE OF
SHOULDER JOINT

POST. & MED. CORDS
OF BRACHIAL PLEXUS

HEAD OF
HUMERUS

SERRATUS ANT. M.

TERES
MINOR TENDON

SUBSCAPULARIS TENDON

SHORT HEAD OF
BICEPS BRACHII &
CORACOBRACHIALIS M.

SUBSCAPULARIS M.

GLENOID LABRUM

DELTOID M.

NECK OF SCAPULA

SYNOVIAL CAVITY

INFRASPINATUS M.

SUPRASCAPULAR VESSELS

CEPHALIC V.

PECTORALIS
MINOR M.

SHORT HEAD OF BICEPS BRACHII
& CORACOBRACHIALIS M.

PECTORALIS
MAJOR M.

THORACOACROMIAL A.

TENDON OF LONG HEAD
OF BICEPS BRACHII M.

DELTOID M.

AXILLARY V. (WALL)

GREATER TUBERCLE

AXILLARY A.

LESSER TUBERCLE

LONG THORACIC N.

HEAD OF HUMERUS

TERES MINOR M.

SERRATUS ANT. M.

SYNOVIAL CAVITY

SUBSCAPULARIS M.

GLENOID LABRUM

DELTOID M.

SUPRASCAPULAR A.

SUBSCAPULARIS TENDON

NECK OF SCAPULA

INFRASPINATUS M.

LAT. CORD OF
BRACHIAL PLEXUS

POST. & MED. CORDS
OF BRACHIAL PLEXUS

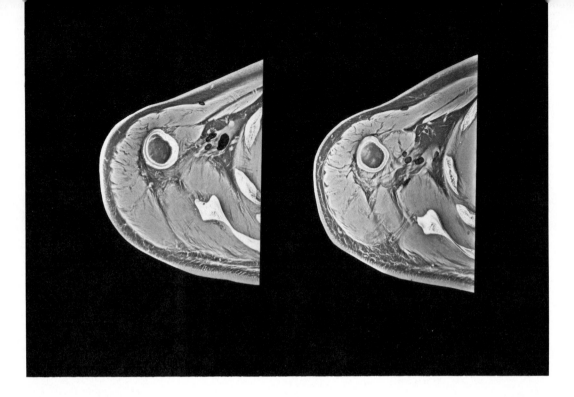

of the axillary artery. The lateral thoracic (seen in these illustrations) and the thoracoacromial arteries (Section 7–5) stem from the second portion of the axillary artery. The third portion of the axillary artery gives rise to three arteries: the anterior humeral circumflex, posterior humeral circumflex, and subscapular. They can be observed in these sections.

The axillary artery and its branches supply the muscles that form the walls of the axilla, the muscles of the shoulder and lateral thoracic wall, the shoulder joint, and the mammary gland; they also participate in anastomoses around the head of the humerus and around the scapula.

The axillary nerve can be seen in Section 7–6. This nerve, along with the posterior humeral circumflex vessels, passes through the quadrangular space of the shoulder. This space is bounded superiorly by the subscapularis, which lies anterior, and the teres minor, which lies posterior; inferiorly by the teres major; medially by the long head of the triceps; and laterally by the surgical neck of the humerus. The axillary nerve is in direct contact with the humerus at the surgical neck. This is one of the three locations where nerves are intimately related to the humerus. The radial nerve in the spiral groove (Section 7–12) and the ulnar nerve at the medial epicondyle (Section 7–16) are the two other examples.

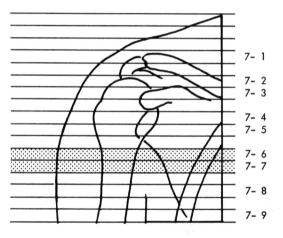

SECTION 7–6

Through the shaft of the humerus, 2 cm below the preceding section

SECTION 7–7

Through the shaft of the humerus, 1 cm below the preceding section

Anatomic Considerations

The axillary artery and several of its branches can be seen in these illustrations. The axillary artery begins at the outer border of the first rib as a continuation of the subclavian artery, traverses the axilla, and terminates at the outer border of the teres major muscle, where it becomes continuous with the brachial artery. The axillary artery is divided into three parts by the pectoralis minor muscle, which crosses anterior to the middle portion of the artery. The three parts are located (1) above, (2) behind, and (3) below the muscle, respectively. The number of branches each part provides is indicated by its number. The superior (supreme) thoracic artery arises from the first part

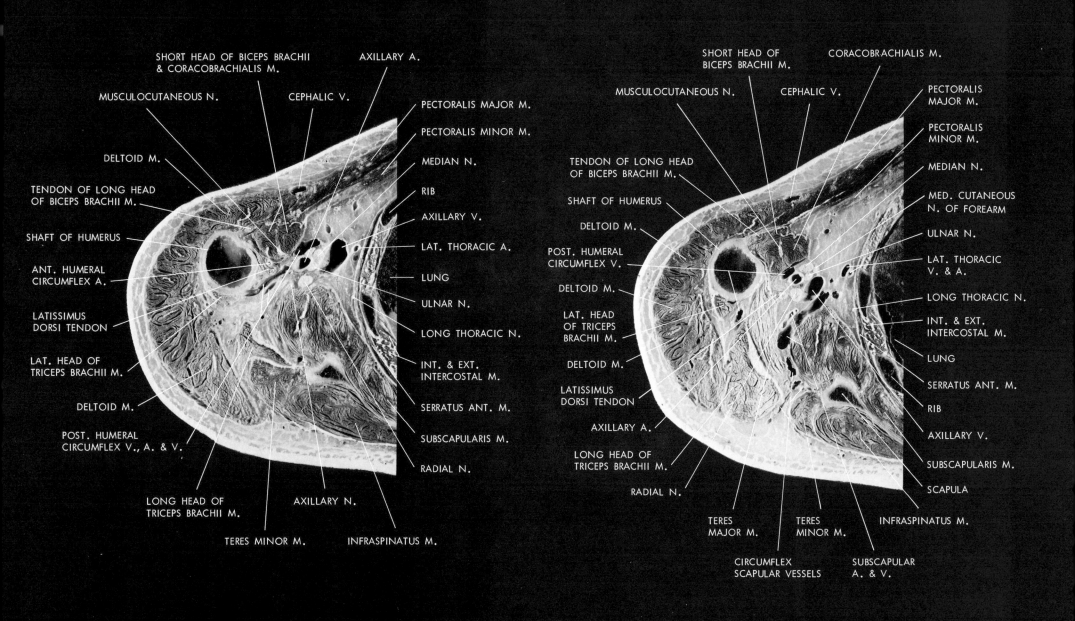

SHORT HEAD OF BICEPS BRACHII & CORACOBRACHIALIS M.

AXILLARY A.

MUSCULOCUTANEOUS N.

CEPHALIC V.

PECTORALIS MAJOR M.

PECTORALIS MINOR M.

DELTOID M.

MEDIAN N.

TENDON OF LONG HEAD OF BICEPS BRACHII M.

RIB

AXILLARY V.

SHAFT OF HUMERUS

LAT. THORACIC A.

ANT. HUMERAL CIRCUMFLEX A.

LUNG

ULNAR N.

LATISSIMUS DORSI TENDON

LONG THORACIC N.

LAT. HEAD OF TRICEPS BRACHII M.

INT. & EXT. INTERCOSTAL M.

DELTOID M.

SERRATUS ANT. M.

POST. HUMERAL CIRCUMFLEX V., A. & V.

SUBSCAPULARIS M.

RADIAL N.

LONG HEAD OF TRICEPS BRACHII M.

AXILLARY N.

TERES MINOR M.

INFRASPINATUS M.

SHORT HEAD OF BICEPS BRACHII M.

CORACOBRACHIALIS M.

MUSCULOCUTANEOUS N.

CEPHALIC V.

PECTORALIS MAJOR M.

PECTORALIS MINOR M.

TENDON OF LONG HEAD OF BICEPS BRACHII M.

MEDIAN N.

MED. CUTANEOUS N. OF FOREARM

SHAFT OF HUMERUS

DELTOID M.

ULNAR N.

POST. HUMERAL CIRCUMFLEX V.

LAT. THORACIC V. & A.

DELTOID M.

LONG THORACIC N.

LAT. HEAD OF TRICEPS BRACHII M.

INT. & EXT. INTERCOSTAL M.

DELTOID M.

LUNG

LATISSIMUS DORSI TENDON

SERRATUS ANT. M.

AXILLARY A.

RIB

LONG HEAD OF TRICEPS BRACHII M.

AXILLARY V.

RADIAL N.

SUBSCAPULARIS M.

SCAPULA

TERES MAJOR M.

TERES MINOR M.

INFRASPINATUS M.

CIRCUMFLEX SCAPULAR VESSELS

SUBSCAPULAR A. & V.

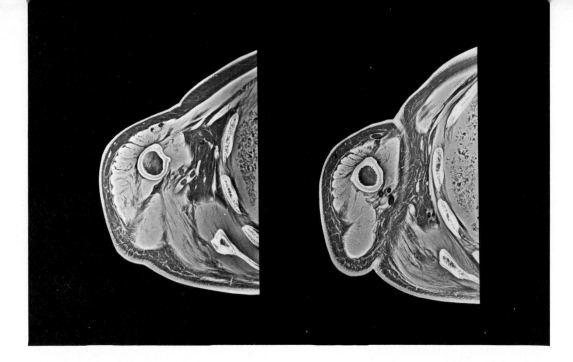

the axillary space. The base or floor of the axilla is formed by the axillary fascia. The anterior wall is formed by the pectoralis major and minor muscles; the posterior wall by the latissimus dorsi, teres major, and subscapularis muscles; the medial wall by the serratus anterior muscle; and the lateral wall by the intertubercular groove of the humerus.

The structures within the axilla are the axillary artery and vein, branches of the brachial plexus, axillary lymph nodes, tendons of the long and short heads of the biceps, and the coracobrachialis muscles. With the exception of lymph nodes, the contents of the axilla can be observed in these sections. The branches of the axillary artery were considered with Sections 7–6 and 7–7.

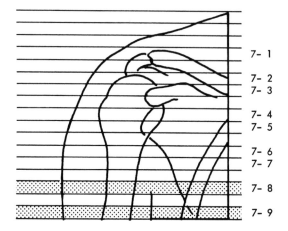

SECTION
7–8

Through the shaft of the humerus, 2 cm below the preceding section

Anatomic Considerations

The axilla can be followed from Section 7–4 to Section 7–9. It is at the junction of the upper limb and the chest and is described as consisting of an apex, base, and four walls. The apex is located between the first rib, clavicle, and base of the coracoid process. All the neurovascular structures pass through the apex to

SECTION
7–9

Through the shaft of the humerus, 2 cm below the preceding section

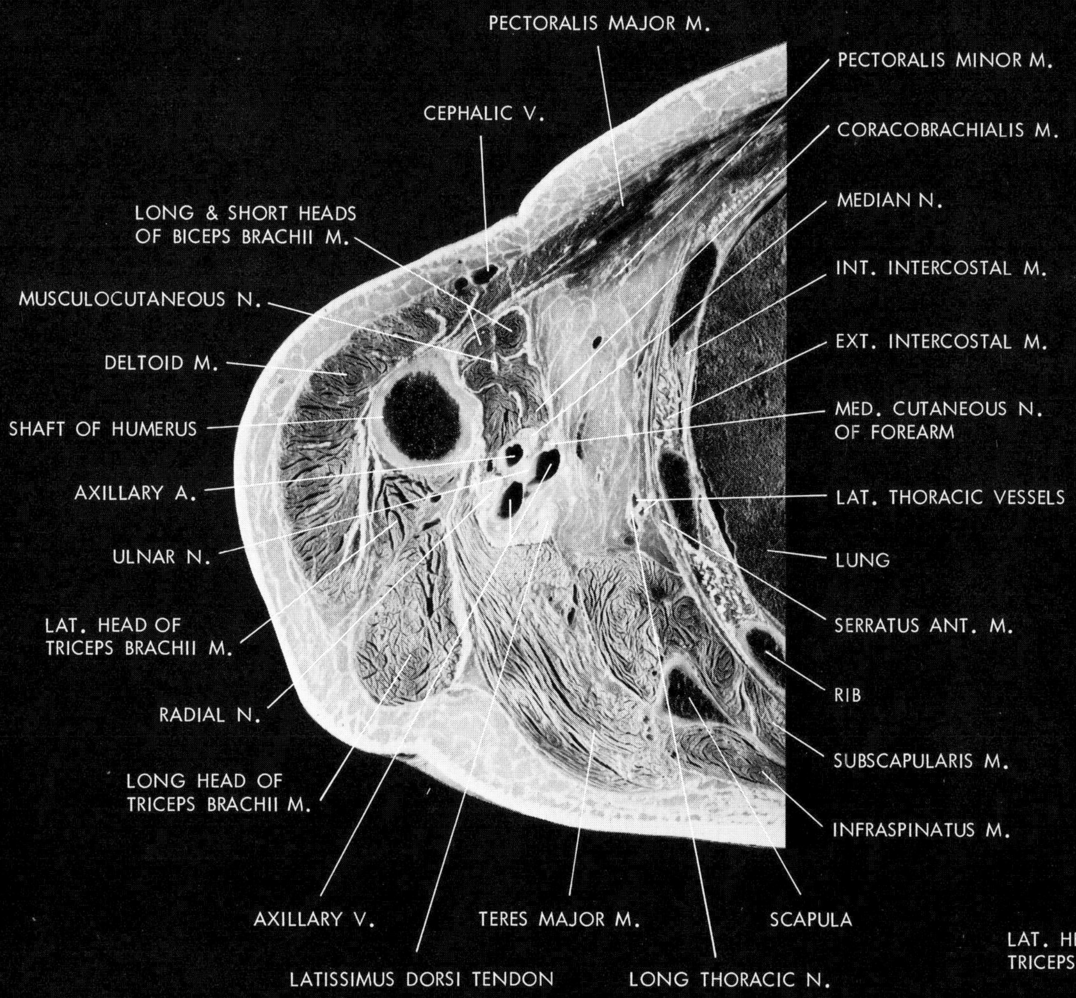

PECTORALIS MAJOR M.

PECTORALIS MINOR M.

CEPHALIC V.

CORACOBRACHIALIS M.

MEDIAN N.

LONG & SHORT HEADS
OF BICEPS BRACHII M.

INT. INTERCOSTAL M.

MUSCULOCUTANEOUS N.

EXT. INTERCOSTAL M.

DELTOID M.

MED. CUTANEOUS N.
OF FOREARM

SHAFT OF HUMERUS

LAT. THORACIC VESSELS

AXILLARY A.

LUNG

ULNAR N.

SERRATUS ANT. M.

LAT. HEAD OF
TRICEPS BRACHII M.

RIB

RADIAL N.

SUBSCAPULARIS M.

LONG HEAD OF
TRICEPS BRACHII M.

INFRASPINATUS M.

AXILLARY V.   TERES MAJOR M.   SCAPULA

LATISSIMUS DORSI TENDON   LONG THORACIC N.

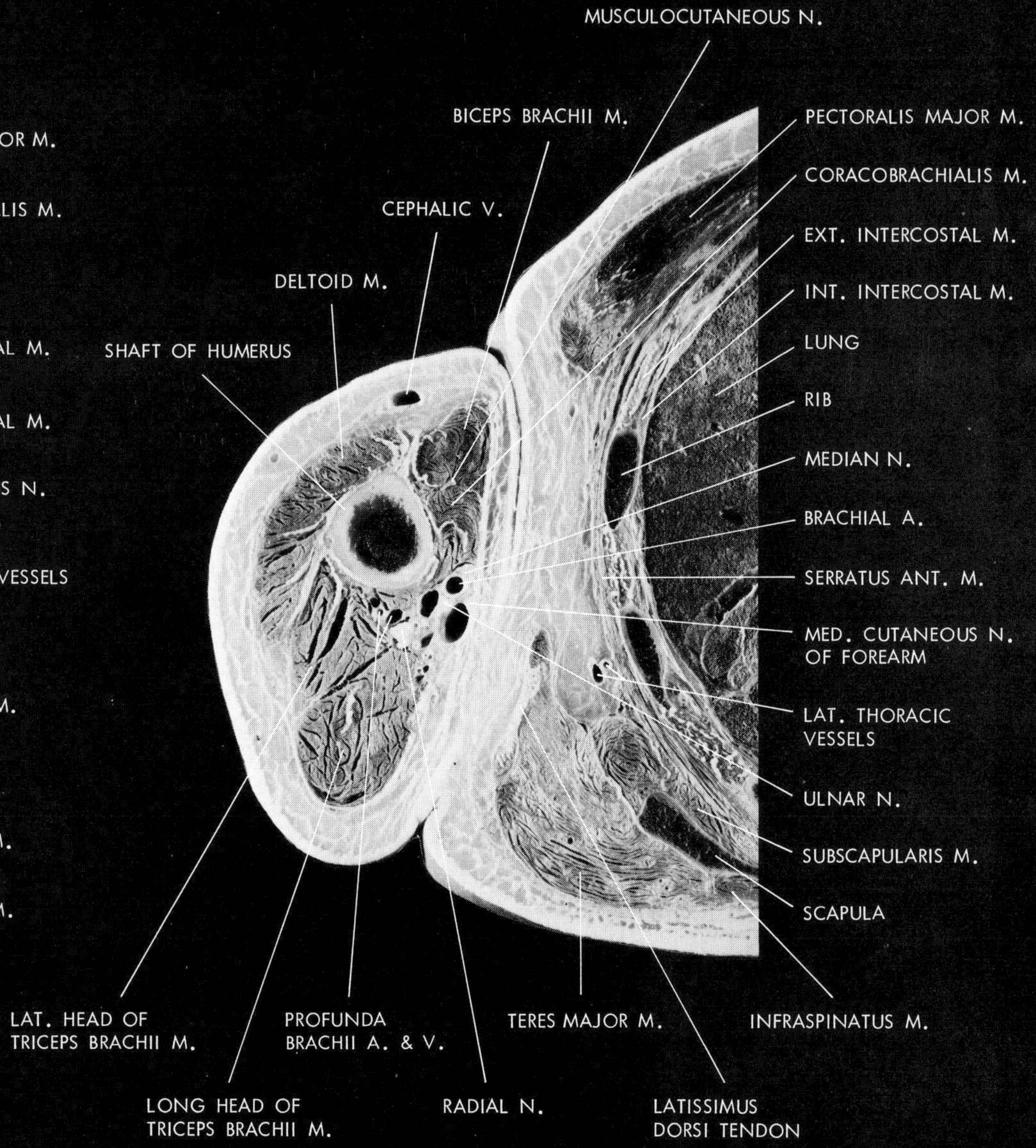

MUSCULOCUTANEOUS N.

BICEPS BRACHII M.

PECTORALIS MAJOR M.

CEPHALIC V.

CORACOBRACHIALIS M.

EXT. INTERCOSTAL M.

DELTOID M.

INT. INTERCOSTAL M.

LUNG

SHAFT OF HUMERUS

RIB

MEDIAN N.

BRACHIAL A.

SERRATUS ANT. M.

MED. CUTANEOUS N.
OF FOREARM

LAT. THORACIC
VESSELS

ULNAR N.

SUBSCAPULARIS M.

SCAPULA

INFRASPINATUS M.

LAT. HEAD OF
TRICEPS BRACHII M.

PROFUNDA
BRACHII A. & V.

TERES MAJOR M.

LATISSIMUS
DORSI TENDON

LONG HEAD OF
TRICEPS BRACHII M.

RADIAL N.

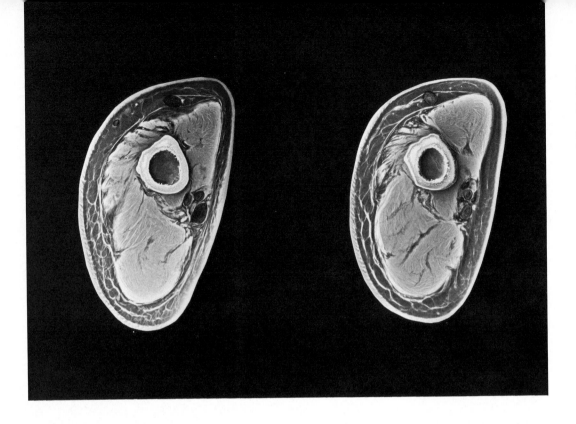

those of Sections 7–14 and 7–15. Note the position of the radial nerve and profunda (deep) brachial vessels between the medial and lateral heads of the triceps. The radial nerve and deep brachial vessels are the innervation and blood vasculature of the posterior compartment of the arm.

The insertions of both the deltoid and the coracobrachialis occur here (Section 7–11). At lower levels, the brachialis muscle occupies the position of these two muscles.

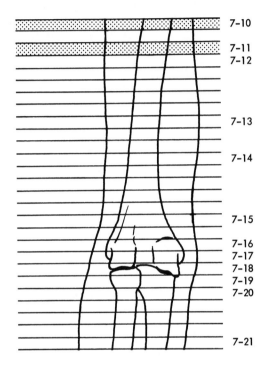

SECTION
7–10

Through the shaft of the humerus, 1 cm below the preceding section

SECTION
7–11

Through the shaft of the humerus, 2 cm below the preceding section

Anatomic Considerations

The three heads of the triceps brachii muscle, the long, lateral, and medial heads, are shown in these illustrations. The triceps lies in the posterior compartment of the arm and is the major extensor of the forearm. At the levels shown here, the triceps forms the bulk of the musculature of the arm, whereas, at a lower level, the musculature of the anterior compartment is equally prominent. Compare the relative size of the triceps in these illustrations with

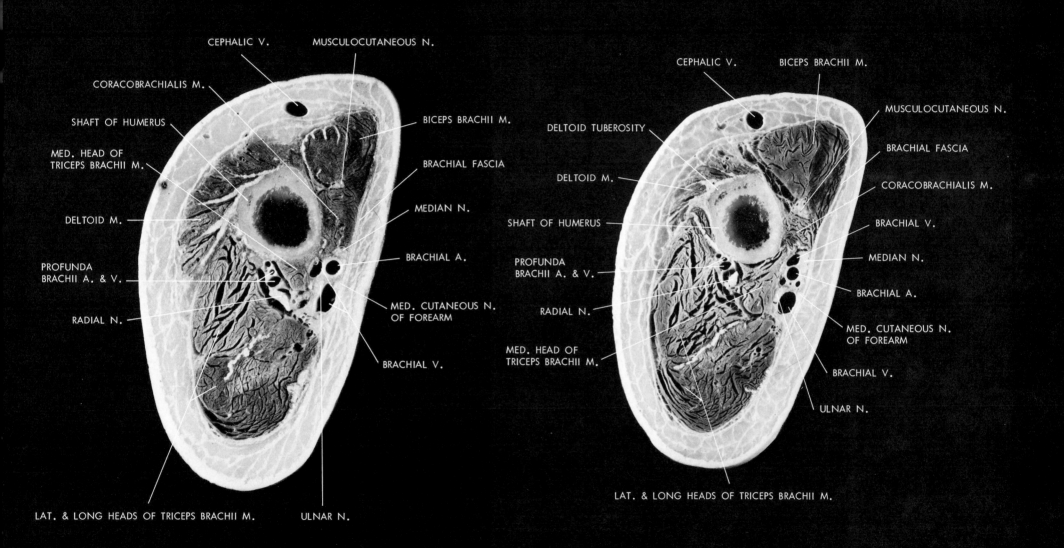

CEPHALIC V.   MUSCULOCUTANEOUS N.

CORACOBRACHIALIS M.

SHAFT OF HUMERUS   BICEPS BRACHII M.

MED. HEAD OF
TRICEPS BRACHII M.   BRACHIAL FASCIA

DELTOID M.   MEDIAN N.

PROFUNDA   BRACHIAL A.
BRACHII A. & V.

                                                    MED. CUTANEOUS N.
RADIAL N.   OF FOREARM

                                                    BRACHIAL V.

LAT. & LONG HEADS OF TRICEPS BRACHII M.   ULNAR N.

CEPHALIC V.   BICEPS BRACHII M.

DELTOID TUBEROSITY   MUSCULOCUTANEOUS N.

                                                    BRACHIAL FASCIA
DELTOID M.

                                                    CORACOBRACHIALIS M.
SHAFT OF HUMERUS

                                                    BRACHIAL V.

PROFUNDA   MEDIAN N.
BRACHII A. & V.

RADIAL N.   BRACHIAL A.

                                                    MED. CUTANEOUS N.
MED. HEAD OF   OF FOREARM
TRICEPS BRACHII M.

                                                    BRACHIAL V.

                                                    ULNAR N.

LAT. & LONG HEADS OF TRICEPS BRACHII M.

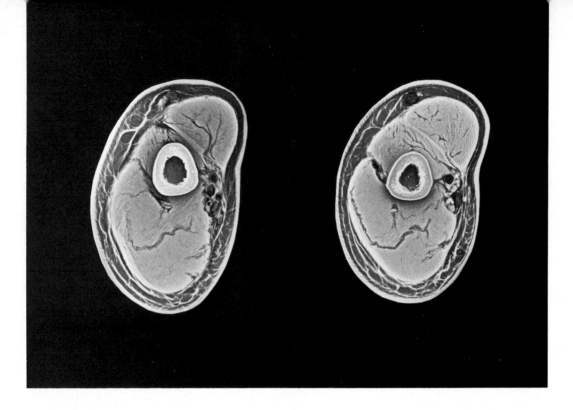

of these muscles are innervated by the musculocutaneous nerve. Additionally, the distal portion of the brachialis is innervated by the radial nerve. In these sections the musculocutaneous nerve lies between the biceps and the brachialis. At a higher level (Section 7–10), this nerve is located between the biceps and the coracobrachialis.

In the illustrations shown here, the radial nerve lies in the spiral groove of the humerus. During a part of their courses, the radial, axillary, and ulnar nerves lie in direct contact with the humerus.

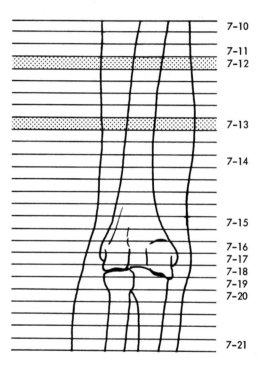

SECTION
7–12

Through the shaft of the humerus, 1 cm below the preceding section

SECTION
7–13

Through the humerus, 5 cm below the preceding section

Anatomic Considerations

The muscles located in the anterior compartment of the arm are the biceps brachii, brachialis, and coracobrachialis. Since the biceps crosses the shoulder and elbow joints on their flexor sides, it serves to flex both the arm and the forearm. The coracobrachialis, which inserts just proximal to the level shown in Section 7–12, flexes the arm. The brachialis, which originates from the humerus at the levels shown here, is the major flexor of the forearm. All three

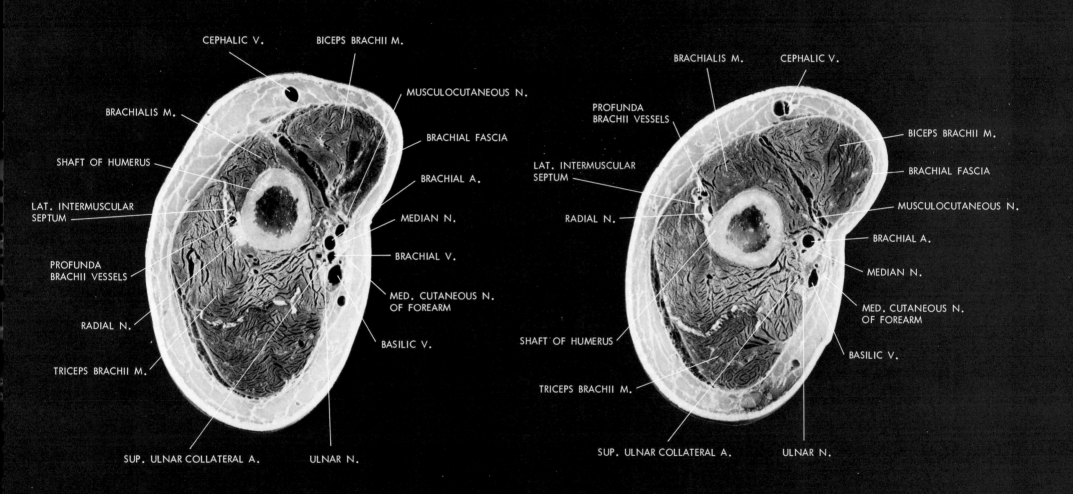

CEPHALIC V.   BICEPS BRACHII M.

MUSCULOCUTANEOUS N.

BRACHIALIS M.

BRACHIAL FASCIA

SHAFT OF HUMERUS

BRACHIAL A.

LAT. INTERMUSCULAR
SEPTUM

MEDIAN N.

BRACHIAL V.

PROFUNDA
BRACHII VESSELS

MED. CUTANEOUS N.
OF FOREARM

RADIAL N.

BASILIC V.

TRICEPS BRACHII M.

SUP. ULNAR COLLATERAL A.   ULNAR N.

BRACHIALIS M.   CEPHALIC V.

PROFUNDA
BRACHII VESSELS

BICEPS BRACHII M.

BRACHIAL FASCIA

LAT. INTERMUSCULAR
SEPTUM

MUSCULOCUTANEOUS N.

RADIAL N.

BRACHIAL A.

MEDIAN N.

MED. CUTANEOUS N.
OF FOREARM

SHAFT OF HUMERUS

BASILIC V.

TRICEPS BRACHII M.

SUP. ULNAR COLLATERAL A.   ULNAR N.

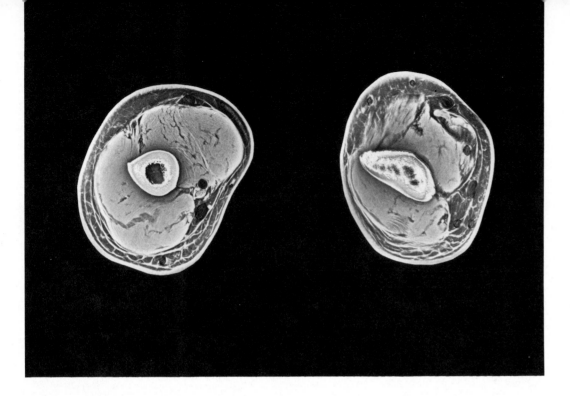

and median nerves. In the lower portion, it is closely related to the median nerve. At the elbow joint, the median nerve is medial to the artery and the tendon of the biceps brachii muscle is lateral to it.

Some of the branches of the brachial artery can be observed in these illustrations. The largest branch, the profunda brachii (Sections 7–9 to 7–13) can be observed. One of its branches follows the radial nerve. The superior ulnar collateral branch of the brachial artery pierces the intermuscular system and descends with the ulnar nerve, taking part in the anastomoses around the elbow joint. The inferior ulnar collateral branch of the brachial artery, not observed in these sections, also takes part in the arterial anastomoses around the elbow joint.

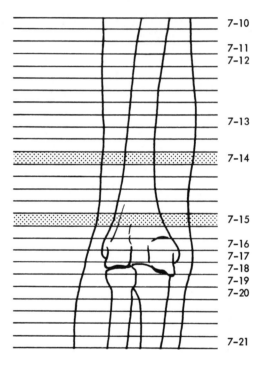

SECTION
7–14

Through the shaft of the humerus, 3 cm below the preceding section

SECTION
7–15

Through the epicondyles of the humerus, 5 cm below the preceding section

Anatomic Considerations

The brachial artery is a continuation of the axillary artery; it begins at the lower border of the teres major muscle and terminates opposite the neck of the radius by dividing into radial and ulnar branches. The course of the brachial artery can be followed from Section 7–9 to Section 7–18; in Section 7–19, the radial and ulnar arteries can be observed.

In the proximal portion of the arm, the brachial artery lies medial to the humerus; distally, it passes anterior to the humerus before crossing the elbow joint to its termination.

As can be seen in the illustrations, the artery in the upper portion of the arm is related to the medial cutaneous nerve of the forearm and to the ulnar

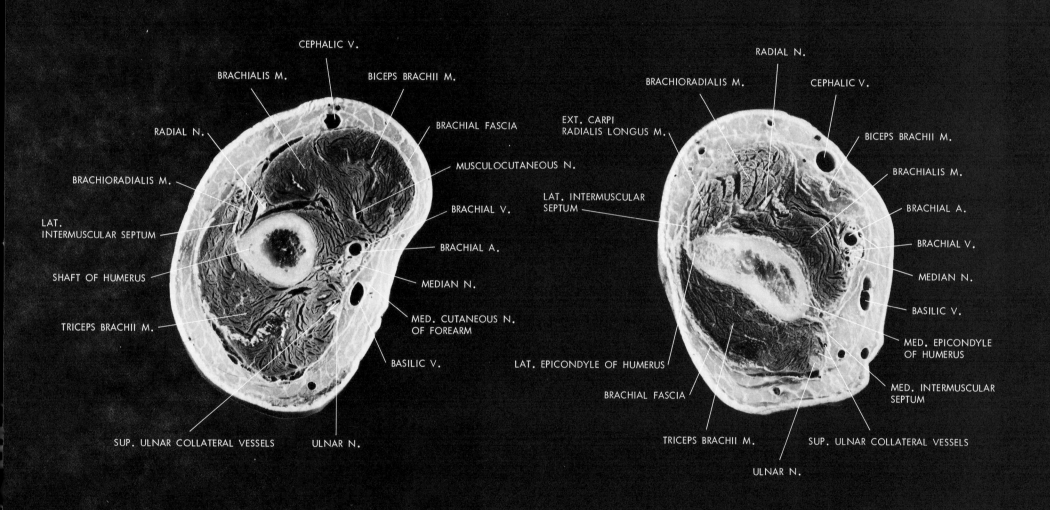

CEPHALIC V.

BRACHIALIS M.

BICEPS BRACHII M.

RADIAL N.

BRACHIAL FASCIA

BRACHIORADIALIS M.

MUSCULOCUTANEOUS N.

LAT.
INTERMUSCULAR SEPTUM

BRACHIAL V.

SHAFT OF HUMERUS

BRACHIAL A.

MEDIAN N.

TRICEPS BRACHII M.

MED. CUTANEOUS N.
OF FOREARM

BASILIC V.

SUP. ULNAR COLLATERAL VESSELS

ULNAR N.

RADIAL N.

BRACHIORADIALIS M.

CEPHALIC V.

EXT. CARPI
RADIALIS LONGUS M.

BICEPS BRACHII M.

BRACHIALIS M.

LAT. INTERMUSCULAR
SEPTUM

BRACHIAL A.

BRACHIAL V.

MEDIAN N.

BASILIC V.

LAT. EPICONDYLE OF HUMERUS

MED. EPICONDYLE
OF HUMERUS

BRACHIAL FASCIA

MED. INTERMUSCULAR
SEPTUM

TRICEPS BRACHII M.

SUP. ULNAR COLLATERAL VESSELS

ULNAR N.

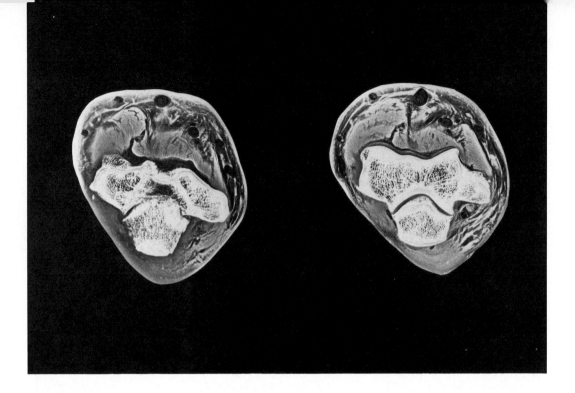

The cubital fossa can be seen in these sections. This is the triangular area in front of the elbow that is bounded laterally by the brachioradialis and medially by the pronator teres. The floor of the fossa is formed mainly by the brachialis. The relationships of the structures in the cubital fossa can be seen in the illustration. The tendon of the biceps lies lateral to the brachial artery, and the median nerve lies medial to the artery.

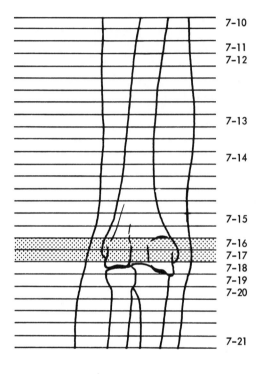

SECTION
7–16

Through the elbow joint

SECTION
7–17

Through the elbow joint, 1 cm below the preceding section

Anatomic Considerations

The elbow joint consists of an articulation between the trochlea of the humerus and the trochlear notch of the ulna and between the capitulum of the humerus and the head of the radius. It is a hinge type of synovial joint with flexion and extension being the only types of movement that occur. The synovial membrane of the elbow joint is continuous with that of the superior radioulnar joint (Section 7–18).

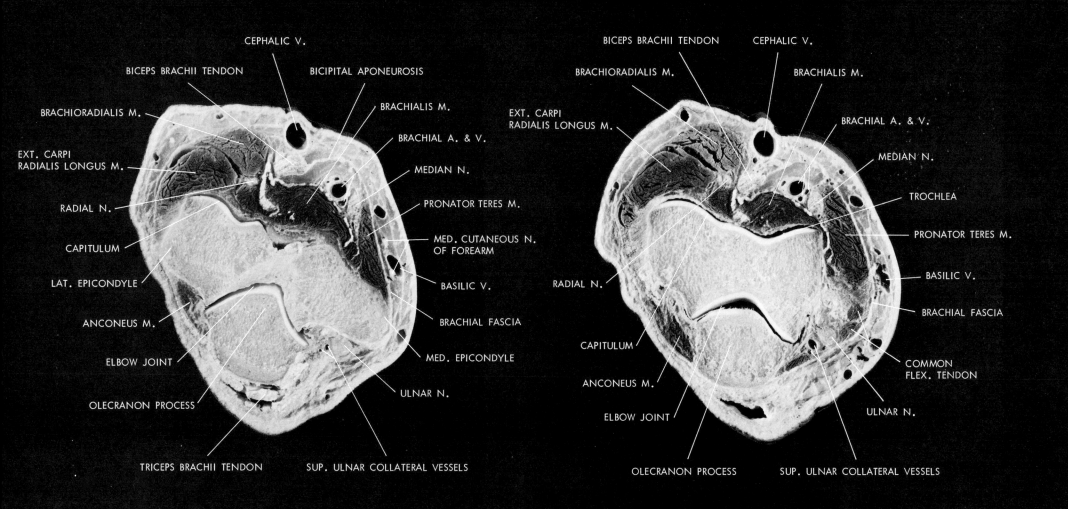

CEPHALIC V.

BICEPS BRACHII TENDON

BICIPITAL APONEUROSIS

BRACHIALIS M.

BRACHIORADIALIS M.

BRACHIAL A. & V.

EXT. CARPI
RADIALIS LONGUS M.

MEDIAN N.

RADIAL N.

PRONATOR TERES M.

CAPITULUM

MED. CUTANEOUS N.
OF FOREARM

LAT. EPICONDYLE

BASILIC V.

ANCONEUS M.

BRACHIAL FASCIA

ELBOW JOINT

MED. EPICONDYLE

OLECRANON PROCESS

ULNAR N.

TRICEPS BRACHII TENDON

SUP. ULNAR COLLATERAL VESSELS

BICEPS BRACHII TENDON

CEPHALIC V.

BRACHIORADIALIS M.

BRACHIALIS M.

EXT. CARPI
RADIALIS LONGUS M.

BRACHIAL A. & V.

MEDIAN N.

TROCHLEA

PRONATOR TERES M.

RADIAL N.

BASILIC V.

CAPITULUM

BRACHIAL FASCIA

ANCONEUS M.

COMMON
FLEX. TENDON

ELBOW JOINT

ULNAR N.

OLECRANON PROCESS

SUP. ULNAR COLLATERAL VESSELS

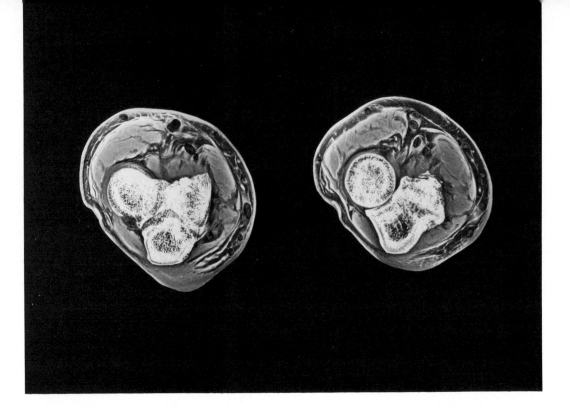

ligament is a strong band that surrounds the head of the radius and attaches to the ulna at points just anterior and posterior to the notch.

The communications of the cephalic vein in this specimen differed from the general pattern usually seen. After the cephalic vein ascended in the forearm, it went deep to terminate in the deep veins accompanying the radial artery. A separate cephalic vein arose at a slightly higher level from these deep veins (Section 7–19) but thereafter followed a typical course to terminate in the axillary vein.

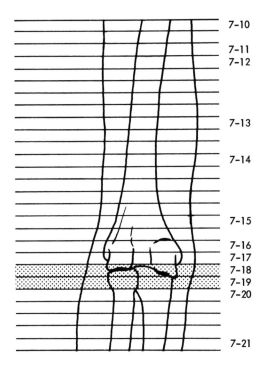

SECTION
7–18

Through the superior radioulnar joint, 1 cm below the preceding section

Anatomic Considerations

The superior, or proximal, radioulnar joint, which can be seen in the illustrations, consists of an articulation between the head of the radius and the radial notch of the ulna. The head of the radius glides in this ulnar notch during pronation and supination, the movements that take place at the two (superior and inferior) radioulnar joints. The head of the radius is held in place by the annular ligament, which can be seen in these illustrations. The annular

SECTION
7–19

Through the superior radioulnar joint, 1 cm below the preceding section

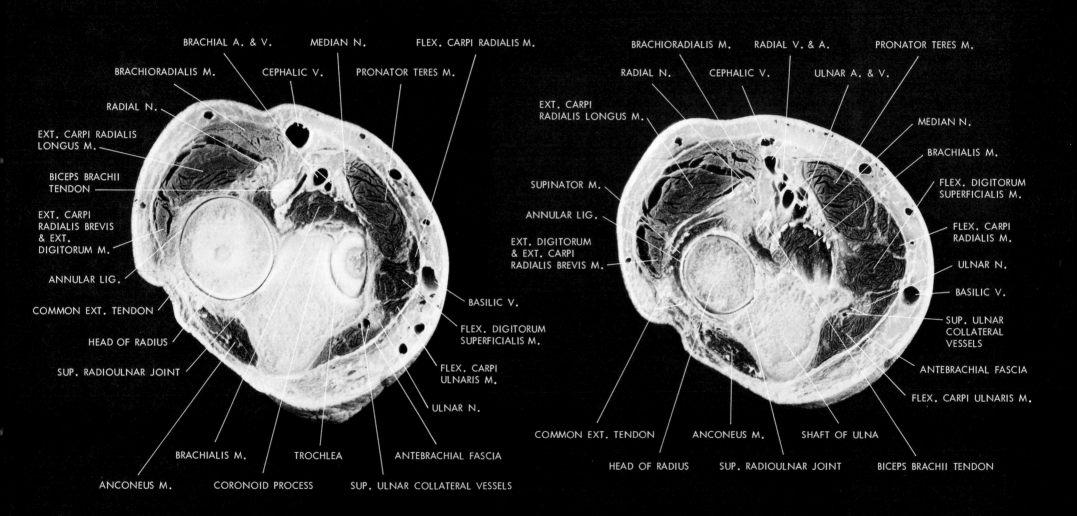

BRACHIAL A. & V.　　MEDIAN N.　　FLEX. CARPI RADIALIS M.

BRACHIORADIALIS M.　　CEPHALIC V.　　PRONATOR TERES M.

RADIAL N.

EXT. CARPI RADIALIS
LONGUS M.

BICEPS BRACHII
TENDON

EXT. CARPI
RADIALIS BREVIS
& EXT.
DIGITORUM M.

ANNULAR LIG.

COMMON EXT. TENDON

HEAD OF RADIUS

SUP. RADIOULNAR JOINT

BASILIC V.

FLEX. DIGITORUM
SUPERFICIALIS M.

FLEX. CARPI
ULNARIS M.

ULNAR N.

ANTEBRACHIAL FASCIA

BRACHIALIS M.　　TROCHLEA　　SUP. ULNAR COLLATERAL VESSELS

ANCONEUS M.　　CORONOID PROCESS

BRACHIORADIALIS M.　　RADIAL V. & A.　　PRONATOR TERES M.

RADIAL N.　　CEPHALIC V.　　ULNAR A. & V.

EXT. CARPI
RADIALIS LONGUS M.

SUPINATOR M.

ANNULAR LIG.

EXT. DIGITORUM
& EXT. CARPI
RADIALIS BREVIS M.

MEDIAN N.

BRACHIALIS M.

FLEX. DIGITORUM
SUPERFICIALIS M.

FLEX. CARPI
RADIALIS M.

ULNAR N.

BASILIC V.

SUP. ULNAR
COLLATERAL
VESSELS

ANTEBRACHIAL FASCIA

FLEX. CARPI ULNARIS M.

COMMON EXT. TENDON　　ANCONEUS M.　　SHAFT OF ULNA

HEAD OF RADIUS　　SUP. RADIOULNAR JOINT　　BICEPS BRACHII TENDON

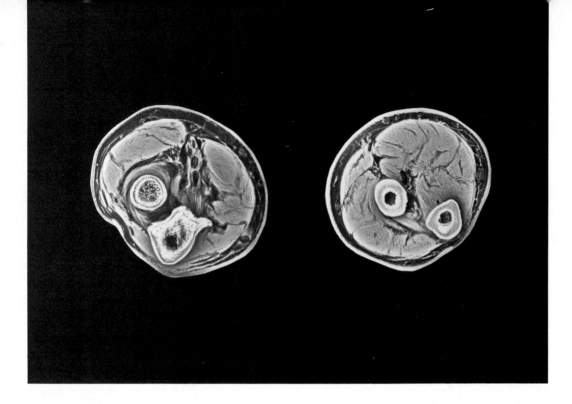

abductor pollicis longus, extensor pollicis brevis, extensor pollicis longus, and extensor indicis. The supinator arises from the lateral epicondyle; the remaining muscles arise either from the radius and interosseous membrane (abductor pollicis longus and extensor pollicis brevis) or from the ulna and interosseous membrane (extensor pollicis longus and extensor indicis). Although these muscles are in the deep group, they become superficial as they approach their insertion.

These muscles can be seen from Sections 7–14 to 7–31.

The radial nerve can be followed from Sections 7–6 to 7–19, and in Sections 7–20 and 7–21 the superficial and deep branches of the radial nerve can be observed. All these postaxial muscles are innervated by the deep branch of the radial nerve.

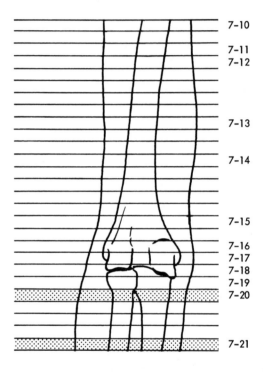

SECTION
7–20

Through the proximal end of the radius and ulna, 1 cm below the preceding section

SECTION
7–21

Through the shafts of the radius and ulna, 4 cm below the preceding section

Anatomic Considerations

The muscles of the extensor region of the forearm are more numerous than those on the flexor side. These are postaxial muscles and can be divided into superficial and deep groups.

From the lateral to the medial border of the forearm, the superficial group consists of the following muscles: brachioradialis, extensor carpi radialis longus, extensor carpi radialis brevis, extensor digitorum, extensor digiti minimi, extensor carpi ulnaris, and anconeus. They all have a common origin from the lateral epicondyle, except the brachioradialis and extensor carpi radialis longus, which arise from the supracondylar ridge of the humerus.

The deep group of muscles, from proximal to distal, are the supinator,

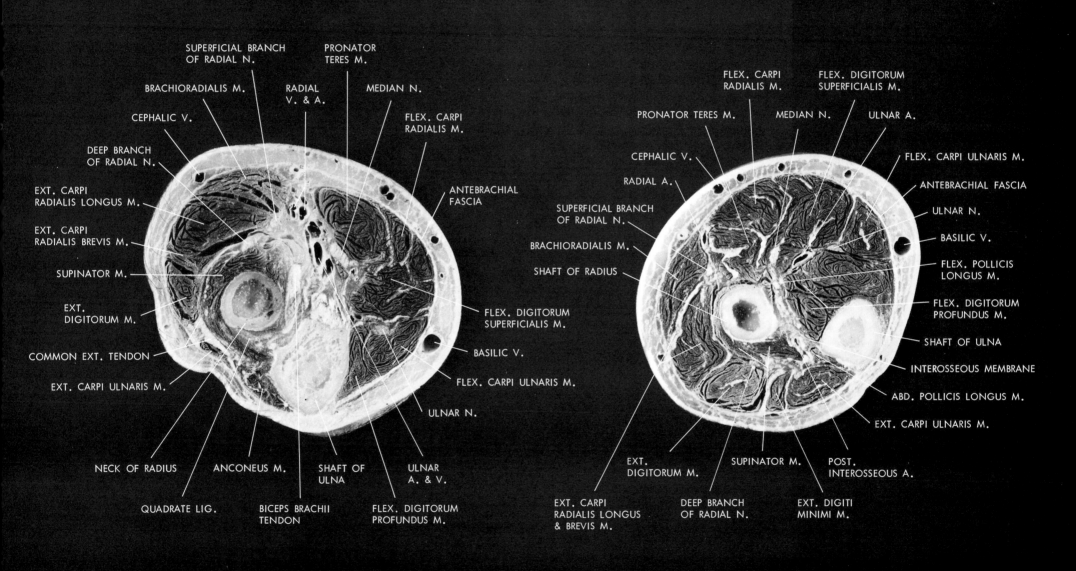

SUPERFICIAL BRANCH
OF RADIAL N.

PRONATOR
TERES M.

BRACHIORADIALIS M.

RADIAL
V. & A.

MEDIAN N.

CEPHALIC V.

FLEX. CARPI
RADIALIS M.

DEEP BRANCH
OF RADIAL N.

EXT. CARPI
RADIALIS LONGUS M.

ANTEBRACHIAL
FASCIA

EXT. CARPI
RADIALIS BREVIS M.

SUPINATOR M.

EXT.
DIGITORUM M.

FLEX. DIGITORUM
SUPERFICIALIS M.

COMMON EXT. TENDON

BASILIC V.

EXT. CARPI ULNARIS M.

FLEX. CARPI ULNARIS M.

ULNAR N.

NECK OF RADIUS

ANCONEUS M.

SHAFT OF
ULNA

ULNAR
A. & V.

QUADRATE LIG.

BICEPS BRACHII
TENDON

FLEX. DIGITORUM
PROFUNDUS M.

FLEX. CARPI
RADIALIS M.

FLEX. DIGITORUM
SUPERFICIALIS M.

PRONATOR TERES M.

MEDIAN N.

ULNAR A.

CEPHALIC V.

FLEX. CARPI ULNARIS M.

RADIAL A.

ANTEBRACHIAL FASCIA

SUPERFICIAL BRANCH
OF RADIAL N.

ULNAR N.

BRACHIORADIALIS M.

BASILIC V.

SHAFT OF RADIUS

FLEX. POLLICIS
LONGUS M.

FLEX. DIGITORUM
PROFUNDUS M.

SHAFT OF ULNA

INTEROSSEOUS MEMBRANE

ABD. POLLICIS LONGUS M.

EXT. CARPI ULNARIS M.

EXT.
DIGITORUM M.

SUPINATOR M.

POST.
INTEROSSEOUS A.

EXT. CARPI
RADIALIS LONGUS
& BREVIS M.

DEEP BRANCH
OF RADIAL N.

EXT. DIGITI
MINIMI M.

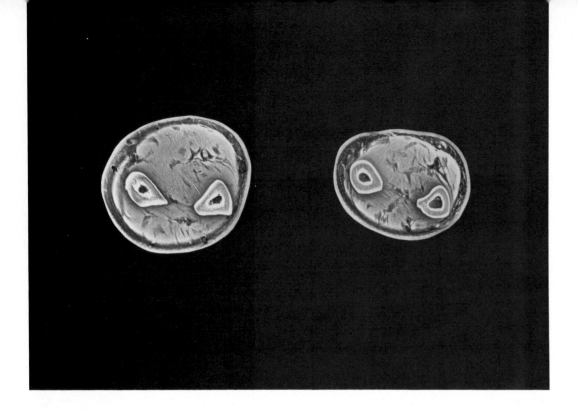

The median and ulnar nerves and their relationships to adjacent muscles can be seen in these and accompanying illustrations. In the cubital fossa, the median nerve gives off branches to the pronator teres, flexor carpi radialis, palmaris longus, and flexor digitorum superficialis. The anterior interosseous nerve, which arises from the median nerve, innervates the lateral half of the flexor digitorum profundus, flexor pollicis longus, and pronator quadratus.

The ulnar nerve gives branches to the flexor carpi ulnaris and the medial half of the flexor digitorum profundus.

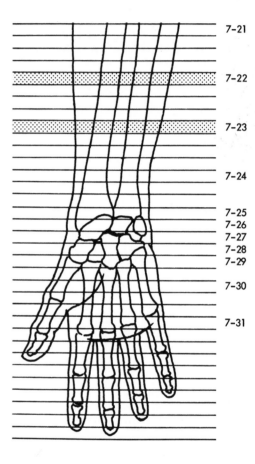

SECTION 7-22

Through the shafts of the radius and ulna, 4 cm below the preceding section

SECTION 7-23

Through the shafts of the radius and ulna, 4 cm below the preceding section

Anatomic Considerations

The muscles of the front of the forearm can be seen in these and the accompanying sections. They are the flexors of the wrist and digits and pronators of the forearm; the muscles are divided into a superficial and a deep group.

From lateral to medial, the superficial group consists of the pronator teres, flexor carpi radialis, palmaris longus (not observed), and flexor carpi ulnaris; the flexor digitorum superficialis is at a deeper plane than are the other muscles. All of these muscles have at least one common origin from the front of the medial epicondyle.

In the deep group there are only three muscles. The flexor digitorum profundus is related to the ulna, the flexor pollicis longus to the radius, and the pronator quadratus to both bones.

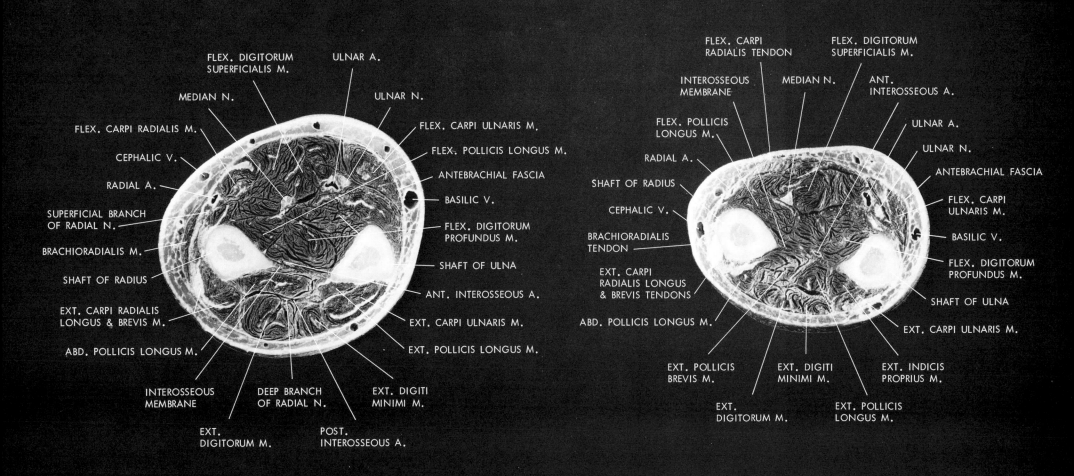

FLEX. DIGITORUM SUPERFICIALIS M.

ULNAR A.

MEDIAN N.

ULNAR N.

FLEX. CARPI RADIALIS M.

FLEX. CARPI ULNARIS M.

CEPHALIC V.

FLEX. POLLICIS LONGUS M.

RADIAL A.

ANTEBRACHIAL FASCIA

SUPERFICIAL BRANCH OF RADIAL N.

BASILIC V.

BRACHIORADIALIS M.

FLEX. DIGITORUM PROFUNDUS M.

SHAFT OF RADIUS

SHAFT OF ULNA

EXT. CARPI RADIALIS LONGUS & BREVIS M.

ANT. INTEROSSEOUS A.

ABD. POLLICIS LONGUS M.

EXT. CARPI ULNARIS M.

EXT. POLLICIS LONGUS M.

INTEROSSEOUS MEMBRANE

DEEP BRANCH OF RADIAL N.

EXT. DIGITI MINIMI M.

EXT. DIGITORUM M.

POST. INTEROSSEOUS A.

FLEX. CARPI RADIALIS TENDON

FLEX. DIGITORUM SUPERFICIALIS M.

INTEROSSEOUS MEMBRANE

MEDIAN N.

ANT. INTEROSSEOUS A.

FLEX. POLLICIS LONGUS M.

ULNAR A.

RADIAL A.

ULNAR N.

SHAFT OF RADIUS

ANTEBRACHIAL FASCIA

CEPHALIC V.

FLEX. CARPI ULNARIS M.

BRACHIORADIALIS TENDON

BASILIC V.

EXT. CARPI RADIALIS LONGUS & BREVIS TENDONS

FLEX. DIGITORUM PROFUNDUS M.

ABD. POLLICIS LONGUS M.

SHAFT OF ULNA

EXT. CARPI ULNARIS M.

EXT. POLLICIS BREVIS M.

EXT. DIGITI MINIMI M.

EXT. INDICIS PROPRIUS M.

EXT. DIGITORUM M.

EXT. POLLICIS LONGUS M.

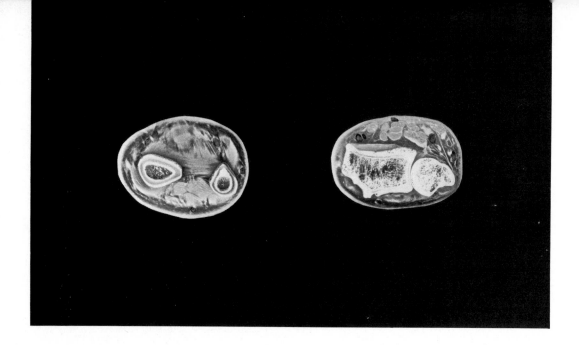

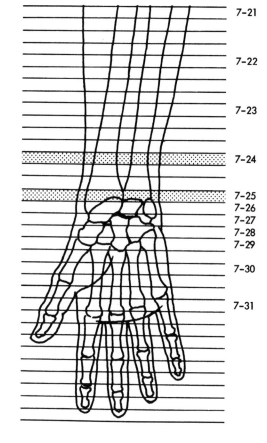

	7-21
	7-22
	7-23
	7-24
	7-25
	7-26
	7-27
	7-28
	7-29
	7-30
	7-31

SECTION 7-24

Through the shafts of the radius and ulna, 4 cm below the preceding section

SECTION 7-25

Through the inferior radioulnar joint, 3 cm below the preceding section

Anatomic Considerations

The inferior (distal) radioulnar joint, shown in Section 7–25, is a uniaxial pivot type of synovial joint between the distal extremity of the radius and the head of the ulna. The pronation and supination of the hand take place at the superior and inferior radioulnar joints. The pronator quadratus, shown in these illustrations, is responsible for eliciting pronation under many conditions. The pronator teres aids in rapid movement and movement against resistance. Supination is elicited by the supinator in slow movement and when the elbow is extended. The biceps brachii greatly assists when the elbow is flexed, especially against resistance.

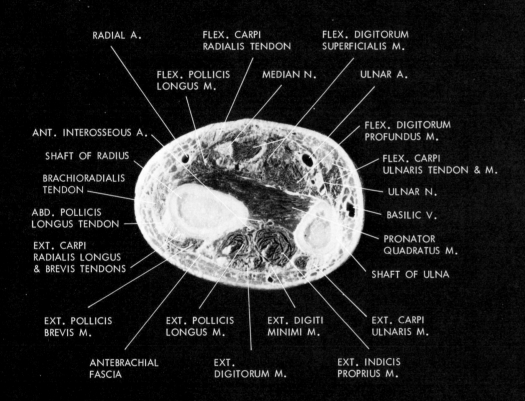

RADIAL A.

FLEX. CARPI
RADIALIS TENDON

FLEX. DIGITORUM
SUPERFICIALIS M.

FLEX. POLLICIS
LONGUS M.

MEDIAN N.

ULNAR A.

ANT. INTEROSSEOUS A.

FLEX. DIGITORUM
PROFUNDUS M.

SHAFT OF RADIUS

FLEX. CARPI
ULNARIS TENDON & M.

BRACHIORADIALIS
TENDON

ULNAR N.

ABD. POLLICIS
LONGUS TENDON

BASILIC V.

EXT. CARPI
RADIALIS LONGUS
& BREVIS TENDONS

PRONATOR
QUADRATUS M.

SHAFT OF ULNA

EXT. POLLICIS
BREVIS M.

EXT. POLLICIS
LONGUS M.

EXT. DIGITI
MINIMI M.

EXT. CARPI
ULNARIS M.

ANTEBRACHIAL
FASCIA

EXT.
DIGITORUM M.

EXT. INDICIS
PROPRIUS M.

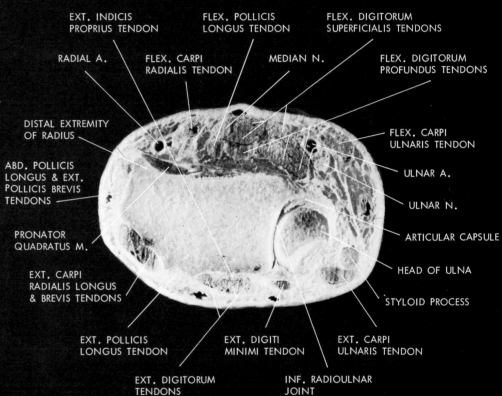

EXT. INDICIS
PROPRIUS TENDON

FLEX. POLLICIS
LONGUS TENDON

FLEX. DIGITORUM
SUPERFICIALIS TENDONS

RADIAL A.

FLEX. CARPI
RADIALIS TENDON

MEDIAN N.

FLEX. DIGITORUM
PROFUNDUS TENDONS

DISTAL EXTREMITY
OF RADIUS

FLEX. CARPI
ULNARIS TENDON

ABD. POLLICIS
LONGUS & EXT.
POLLICIS BREVIS
TENDONS

ULNAR A.

ULNAR N.

PRONATOR
QUADRATUS M.

ARTICULAR CAPSULE

EXT. CARPI
RADIALIS LONGUS
& BREVIS TENDONS

HEAD OF ULNA

STYLOID PROCESS

EXT. POLLICIS
LONGUS TENDON

EXT. DIGITI
MINIMI TENDON

EXT. CARPI
ULNARIS TENDON

EXT. DIGITORUM
TENDONS

INF. RADIOULNAR
JOINT

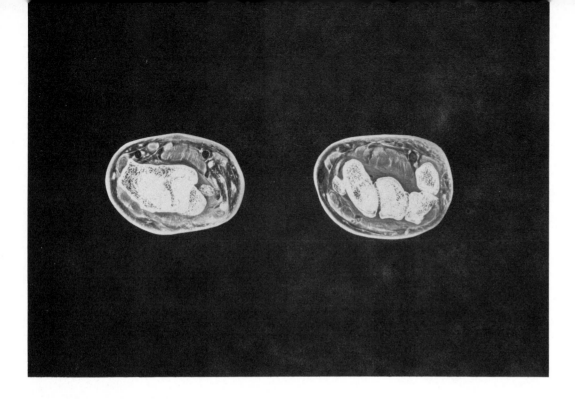

tendons between the extensor retinaculum and bone. From lateral to medial, the first compartment contains the tendons of the abductor pollicis longus and extensor pollicis brevis, the second compartment contains the tendons of the extensor carpi radialis longus and brevis, the third compartment contains only the tendon of the extensor pollicis longus, the fourth compartment is traversed by the extensor indicis and extensor digitorum, the fifth compartment contains the extensor digiti minimi, and the sixth compartment contains the extensor carpi ulnaris.

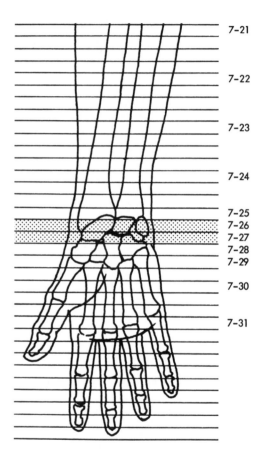

SECTION 7–26

Through the carpal bones, 1 cm below the preceding section

SECTION 7–27

Through the carpal bones, 1 cm below the preceding section

Anatomic Considerations

The wrist joint is classified as a condylar articulation between the forearm and the hand. The proximal articulating surface is composed of the distal end of the radius and the articular disc, which excludes the ulna from this joint. The distal articulating surface consists primarily of the scaphoid and lunate bones (Section 7–26); the triangular bone forms a small part of this surface. The joint is surrounded by a fibrous capsule that is strengthened by the volar and dorsal radiocarpal ligaments and on each side by the ulnar and radial collateral ligaments. The capsule is stronger at the medial and lateral sides than it is dorsally and ventrally. The movements that take place at the joint are flexion, extension, abduction, adduction, and circumduction.

In these illustrations the compartments on the dorsal side of the wrist can be observed. Each compartment transmits either one or two tendons and is lined by a synovial membrane. The membrane facilitates the movement of the

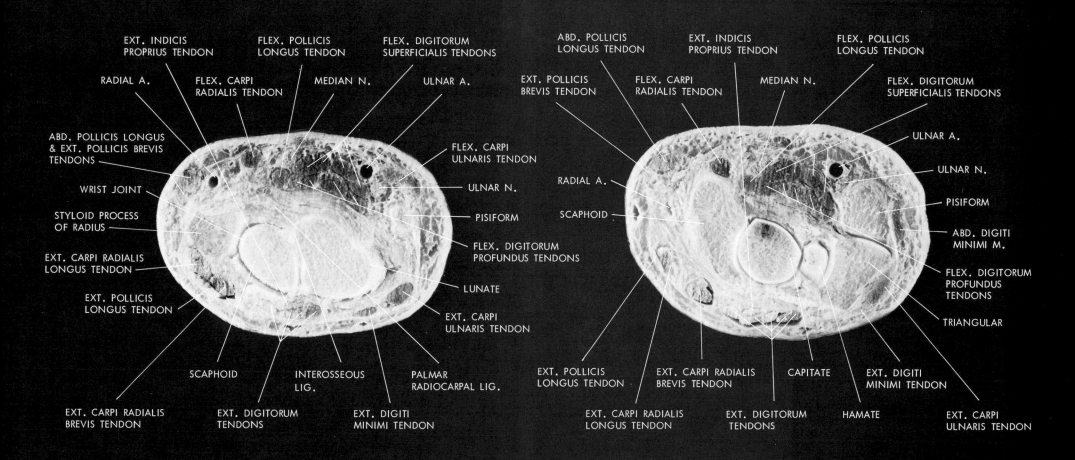

EXT. INDICIS PROPRIUS TENDON
FLEX. POLLICIS LONGUS TENDON
FLEX. DIGITORUM SUPERFICIALIS TENDONS
RADIAL A.
FLEX. CARPI RADIALIS TENDON
MEDIAN N.
ULNAR A.
ABD. POLLICIS LONGUS & EXT. POLLICIS BREVIS TENDONS
FLEX. CARPI ULNARIS TENDON
WRIST JOINT
ULNAR N.
STYLOID PROCESS OF RADIUS
PISIFORM
EXT. CARPI RADIALIS LONGUS TENDON
FLEX. DIGITORUM PROFUNDUS TENDONS
EXT. POLLICIS LONGUS TENDON
LUNATE
EXT. CARPI ULNARIS TENDON
SCAPHOID
INTEROSSEOUS LIG.
PALMAR RADIOCARPAL LIG.
EXT. CARPI RADIALIS BREVIS TENDON
EXT. DIGITORUM TENDONS
EXT. DIGITI MINIMI TENDON

ABD. POLLICIS LONGUS TENDON
EXT. INDICIS PROPRIUS TENDON
FLEX. POLLICIS LONGUS TENDON
EXT. POLLICIS BREVIS TENDON
FLEX. CARPI RADIALIS TENDON
MEDIAN N.
FLEX. DIGITORUM SUPERFICIALIS TENDONS
ULNAR A.
RADIAL A.
ULNAR N.
SCAPHOID
PISIFORM
ABD. DIGITI MINIMI M.
FLEX. DIGITORUM PROFUNDUS TENDONS
TRIANGULAR
EXT. POLLICIS LONGUS TENDON
EXT. CARPI RADIALIS BREVIS TENDON
CAPITATE
EXT. DIGITI MINIMI TENDON
EXT. CARPI RADIALIS LONGUS TENDON
EXT. DIGITORUM TENDONS
HAMATE
EXT. CARPI ULNARIS TENDON

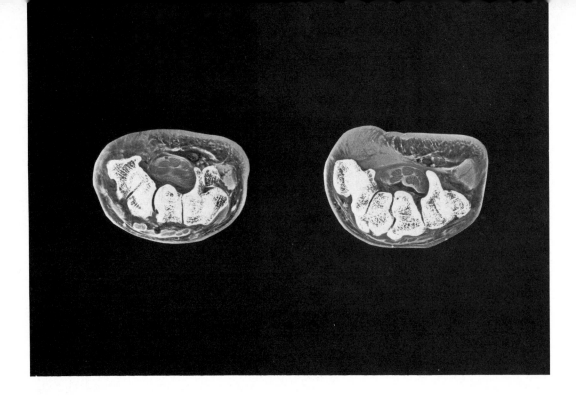

the flexor pollicis longus lies lateral, and the median nerve is superficial (anterior). The tendons of the flexor digitorum profundus lie deep to the tendons of the flexor digitorum superficialis; there is a superficial and deep tendon for each of the four medial digits. The relationship of the ulnar artery to the ulnar nerve should be noted. As can be seen in the sections, both of these structures lie outside the carpal tunnel.

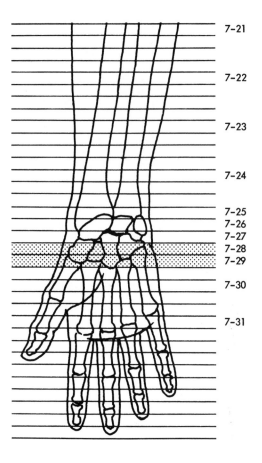

SECTION 7–28

Through the carpal bones, 1 cm below the preceding section

SECTION 7–29

Through the heads of the metacarpals, 1 cm below the preceding section

Anatomic Considerations

The flexor retinaculum can be seen in these illustrations. It is a localized modification of the antebrachial (deep) fascia that forms a strong fibrous band that crosses in front of the carpal bones and converts its anterior concavity into a carpal tunnel through which the long flexor tendons and median nerve pass to the hand. The flexor retinaculum is attached medially to the pisiform bone and the hook of the hamate. Laterally, it splits to form two laminae. The superficial one is attached to the tubercles of the scaphoid and trapezium, and the deep lamina is attached to the trapezium. The tendon of the flexor carpi radialis lies between the two laminae. The relationships of the structures to each other in the carpal tunnel can be seen in the illustrations. The tendon of

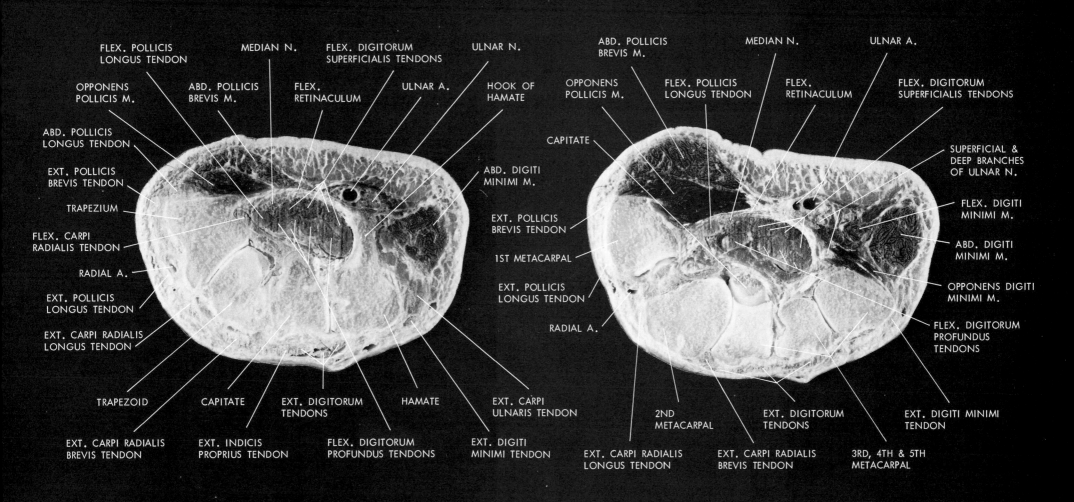

FLEX. POLLICIS
LONGUS TENDON

MEDIAN N.

FLEX. DIGITORUM
SUPERFICIALIS TENDONS

ULNAR N.

ABD. POLLICIS
BREVIS M.

MEDIAN N.

ULNAR A.

OPPONENS
POLLICIS M.

ABD. POLLICIS
BREVIS M.

FLEX.
RETINACULUM

ULNAR A.

HOOK OF
HAMATE

OPPONENS
POLLICIS M.

FLEX. POLLICIS
LONGUS TENDON

FLEX.
RETINACULUM

FLEX. DIGITORUM
SUPERFICIALIS TENDONS

ABD. POLLICIS
LONGUS TENDON

CAPITATE

SUPERFICIAL &
DEEP BRANCHES
OF ULNAR N.

EXT. POLLICIS
BREVIS TENDON

ABD. DIGITI
MINIMI M.

FLEX. DIGITI
MINIMI M.

TRAPEZIUM

EXT. POLLICIS
BREVIS TENDON

ABD. DIGITI
MINIMI M.

FLEX. CARPI
RADIALIS TENDON

1ST METACARPAL

OPPONENS DIGITI
MINIMI M.

RADIAL A.

EXT. POLLICIS
LONGUS TENDON

EXT. POLLICIS
LONGUS TENDON

FLEX. DIGITORUM
PROFUNDUS
TENDONS

EXT. CARPI RADIALIS
LONGUS TENDON

RADIAL A.

TRAPEZOID

CAPITATE

EXT. DIGITORUM
TENDONS

HAMATE

EXT. CARPI
ULNARIS TENDON

2ND
METACARPAL

EXT. DIGITORUM
TENDONS

EXT. DIGITI MINIMI
TENDON

EXT. CARPI RADIALIS
BREVIS TENDON

EXT. INDICIS
PROPRIUS TENDON

FLEX. DIGITORUM
PROFUNDUS TENDONS

EXT. DIGITI
MINIMI TENDON

EXT. CARPI RADIALIS
LONGUS TENDON

EXT. CARPI RADIALIS
BREVIS TENDON

3RD, 4TH & 5TH
METACARPAL

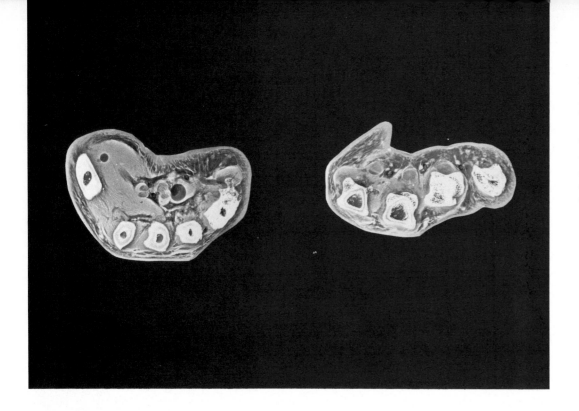

The interosseous-adductor compartment is the deepest of the four compartments and is enclosed by the dorsal interosseous fascia and palmar interosseous fascia. The muscles in this compartment are the adductor pollicis and the palmar and dorsal interosseous muscles (Section 7–30). These are innervated by the ulnar nerve.

In Section 7–31, the fibrous sheath that surrounds the flexor tendons can be seen. Each sheath, along with the phalanges and the palmar ligaments of the joints, forms an osteofibrous canal that contains the tendons that are enclosed by a synovial sheath. In the fingers, each canal contains the tendons of the flexor digitorum superficialis and profundus, and in the thumb the canal contains the flexor pollicis longus.

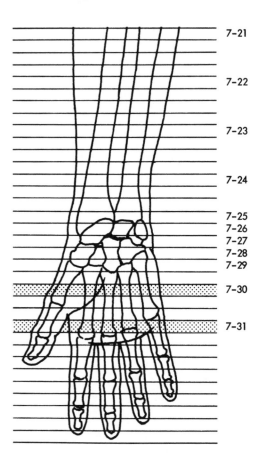

SECTION
7–30

Through the shafts of the metacarpal bones, 2 cm below the preceding section

SECTION
7–31

Through the hand, 3 cm below the preceding section

Anatomic Considerations

Owing to the divisions of the deep fascia, the hand can be divided into fascial compartments that correspond to muscle groups. The thenar compartment consists of the abductor pollicis brevis, the flexor pollicis brevis, and the opponens pollicis (Sections 7–29 and 7–30). The median nerve (Section 7–30) innervates these muscles.

The muscles of the hypothenar compartment are the abductor digiti minimi, the flexor digiti minimi brevis, and the opponens digiti minimi (Sections 7–29 and 7–30). The ulnar nerve (Section 7–29) innervates these muscles. The muscles found in the central compartment, which is between the palmar aponeurosis and the fascial membrane deep to the long flexor tendons and between the thenar and hypothenar fascial septa, are the flexor digitorum superficialis and profundus and the lumbricales (Section 7–30). The nerves of this compartment are the terminal branches of the median and ulnar; the median nerve innervates the two radial lumbricales, and the ulnar nerve innervates the two ulnar muscles.

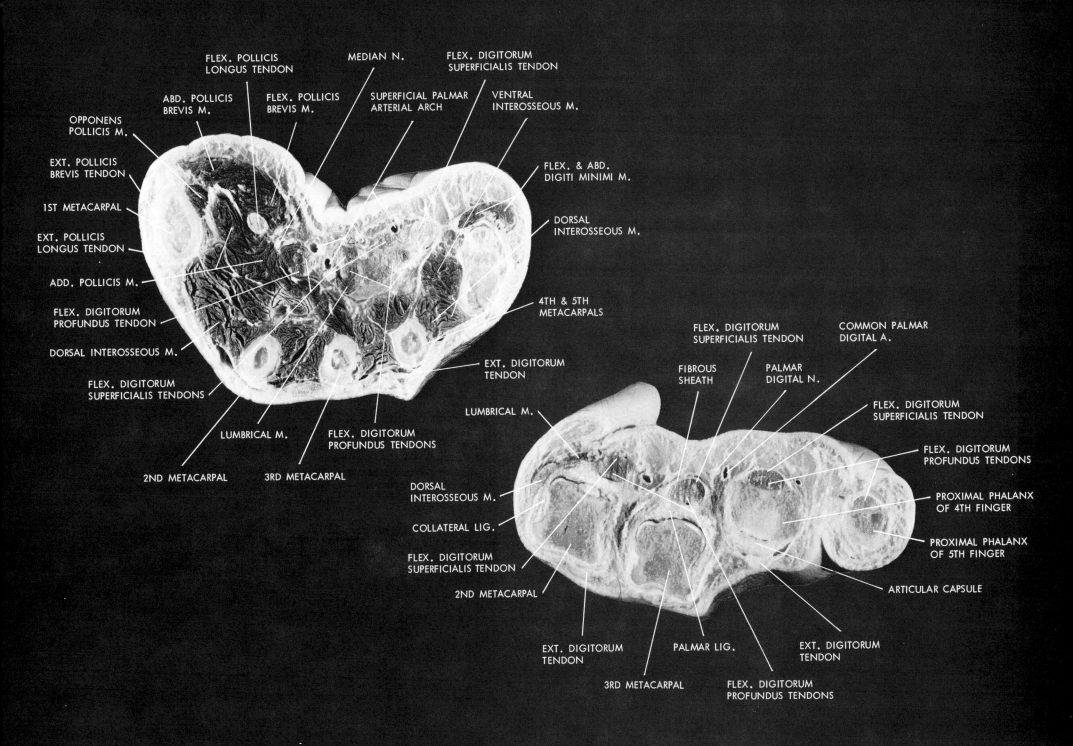

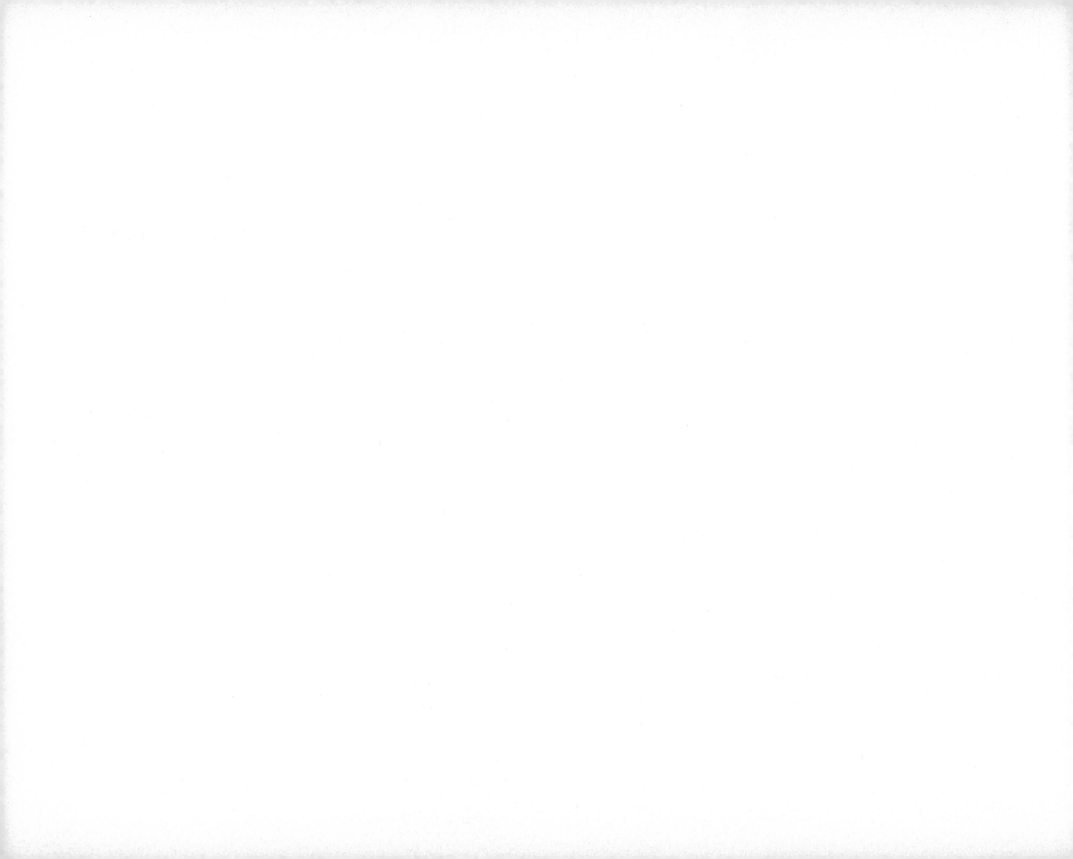

Appendix

One female and two male specimens were used to prepare the sagittal sections in this appendix. Six sections (A–1 through A–6) were used for the head and neck, 12 sections (A–7 through A–18) for the thorax and abdomen, six sections (A–19 through A–24) for the female pelvis, and four sections (A–25 through A–28) for the male pelvis.

All the sagittal sections, which are 1 cm thick, are viewed from the right side. The sketch that accompanies each illustration indicates the position of the section.

All the sections were 1 cm apart except for Sections A–17 and A–18, which were 2 cm apart.

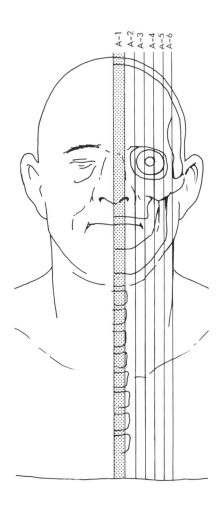

A-1
A-2
A-3
A-4
A-5
A-6

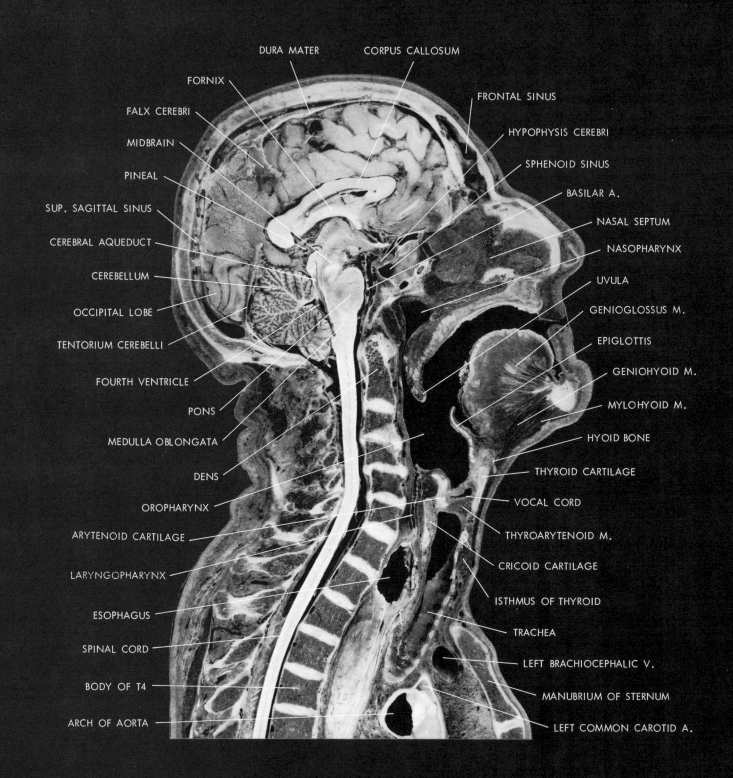

DURA MATER
CORPUS CALLOSUM
FORNIX
FRONTAL SINUS
FALX CEREBRI
HYPOPHYSIS CEREBRI
MIDBRAIN
SPHENOID SINUS
PINEAL
BASILAR A.
SUP. SAGITTAL SINUS
NASAL SEPTUM
CEREBRAL AQUEDUCT
NASOPHARYNX
CEREBELLUM
UVULA
OCCIPITAL LOBE
GENIOGLOSSUS M.
TENTORIUM CEREBELLI
EPIGLOTTIS
GENIOHYOID M.
FOURTH VENTRICLE
MYLOHYOID M.
PONS
HYOID BONE
MEDULLA OBLONGATA
THYROID CARTILAGE
DENS
VOCAL CORD
OROPHARYNX
THYROARYTENOID M.
ARYTENOID CARTILAGE
CRICOID CARTILAGE
LARYNGOPHARYNX
ISTHMUS OF THYROID
ESOPHAGUS
TRACHEA
SPINAL CORD
LEFT BRACHIOCEPHALIC V.
BODY OF T4
MANUBRIUM OF STERNUM
ARCH OF AORTA
LEFT COMMON CAROTID A.

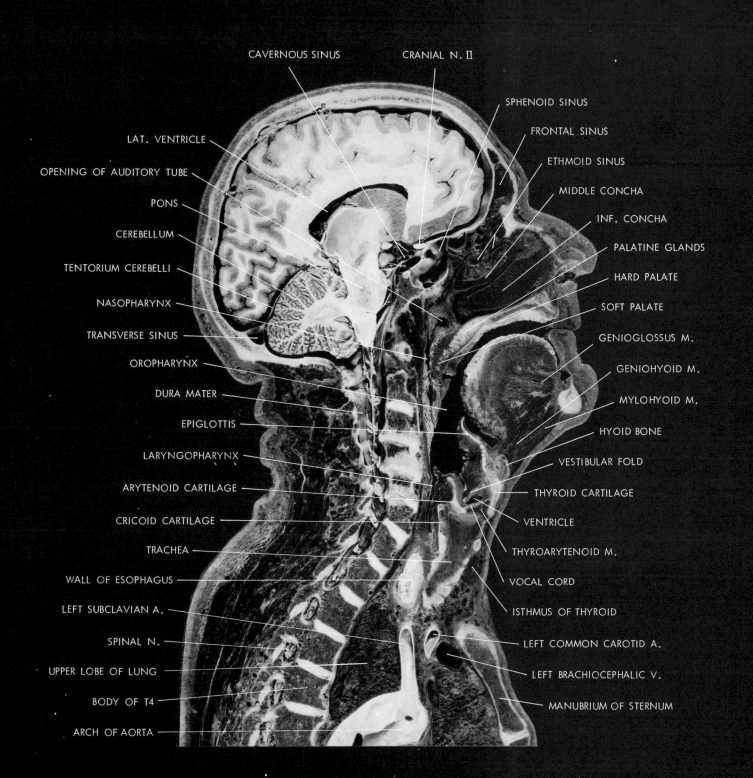

CAVERNOUS SINUS

CRANIAL N. II

LAT. VENTRICLE

OPENING OF AUDITORY TUBE

PONS

CEREBELLUM

TENTORIUM CEREBELLI

NASOPHARYNX

TRANSVERSE SINUS

OROPHARYNX

DURA MATER

EPIGLOTTIS

LARYNGOPHARYNX

ARYTENOID CARTILAGE

CRICOID CARTILAGE

TRACHEA

WALL OF ESOPHAGUS

LEFT SUBCLAVIAN A.

SPINAL N.

UPPER LOBE OF LUNG

BODY OF T4

ARCH OF AORTA

SPHENOID SINUS

FRONTAL SINUS

ETHMOID SINUS

MIDDLE CONCHA

INF. CONCHA

PALATINE GLANDS

HARD PALATE

SOFT PALATE

GENIOGLOSSUS M.

GENIOHYOID M.

MYLOHYOID M.

HYOID BONE

VESTIBULAR FOLD

THYROID CARTILAGE

VENTRICLE

THYROARYTENOID M.

VOCAL CORD

ISTHMUS OF THYROID

LEFT COMMON CAROTID A.

LEFT BRACHIOCEPHALIC V.

MANUBRIUM OF STERNUM

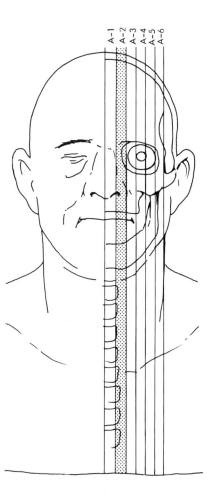

SAGITTAL SECTION
A–2

Head and Neck

A–1
A–2
A–3
A–4
A–5
A–6

SAGITTAL SECTION
A–3

Head and Neck

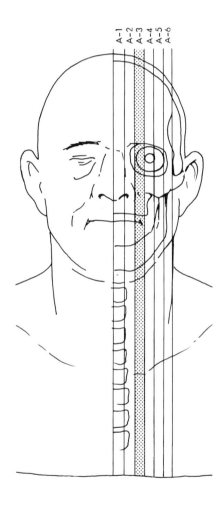

A-1
A-2
A-3
A-4
A-5
A-6

INT. CAROTID A.

CRANIAL N. II

CHOROID PLEXUS

ORBITAL PLATE OF FRONTAL BONE

LAT. VENTRICLE

FRONTAL SINUS

TENTORIUM CEREBELLI

MED. RECTUS M.

SPHENOID SINUS

NASOPHARYNX

MIDDLE & INF. CONCHAE

CEREBELLUM

CARTILAGE & OPENING OF AUDITORY TUBE

TRANSVERSE SINUS

PALATINE GLANDS

TONGUE

VERTEBRAL A.

SUBLINGUAL GLAND

LONGUS CAPITIS M.

MYLOHYOID M.

LINGUAL A.

HYOID BONE

HYOGLOSSUS M.

THYROHYOID M.

THYROID CARTILAGE

STERNOHYOID M.

CRICOID CARTILAGE

THYROID

THYROCERVICAL TRUNK

COMMON CAROTID A.

CLAVICLE

SUBCLAVIAN A.

LEFT BRACHIOCEPHALIC V.

UPPER LOBE OF LUNG

MANUBRIUM OF STERNUM

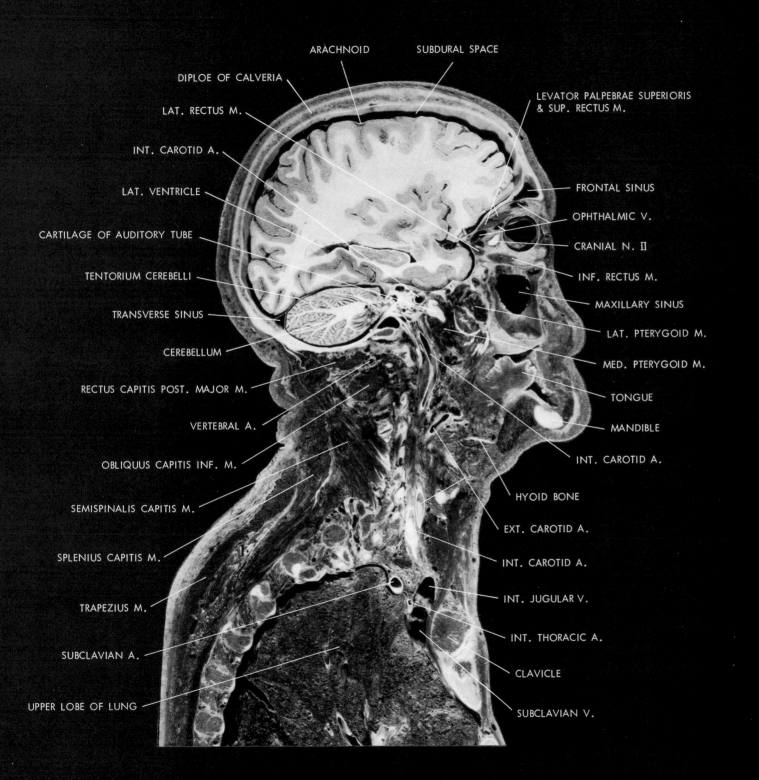

ARACHNOID
SUBDURAL SPACE
DIPLOE OF CALVERIA
LAT. RECTUS M.
INT. CAROTID A.
LAT. VENTRICLE
CARTILAGE OF AUDITORY TUBE
TENTORIUM CEREBELLI
TRANSVERSE SINUS
CEREBELLUM
RECTUS CAPITIS POST. MAJOR M.
VERTEBRAL A.
OBLIQUUS CAPITIS INF. M.
SEMISPINALIS CAPITIS M.
SPLENIUS CAPITIS M.
TRAPEZIUS M.
SUBCLAVIAN A.
UPPER LOBE OF LUNG

LEVATOR PALPEBRAE SUPERIORIS & SUP. RECTUS M.
FRONTAL SINUS
OPHTHALMIC V.
CRANIAL N. II
INF. RECTUS M.
MAXILLARY SINUS
LAT. PTERYGOID M.
MED. PTERYGOID M.
TONGUE
MANDIBLE
INT. CAROTID A.
HYOID BONE
EXT. CAROTID A.
INT. CAROTID A.
INT. JUGULAR V.
INT. THORACIC A.
CLAVICLE
SUBCLAVIAN V.

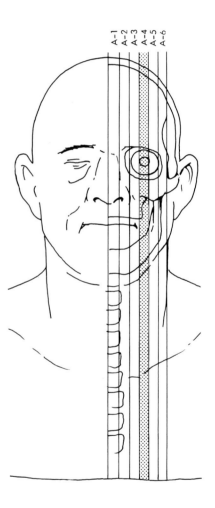

SAGITTAL SECTION
A–4

Head and Neck

A-1 A-2 A-3 A-4 A-5 A-6

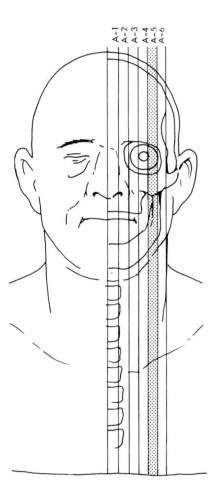

TEMPORAL LOBE

LAT. PTERYGOID M.

INT. JUGULAR V.

LAT. RECTUS M.

ARACHNOID

SCLERA

SUBDURAL SPACE

RETINA

DIPLOE OF CALVERIA

LENS

TENTORIUM CEREBELLI

INF. OBLIQUE M.

CEREBELLUM

MAXILLARY SINUS

TRANSVERSE SINUS

TEMPORALIS M.

SIGMOID SINUS

ORAL VESTIBULE

OCCIPITAL A.

BUCCINATOR M.

SEMISPINALIS CAPITIS M.

MED. PTERYGOID M.

OBLIQUUS CAPITIS SUP. M.

MANDIBLE

SPLENIUS CAPITIS M.

EXT. CAROTID A.

STERNOCLEIDOMASTOID M.

FACIAL A.

OBLIQUUS CAPITIS INF. M.

SUBMANDIBULAR GLAND

STERNOCLEIDOMASTOID M.

TRAPEZIUS M.

INT. JUGULAR V.

LEVATOR SCAPULAE M.

SUBCLAVIAN A.

SCAPULA

CLAVICLE

SUBCLAVIAN V.

UPPER LOBE OF LUNG

INT. THORACIC A.

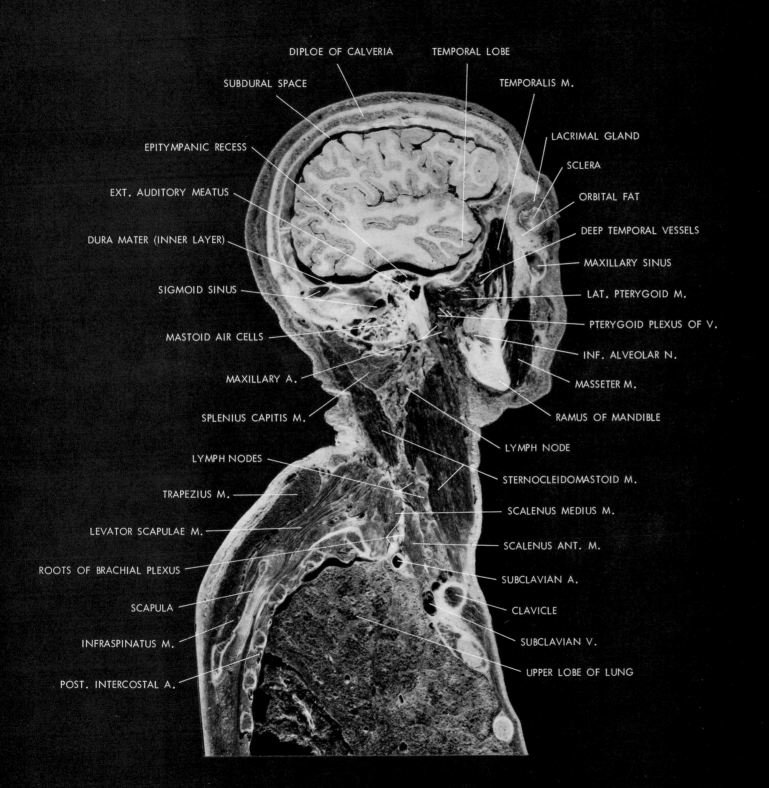

DIPLOE OF CALVERIA

TEMPORAL LOBE

SUBDURAL SPACE

TEMPORALIS M.

EPITYMPANIC RECESS

LACRIMAL GLAND

SCLERA

EXT. AUDITORY MEATUS

ORBITAL FAT

DEEP TEMPORAL VESSELS

DURA MATER (INNER LAYER)

MAXILLARY SINUS

SIGMOID SINUS

LAT. PTERYGOID M.

PTERYGOID PLEXUS OF V.

MASTOID AIR CELLS

INF. ALVEOLAR N.

MAXILLARY A.

MASSETER M.

SPLENIUS CAPITIS M.

RAMUS OF MANDIBLE

LYMPH NODE

LYMPH NODES

STERNOCLEIDOMASTOID M.

TRAPEZIUS M.

SCALENUS MEDIUS M.

LEVATOR SCAPULAE M.

SCALENUS ANT. M.

ROOTS OF BRACHIAL PLEXUS

SUBCLAVIAN A.

SCAPULA

CLAVICLE

INFRASPINATUS M.

SUBCLAVIAN V.

POST. INTERCOSTAL A.

UPPER LOBE OF LUNG

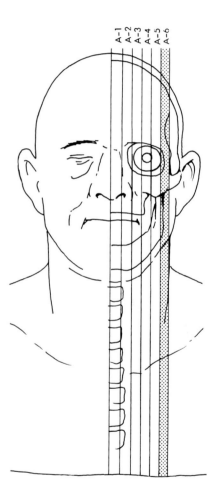

A-1
A-2
A-3
A-4
A-5
A-6

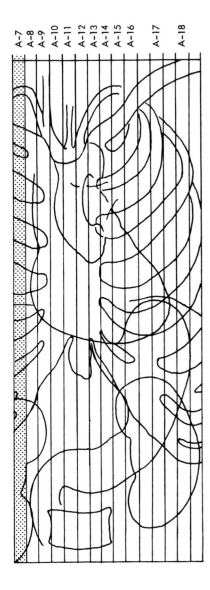

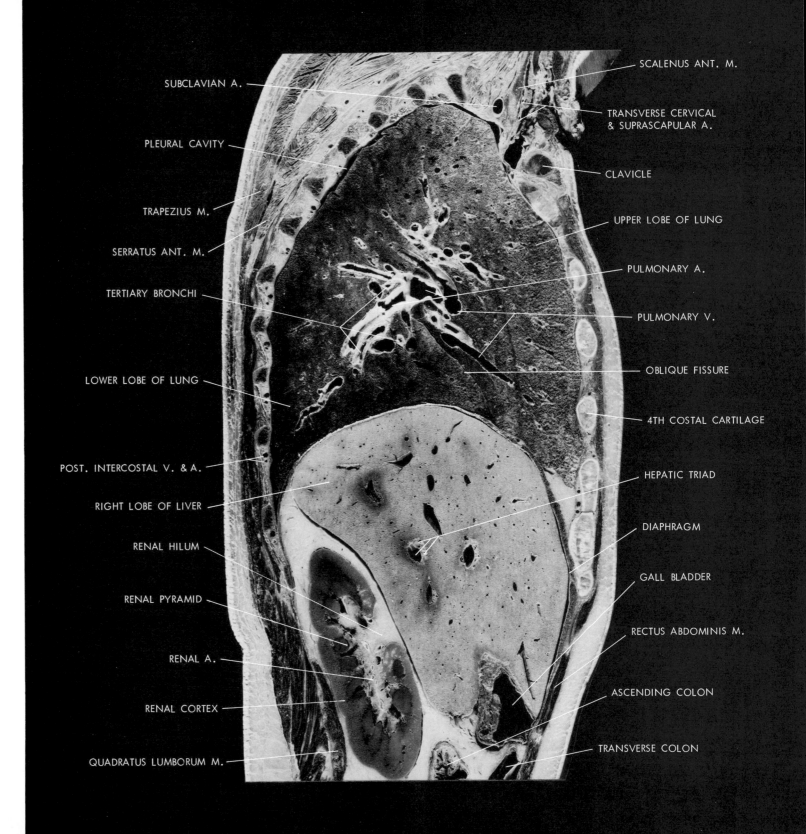

SUBCLAVIAN A.

PLEURAL CAVITY

TRAPEZIUS M.

SERRATUS ANT. M.

TERTIARY BRONCHI

LOWER LOBE OF LUNG

POST. INTERCOSTAL V. & A.

RIGHT LOBE OF LIVER

RENAL HILUM

RENAL PYRAMID

RENAL A.

RENAL CORTEX

QUADRATUS LUMBORUM M.

SCALENUS ANT. M.

TRANSVERSE CERVICAL
& SUPRASCAPULAR A.

CLAVICLE

UPPER LOBE OF LUNG

PULMONARY A.

PULMONARY V.

OBLIQUE FISSURE

4TH COSTAL CARTILAGE

HEPATIC TRIAD

DIAPHRAGM

GALL BLADDER

RECTUS ABDOMINIS M.

ASCENDING COLON

TRANSVERSE COLON

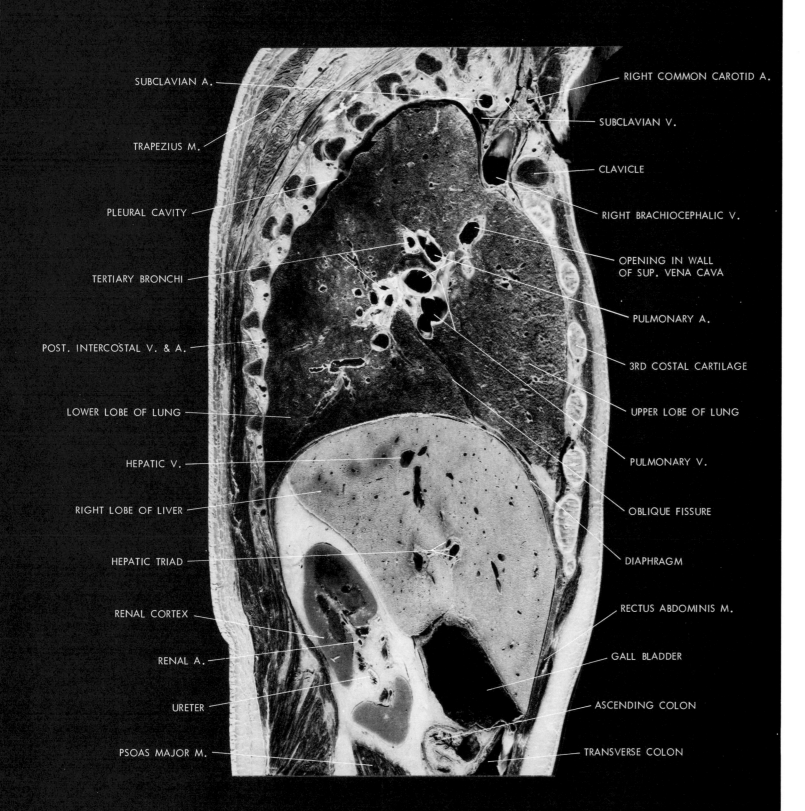

SUBCLAVIAN A.

TRAPEZIUS M.

PLEURAL CAVITY

TERTIARY BRONCHI

POST. INTERCOSTAL V. & A.

LOWER LOBE OF LUNG

HEPATIC V.

RIGHT LOBE OF LIVER

HEPATIC TRIAD

RENAL CORTEX

RENAL A.

URETER

PSOAS MAJOR M.

RIGHT COMMON CAROTID A.

SUBCLAVIAN V.

CLAVICLE

RIGHT BRACHIOCEPHALIC V.

OPENING IN WALL
OF SUP. VENA CAVA

PULMONARY A.

3RD COSTAL CARTILAGE

UPPER LOBE OF LUNG

PULMONARY V.

OBLIQUE FISSURE

DIAPHRAGM

RECTUS ABDOMINIS M.

GALL BLADDER

ASCENDING COLON

TRANSVERSE COLON

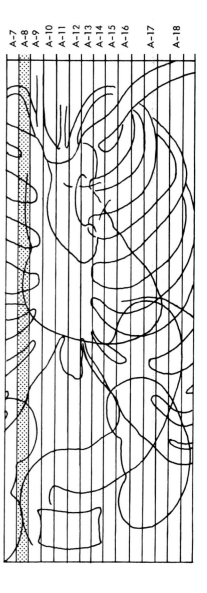

A-7 A-8 A-9 A-10 A-11 A-12 A-13 A-14 A-15 A-16 A-17 A-18

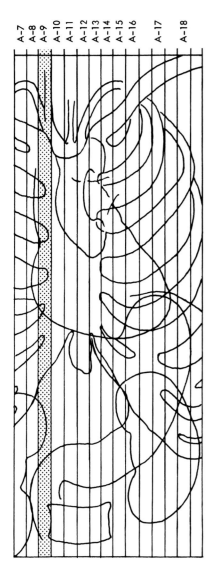

A-7 A-8 A-9 A-10 A-11 A-12 A-13 A-14 A-15 A-16 A-17 A-18

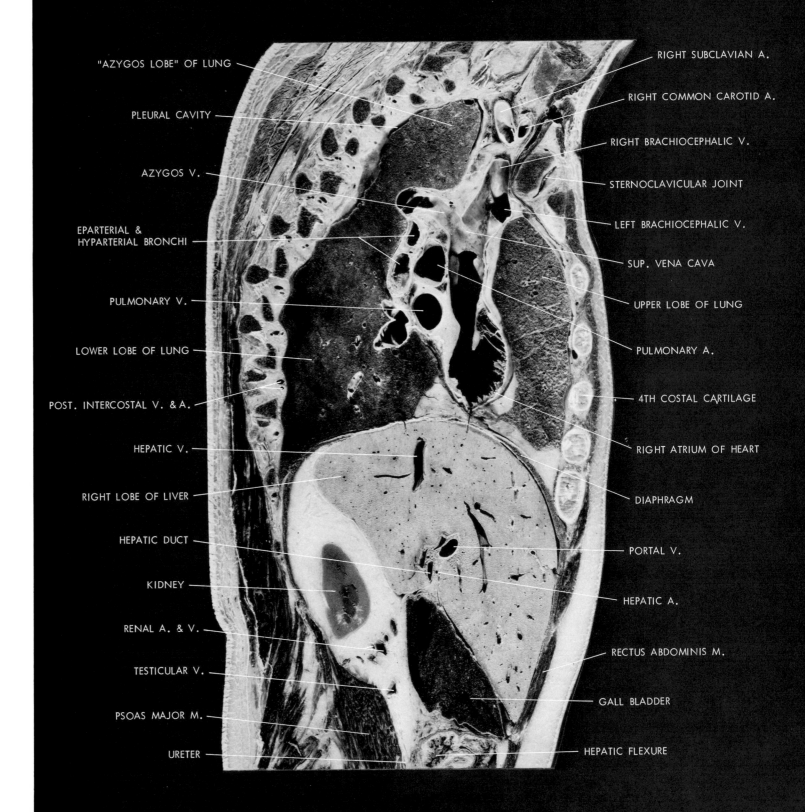

"AZYGOS LOBE" OF LUNG

PLEURAL CAVITY

AZYGOS V.

EPARTERIAL &
HYPARTERIAL BRONCHI

PULMONARY V.

LOWER LOBE OF LUNG

POST. INTERCOSTAL V. & A.

HEPATIC V.

RIGHT LOBE OF LIVER

HEPATIC DUCT

KIDNEY

RENAL A. & V.

TESTICULAR V.

PSOAS MAJOR M.

URETER

RIGHT SUBCLAVIAN A.

RIGHT COMMON CAROTID A.

RIGHT BRACHIOCEPHALIC V.

STERNOCLAVICULAR JOINT

LEFT BRACHIOCEPHALIC V.

SUP. VENA CAVA

UPPER LOBE OF LUNG

PULMONARY A.

4TH COSTAL CARTILAGE

RIGHT ATRIUM OF HEART

DIAPHRAGM

PORTAL V.

HEPATIC A.

RECTUS ABDOMINIS M.

GALL BLADDER

HEPATIC FLEXURE

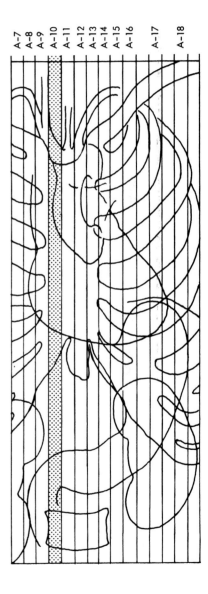

BODY OF TI

"AZYGOS LOBE" OF LUNG

AZYGOS V.

PULMONARY A.

LEFT ATRIUM OF HEART

POST. INTERCOSTAL V. & A.

LOWER LOBE OF LUNG

DIAPHRAGM

SUPRARENAL GLAND

INF. VENA CAVA

RENAL A. & V.

PSOAS MAJOR M.

TRACHEA

BRACHIOCEPHALIC A.

CLAVICLE

LEFT BRACHIOCEPHALIC V.

WALL OF ARCH OF AORTA

SUP. VENA CAVA

UPPER LOBE OF LUNG

3RD COSTAL CARTILAGE

RIGHT ATRIUM OF HEART

HEPATIC V.

CAUDATE LOBE

PORTAL V.

HEPATIC A.

HEPATIC DUCT

CYSTIC DUCT

RECTUS ABDOMINIS M.

GALL BLADDER

DESCENDING PORTION OF DUODENUM

SAGITTAL
SECTION
A–10

*Thorax and
Abdomen*

A-7 A-8 A-9 A-10 A-11 A-12 A-13 A-14 A-15 A-16 A-17 A-18

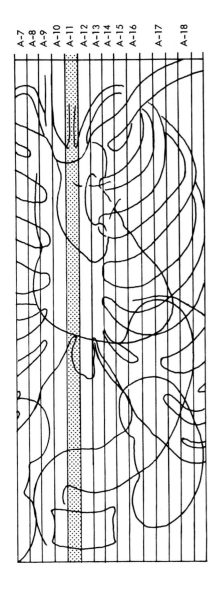

A-7 A-8 A-9 A-10 A-11 A-12 A-13 A-14 A-15 A-16 A-17 A-18

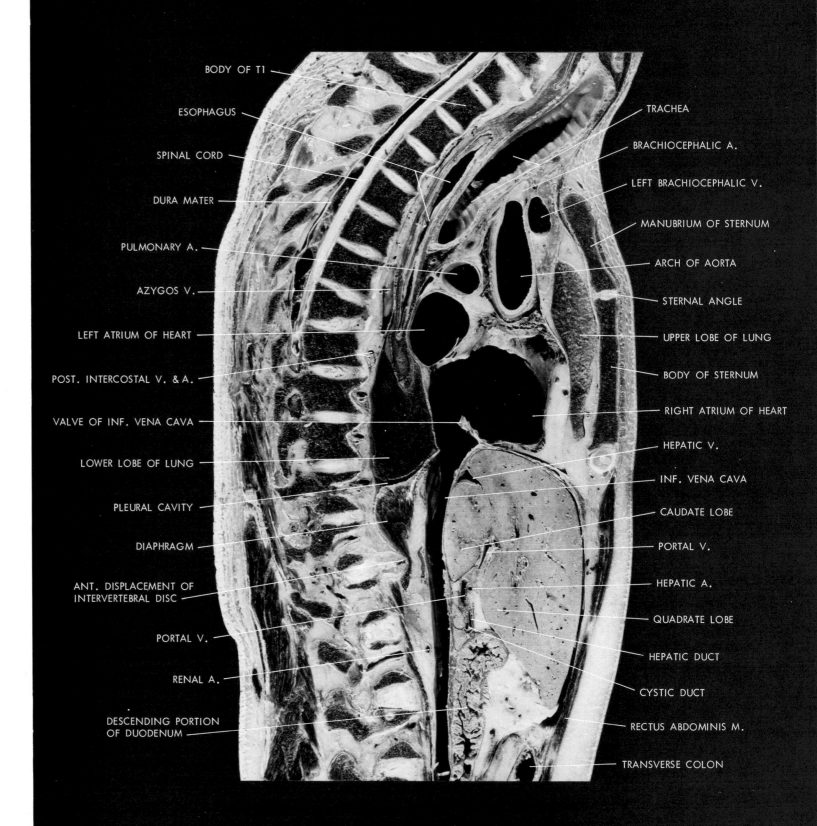

BODY OF T1

ESOPHAGUS

SPINAL CORD

DURA MATER

PULMONARY A.

AZYGOS V.

LEFT ATRIUM OF HEART

POST. INTERCOSTAL V. & A.

VALVE OF INF. VENA CAVA

LOWER LOBE OF LUNG

PLEURAL CAVITY

DIAPHRAGM

ANT. DISPLACEMENT OF
INTERVERTEBRAL DISC

PORTAL V.

RENAL A.

DESCENDING PORTION
OF DUODENUM

TRACHEA

BRACHIOCEPHALIC A.

LEFT BRACHIOCEPHALIC V.

MANUBRIUM OF STERNUM

ARCH OF AORTA

STERNAL ANGLE

UPPER LOBE OF LUNG

BODY OF STERNUM

RIGHT ATRIUM OF HEART

HEPATIC V.

INF. VENA CAVA

CAUDATE LOBE

PORTAL V.

HEPATIC A.

QUADRATE LOBE

HEPATIC DUCT

CYSTIC DUCT

RECTUS ABDOMINIS M.

TRANSVERSE COLON

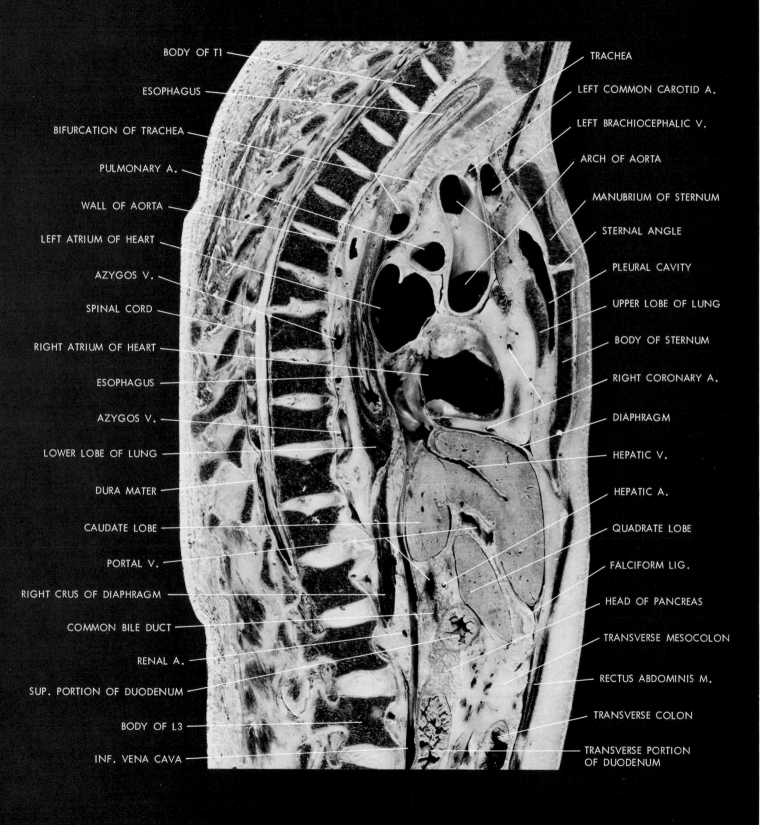

BODY OF T1

ESOPHAGUS

BIFURCATION OF TRACHEA

PULMONARY A.

WALL OF AORTA

LEFT ATRIUM OF HEART

AZYGOS V.

SPINAL CORD

RIGHT ATRIUM OF HEART

ESOPHAGUS

AZYGOS V.

LOWER LOBE OF LUNG

DURA MATER

CAUDATE LOBE

PORTAL V.

RIGHT CRUS OF DIAPHRAGM

COMMON BILE DUCT

RENAL A.

SUP. PORTION OF DUODENUM

BODY OF L3

INF. VENA CAVA

TRACHEA

LEFT COMMON CAROTID A.

LEFT BRACHIOCEPHALIC V.

ARCH OF AORTA

MANUBRIUM OF STERNUM

STERNAL ANGLE

PLEURAL CAVITY

UPPER LOBE OF LUNG

BODY OF STERNUM

RIGHT CORONARY A.

DIAPHRAGM

HEPATIC V.

HEPATIC A.

QUADRATE LOBE

FALCIFORM LIG.

HEAD OF PANCREAS

TRANSVERSE MESOCOLON

RECTUS ABDOMINIS M.

TRANSVERSE COLON

TRANSVERSE PORTION
OF DUODENUM

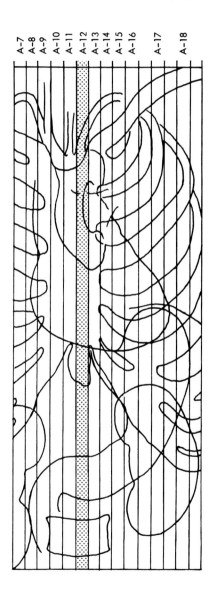

SAGITTAL
SECTION
A–12

*Thorax and
Abdomen*

A-7 A-8 A-9 A-10 A-11 A-12 A-13 A-14 A-15 A-16 A-17 A-18

APPENDIX

327

SAGITTAL SECTION

A–13

Thorax and Abdomen

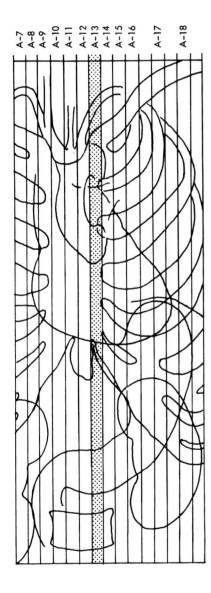

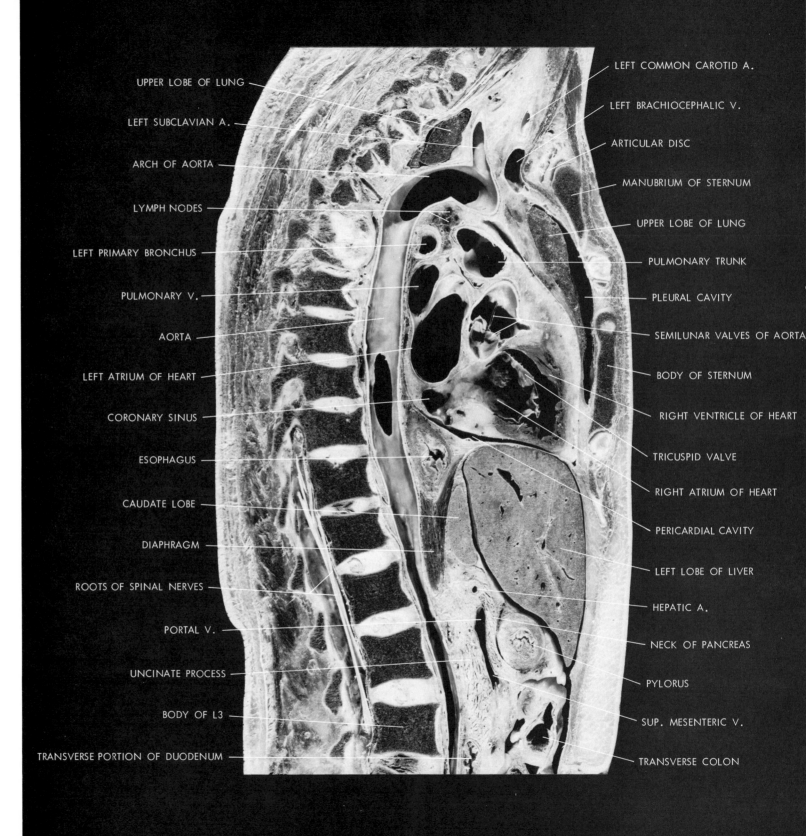

LEFT COMMON CAROTID A.

UPPER LOBE OF LUNG

LEFT BRACHIOCEPHALIC V.

LEFT SUBCLAVIAN A.

ARTICULAR DISC

ARCH OF AORTA

MANUBRIUM OF STERNUM

LYMPH NODES

UPPER LOBE OF LUNG

LEFT PRIMARY BRONCHUS

PULMONARY TRUNK

PULMONARY V.

PLEURAL CAVITY

AORTA

SEMILUNAR VALVES OF AORTA

LEFT ATRIUM OF HEART

BODY OF STERNUM

CORONARY SINUS

RIGHT VENTRICLE OF HEART

ESOPHAGUS

TRICUSPID VALVE

CAUDATE LOBE

RIGHT ATRIUM OF HEART

DIAPHRAGM

PERICARDIAL CAVITY

ROOTS OF SPINAL NERVES

LEFT LOBE OF LIVER

PORTAL V.

HEPATIC A.

UNCINATE PROCESS

NECK OF PANCREAS

BODY OF L3

PYLORUS

TRANSVERSE PORTION OF DUODENUM

SUP. MESENTERIC V.

TRANSVERSE COLON

PLEURAL CAVITY

UPPER LOBE OF LUNG

OBLIQUE FISSURE

LOWER LOBE OF LUNG

ARCH OF AORTA

BRONCHUS

PULMONARY V.

LEFT CORONARY A.

LEFT ATRIUM OF HEART

CORONARY SINUS

WALL OF AORTA

DIAPHRAGM

LEFT GASTRIC A.

SPLENIC A. & V.

RENAL A.

RENAL V.

WALL OF AORTA

SPINAL N. L2

UNCINATE PROCESS

BODY OF L3

INT. JUGULAR V.

SUBCLAVIAN A.

LEFT BRACHIOCEPHALIC V.

CLAVICLE

1ST COSTAL CARTILAGE

PULMONARY A.

INT. THORACIC A.

SEMILUNAR VALVES OF
PULMONARY TRUNK

SEMILUNAR VALVES OF AORTA

LEFT VENTRICLE OF HEART

RIGHT VENTRICLE OF HEART

PERICARDIAL CAVITY

ESOPHAGUS

LEFT LOBE OF LIVER

PORTAL V.

BODY OF PANCREAS

PYLORUS

SUP. MESENTERIC A.

TRANSVERSE COLON

SUP. MESENTERIC V.

TRANSVERSE PORTION OF DUODENUM

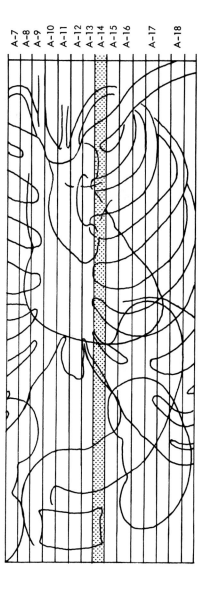

SAGITTAL
SECTION
A–14

**Thorax and
Abdomen**

A-7
A-8
A-9
A-10
A-11
A-12
A-13
A-14
A-15
A-16
A-17
A-18

A-7 A-8 A-9 A-10 A-11 A-12 A-13 A-14 A-15 A-16 A-17 A-18

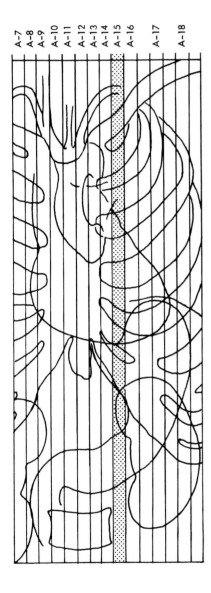

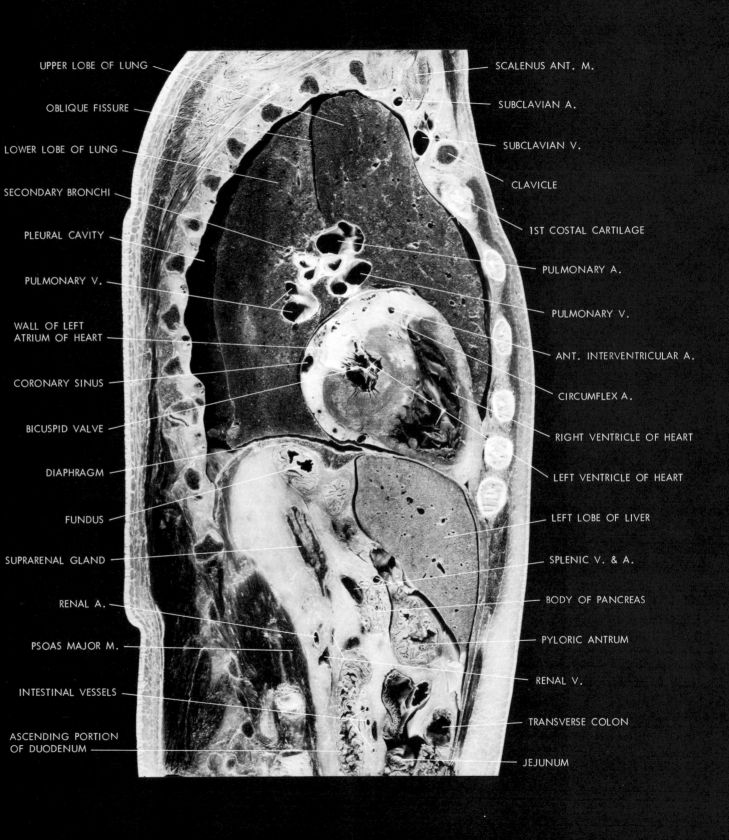

UPPER LOBE OF LUNG

OBLIQUE FISSURE

LOWER LOBE OF LUNG

SECONDARY BRONCHI

PLEURAL CAVITY

PULMONARY V.

WALL OF LEFT
ATRIUM OF HEART

CORONARY SINUS

BICUSPID VALVE

DIAPHRAGM

FUNDUS

SUPRARENAL GLAND

RENAL A.

PSOAS MAJOR M.

INTESTINAL VESSELS

ASCENDING PORTION
OF DUODENUM

SCALENUS ANT. M.

SUBCLAVIAN A.

SUBCLAVIAN V.

CLAVICLE

1ST COSTAL CARTILAGE

PULMONARY A.

PULMONARY V.

ANT. INTERVENTRICULAR A.

CIRCUMFLEX A.

RIGHT VENTRICLE OF HEART

LEFT VENTRICLE OF HEART

LEFT LOBE OF LIVER

SPLENIC V. & A.

BODY OF PANCREAS

PYLORIC ANTRUM

RENAL V.

TRANSVERSE COLON

JEJUNUM

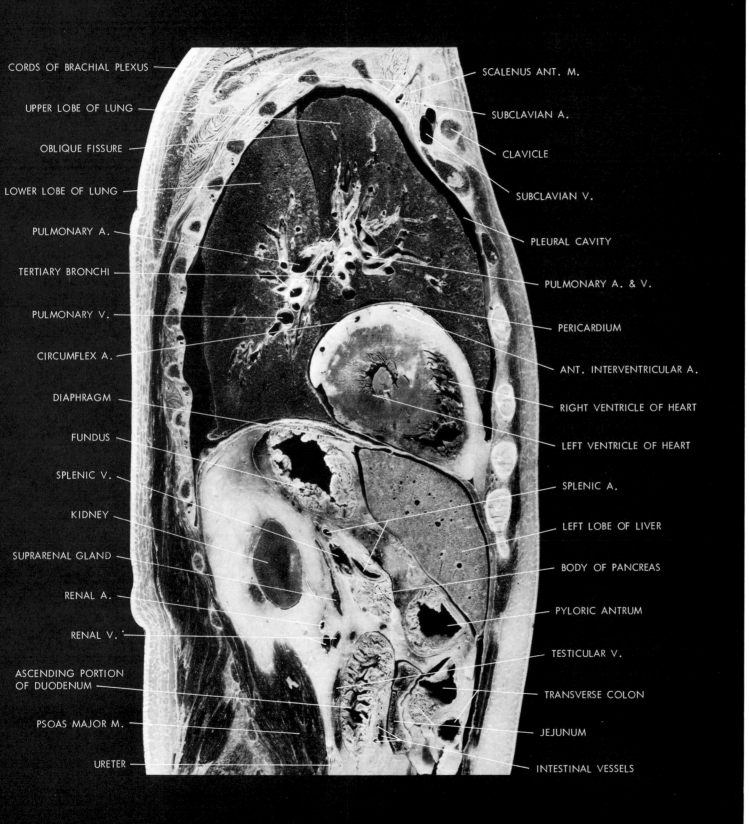

CORDS OF BRACHIAL PLEXUS

UPPER LOBE OF LUNG

OBLIQUE FISSURE

LOWER LOBE OF LUNG

PULMONARY A.

TERTIARY BRONCHI

PULMONARY V.

CIRCUMFLEX A.

DIAPHRAGM

FUNDUS

SPLENIC V.

KIDNEY

SUPRARENAL GLAND

RENAL A.

RENAL V.

ASCENDING PORTION OF DUODENUM

PSOAS MAJOR M.

URETER

SCALENUS ANT. M.

SUBCLAVIAN A.

CLAVICLE

SUBCLAVIAN V.

PLEURAL CAVITY

PULMONARY A. & V.

PERICARDIUM

ANT. INTERVENTRICULAR A.

RIGHT VENTRICLE OF HEART

LEFT VENTRICLE OF HEART

SPLENIC A.

LEFT LOBE OF LIVER

BODY OF PANCREAS

PYLORIC ANTRUM

TESTICULAR V.

TRANSVERSE COLON

JEJUNUM

INTESTINAL VESSELS

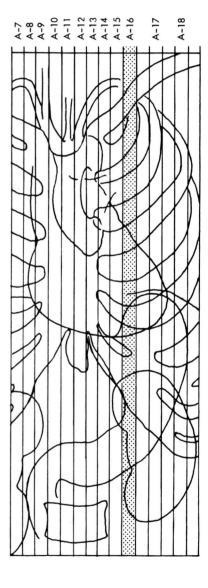

SAGITTAL
SECTION
A–16

Thorax and Abdomen

A-7 A-8 A-9 A-10 A-11 A-12 A-13 A-14 A-15 A-16 A-17 A-18

APPENDIX

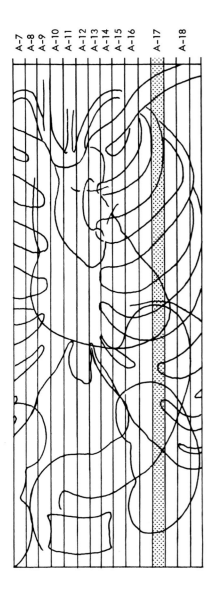

A-7 A-8 A-9 A-10 A-11 A-12 A-13 A-14 A-15 A-16 A-17 A-18

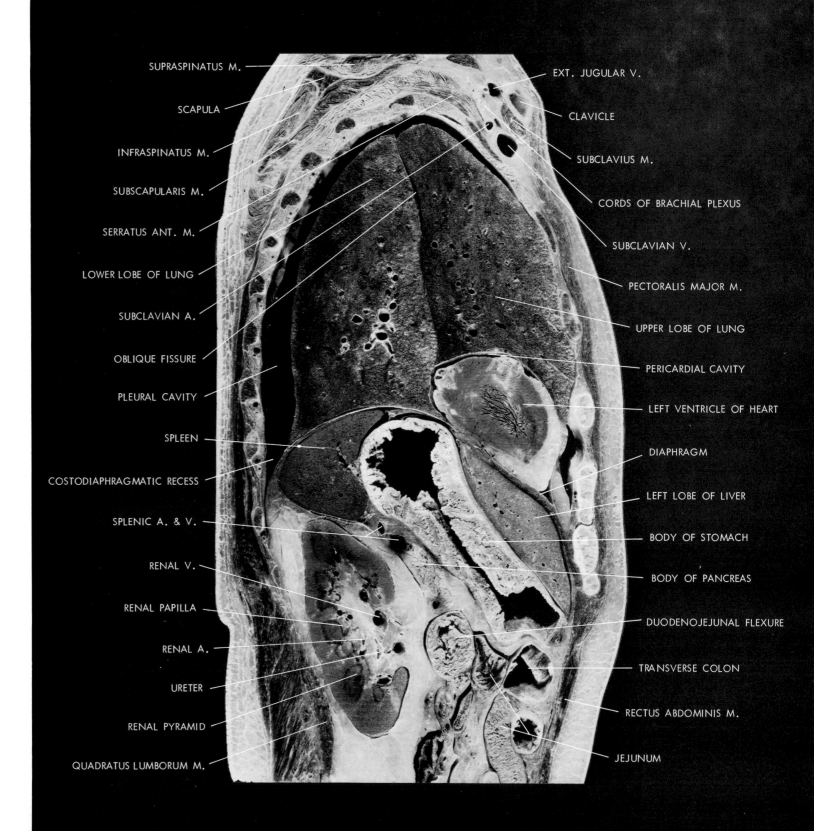

SUPRASPINATUS M.

SCAPULA

INFRASPINATUS M.

SUBSCAPULARIS M.

SERRATUS ANT. M.

LOWER LOBE OF LUNG

SUBCLAVIAN A.

OBLIQUE FISSURE

PLEURAL CAVITY

SPLEEN

COSTODIAPHRAGMATIC RECESS

SPLENIC A. & V.

RENAL V.

RENAL PAPILLA

RENAL A.

URETER

RENAL PYRAMID

QUADRATUS LUMBORUM M.

EXT. JUGULAR V.

CLAVICLE

SUBCLAVIUS M.

CORDS OF BRACHIAL PLEXUS

SUBCLAVIAN V.

PECTORALIS MAJOR M.

UPPER LOBE OF LUNG

PERICARDIAL CAVITY

LEFT VENTRICLE OF HEART

DIAPHRAGM

LEFT LOBE OF LIVER

BODY OF STOMACH

BODY OF PANCREAS

DUODENOJEJUNAL FLEXURE

TRANSVERSE COLON

RECTUS ABDOMINIS M.

JEJUNUM

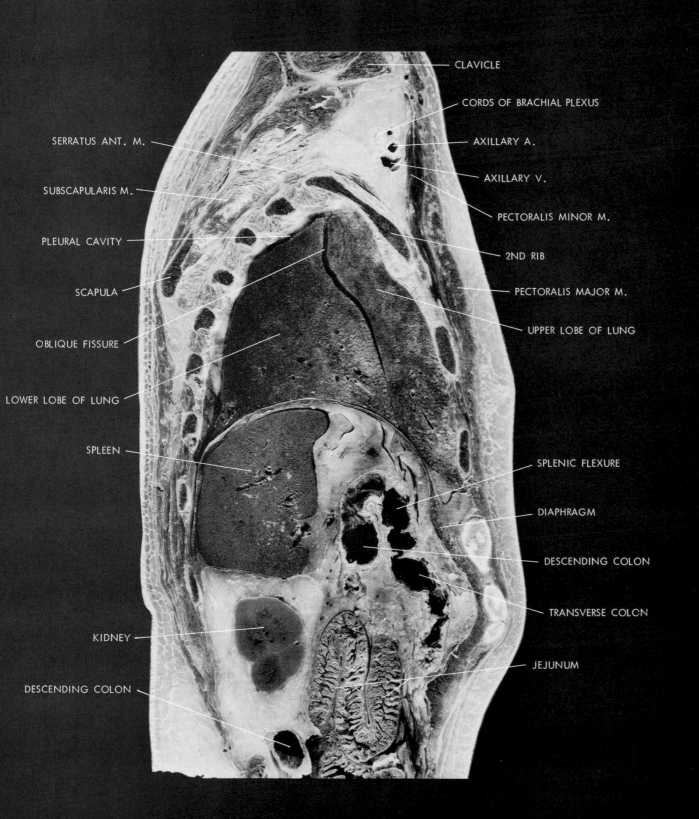

CLAVICLE

CORDS OF BRACHIAL PLEXUS

SERRATUS ANT. M.

AXILLARY A.

AXILLARY V.

SUBSCAPULARIS M.

PECTORALIS MINOR M.

PLEURAL CAVITY

2ND RIB

SCAPULA

PECTORALIS MAJOR M.

OBLIQUE FISSURE

UPPER LOBE OF LUNG

LOWER LOBE OF LUNG

SPLEEN

SPLENIC FLEXURE

DIAPHRAGM

DESCENDING COLON

TRANSVERSE COLON

KIDNEY

JEJUNUM

DESCENDING COLON

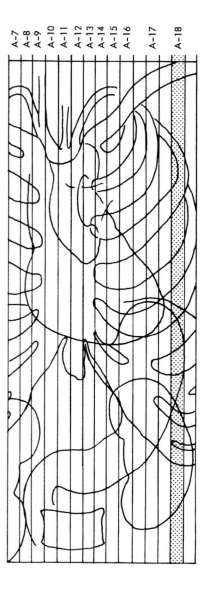

A-7 A-8 A-9 A-10 A-11 A-12 A-13 A-14 A-15 A-16 A-17 A-18

SAGITTAL
SECTION
A–19

Female Pelvis

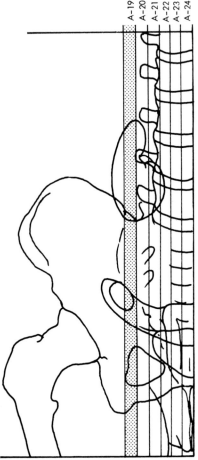

RENAL CORTEX

PSOAS MAJOR M.

SUSPENSORY LIG. OF OVARY

ALA OF SACRUM

SCIATIC N.

PIRIFORMIS M.

GLUTEAL VESSELS

GLUTEUS MAXIMUS M.

ILEUM

RAMUS OF ISCHIUM

ADDUCTOR GROUP OF M.

RIGHT LOBE OF LIVER

HEPATIC FLEXURE

ASCENDING COLON

BRANCHES OF INT. ILIAC VESSELS

OVARY

EXT. ILIAC A.

EXT. ILIAC V.

OVIDUCT

ILIOPECTINEAL EMINENCE

OBTURATOR INTERNUS M.

OBTURATOR EXTERNUS M.

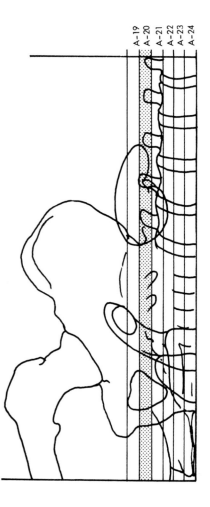

SAGITTAL SECTION
A-20

Female Pelvis

URETER

PSOAS MAJOR M.

COMMON ILIAC V.

INT. ILIAC A.

SACRUM

INT. ILIAC V.

RAMI OF SACRAL PLEXUS

PIRIFORMIS M.

SIGMOID COLON

URETER

GLUTEUS MAXIMUS M.

BASE OF BROAD LIG.

LEVATOR ANI M.

OBTURATOR INTERNUS M.

RAMUS OF ISCHIUM

RIGHT LOBE OF LIVER

RENAL PYRAMID

JEJUNUM

EXT. ILIAC A.

TRANSVERSE COLON

ASCENDING COLON

ILEUM

OVIDUCT

BROAD LIG.

SUP. RAMUS OF PUBIS

OBTURATOR V.

UTERINE A.

OBTURATOR EXTERNUS M.

ADDUCTOR GROUP OF M.

A-19 A-20 A-21 A-22 A-23 A-24

SAGITTAL
SECTION
A–21

Female Pelvis

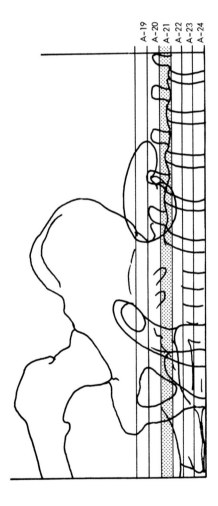

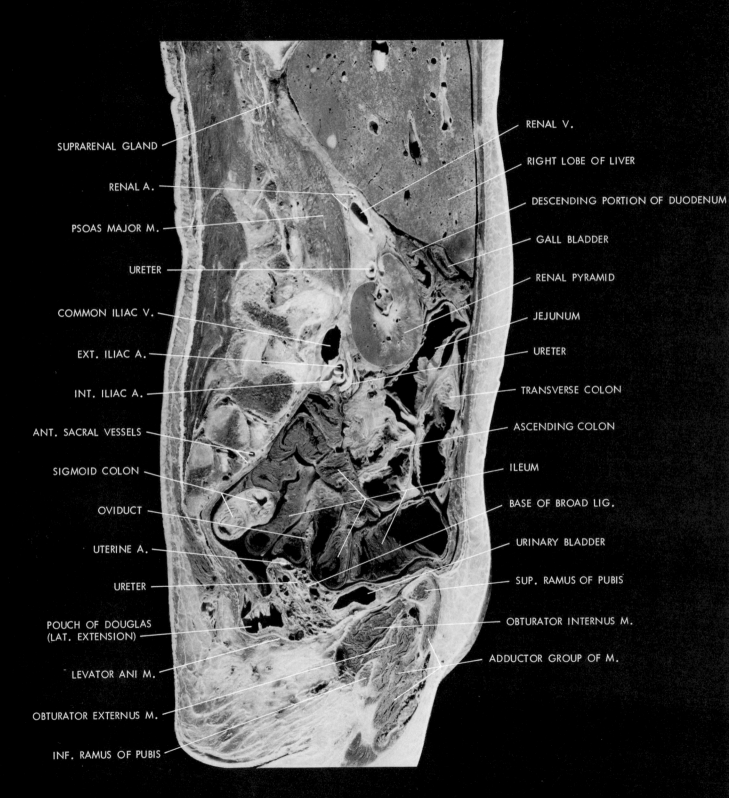

SUPRARENAL GLAND

RENAL A.

PSOAS MAJOR M.

URETER

COMMON ILIAC V.

EXT. ILIAC A.

INT. ILIAC A.

ANT. SACRAL VESSELS

SIGMOID COLON

OVIDUCT

UTERINE A.

URETER

POUCH OF DOUGLAS
(LAT. EXTENSION)

LEVATOR ANI M.

OBTURATOR EXTERNUS M.

INF. RAMUS OF PUBIS

RENAL V.

RIGHT LOBE OF LIVER

DESCENDING PORTION OF DUODENUM

GALL BLADDER

RENAL PYRAMID

JEJUNUM

URETER

TRANSVERSE COLON

ASCENDING COLON

ILEUM

BASE OF BROAD LIG.

URINARY BLADDER

SUP. RAMUS OF PUBIS

OBTURATOR INTERNUS M.

ADDUCTOR GROUP OF M.

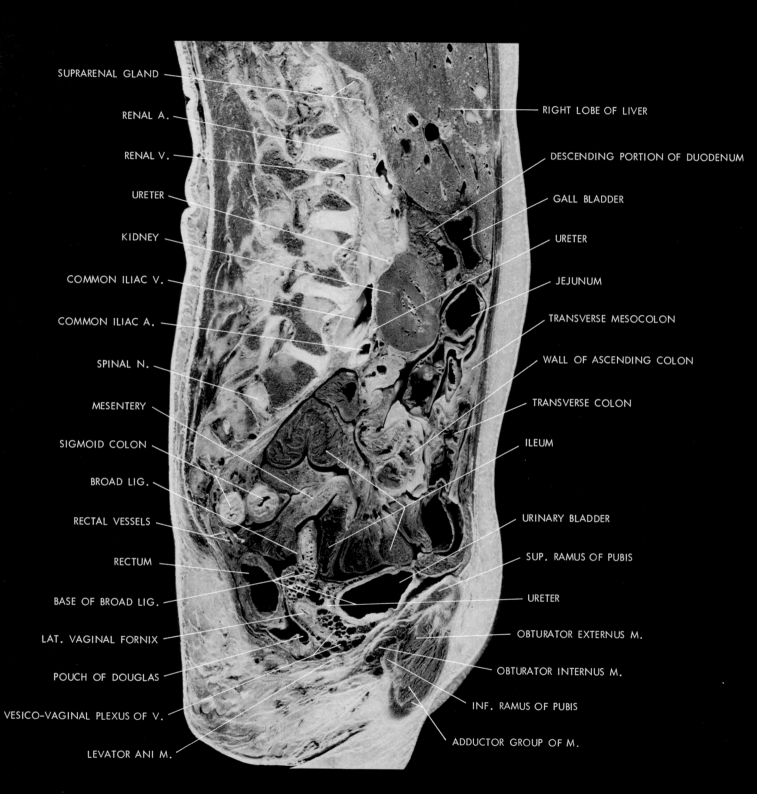

SUPRARENAL GLAND

RENAL A.

RENAL V.

URETER

KIDNEY

COMMON ILIAC V.

COMMON ILIAC A.

SPINAL N.

MESENTERY

SIGMOID COLON

BROAD LIG.

RECTAL VESSELS

RECTUM

BASE OF BROAD LIG.

LAT. VAGINAL FORNIX

POUCH OF DOUGLAS

VESICO-VAGINAL PLEXUS OF V.

LEVATOR ANI M.

RIGHT LOBE OF LIVER

DESCENDING PORTION OF DUODENUM

GALL BLADDER

URETER

JEJUNUM

TRANSVERSE MESOCOLON

WALL OF ASCENDING COLON

TRANSVERSE COLON

ILEUM

URINARY BLADDER

SUP. RAMUS OF PUBIS

URETER

OBTURATOR EXTERNUS M.

OBTURATOR INTERNUS M.

INF. RAMUS OF PUBIS

ADDUCTOR GROUP OF M.

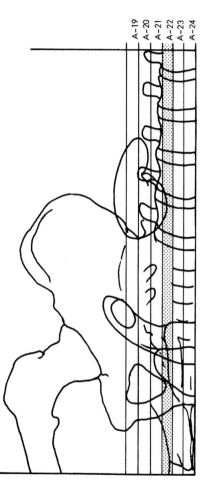

SAGITTAL
SECTION
A–22

Female Pelvis

A–19 A–20 A–21 A–22 A–23 A–24

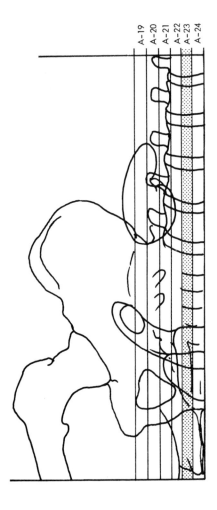

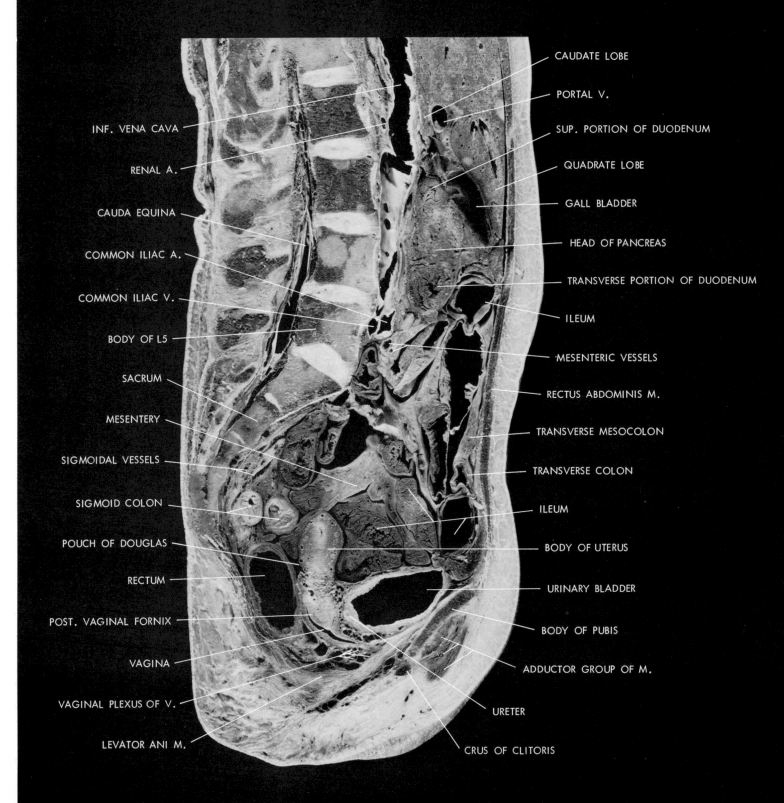

CAUDATE LOBE

PORTAL V.

INF. VENA CAVA

SUP. PORTION OF DUODENUM

RENAL A.

QUADRATE LOBE

CAUDA EQUINA

GALL BLADDER

COMMON ILIAC A.

HEAD OF PANCREAS

COMMON ILIAC V.

TRANSVERSE PORTION OF DUODENUM

BODY OF L5

ILEUM

SACRUM

MESENTERIC VESSELS

MESENTERY

RECTUS ABDOMINIS M.

SIGMOIDAL VESSELS

TRANSVERSE MESOCOLON

SIGMOID COLON

TRANSVERSE COLON

POUCH OF DOUGLAS

ILEUM

RECTUM

BODY OF UTERUS

POST. VAGINAL FORNIX

URINARY BLADDER

VAGINA

BODY OF PUBIS

VAGINAL PLEXUS OF V.

ADDUCTOR GROUP OF M.

LEVATOR ANI M.

URETER

CRUS OF CLITORIS

A-19
A-20
A-21
A-22
A-23
A-24

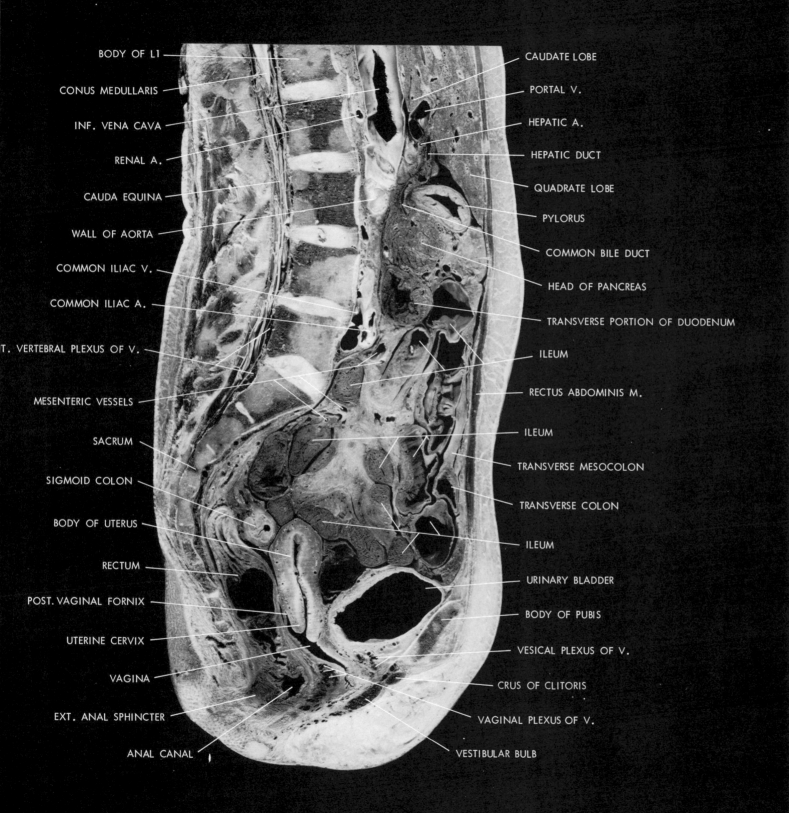

BODY OF L1

CONUS MEDULLARIS

INF. VENA CAVA

RENAL A.

CAUDA EQUINA

WALL OF AORTA

COMMON ILIAC V.

COMMON ILIAC A.

T. VERTEBRAL PLEXUS OF V.

MESENTERIC VESSELS

SACRUM

SIGMOID COLON

BODY OF UTERUS

RECTUM

POST. VAGINAL FORNIX

UTERINE CERVIX

VAGINA

EXT. ANAL SPHINCTER

ANAL CANAL

CAUDATE LOBE

PORTAL V.

HEPATIC A.

HEPATIC DUCT

QUADRATE LOBE

PYLORUS

COMMON BILE DUCT

HEAD OF PANCREAS

TRANSVERSE PORTION OF DUODENUM

ILEUM

RECTUS ABDOMINIS M.

ILEUM

TRANSVERSE MESOCOLON

TRANSVERSE COLON

ILEUM

URINARY BLADDER

BODY OF PUBIS

VESICAL PLEXUS OF V.

CRUS OF CLITORIS

VAGINAL PLEXUS OF V.

VESTIBULAR BULB

SAGITTAL SECTION

A–24

Female Pelvis

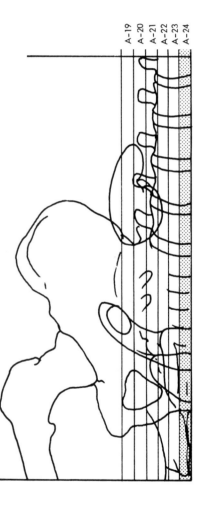

A-19
A-20
A-21
A-22
A-23
A-24

SAGITTAL
SECTION
A-25

Male Pelvis

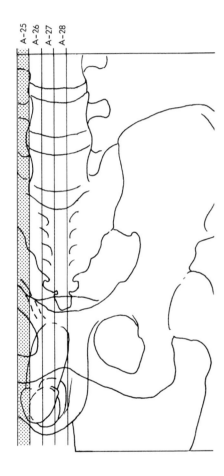

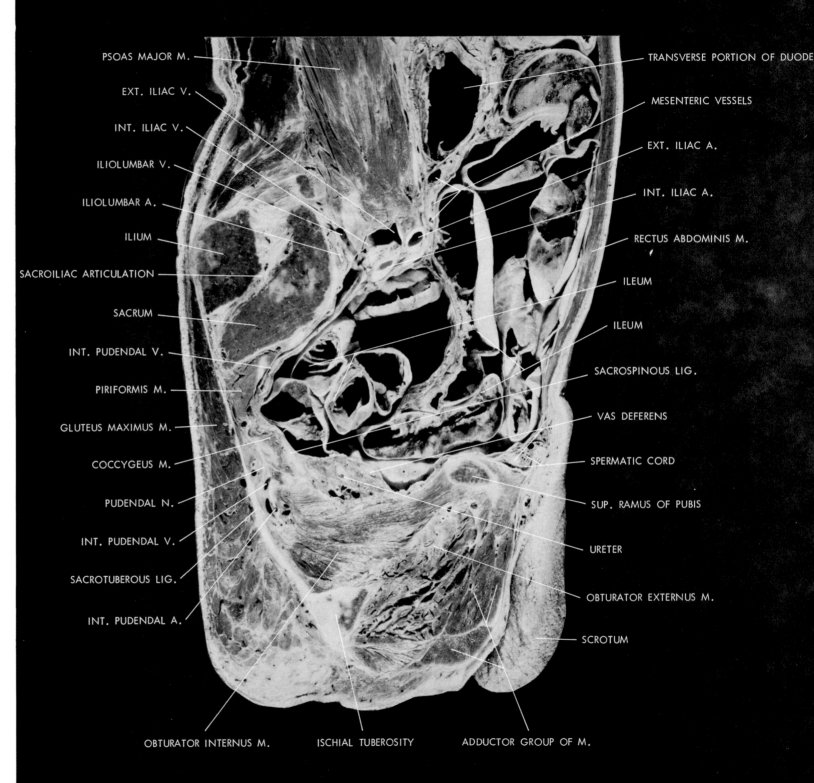

PSOAS MAJOR M.

EXT. ILIAC V.

INT. ILIAC V.

ILIOLUMBAR V.

ILIOLUMBAR A.

ILIUM

SACROILIAC ARTICULATION

SACRUM

INT. PUDENDAL V.

PIRIFORMIS M.

GLUTEUS MAXIMUS M.

COCCYGEUS M.

PUDENDAL N.

INT. PUDENDAL V.

SACROTUBEROUS LIG.

INT. PUDENDAL A.

OBTURATOR INTERNUS M.

ISCHIAL TUBEROSITY

ADDUCTOR GROUP OF M.

TRANSVERSE PORTION OF DUODE

MESENTERIC VESSELS

EXT. ILIAC A.

INT. ILIAC A.

RECTUS ABDOMINIS M.

ILEUM

ILEUM

SACROSPINOUS LIG.

VAS DEFERENS

SPERMATIC CORD

SUP. RAMUS OF PUBIS

URETER

OBTURATOR EXTERNUS M.

SCROTUM

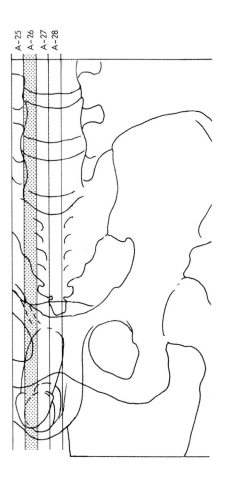

INF. VENA CAVA

COMMON ILIAC V.

SACRUM

INT. ILIAC A.

SPINAL N.

PIRIFORMIS M.

AREOLAR TISSUE

GLUTEUS MAXIMUS M.

COCCYGEUS M.

SEMINAL VESICLE

INF. RECTAL VESSELS

VESICAL PLEXUS OF V.

OBTURATOR INTERNUS M.

RAMUS OF ISCHIUM

TESTIS

SCROTUM

TRANSVERSE PORTION
OF DUODENUM

EXT. ILIAC A.

ILEUM

URETER

SUP. RAMUS OF PUBIS

OBTURATOR EXTERNUS M.

VAS DEFERENS

PAMPINIFORM PLEXUS OF V.

ADDUCTOR GROUP OF M.

VAS DEFERENS

CORPUS CAVERNOSUM

A–25

A–26

A–27

A–28

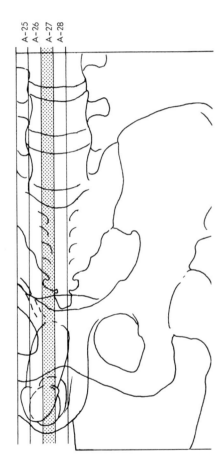

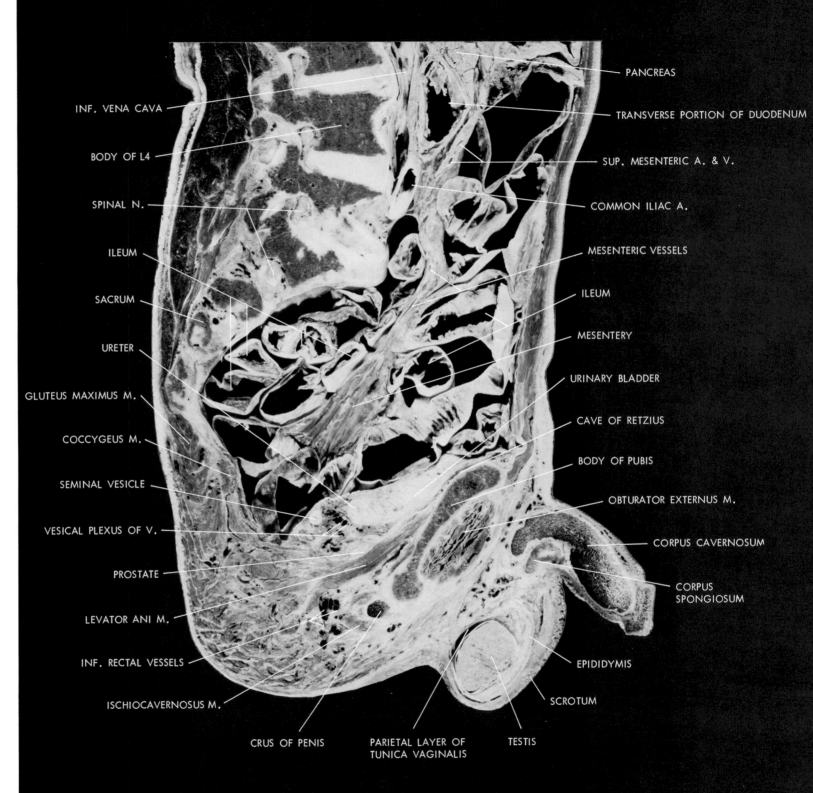

PANCREAS

INF. VENA CAVA

TRANSVERSE PORTION OF DUODENUM

BODY OF L4

SUP. MESENTERIC A. & V.

SPINAL N.

COMMON ILIAC A.

ILEUM

MESENTERIC VESSELS

SACRUM

ILEUM

URETER

MESENTERY

GLUTEUS MAXIMUS M.

URINARY BLADDER

COCCYGEUS M.

CAVE OF RETZIUS

SEMINAL VESICLE

BODY OF PUBIS

VESICAL PLEXUS OF V.

OBTURATOR EXTERNUS M.

PROSTATE

CORPUS CAVERNOSUM

LEVATOR ANI M.

CORPUS
SPONGIOSUM

INF. RECTAL VESSELS

ISCHIOCAVERNOSUS M.

EPIDIDYMIS

SCROTUM

CRUS OF PENIS

PARIETAL LAYER OF
TUNICA VAGINALIS

TESTIS

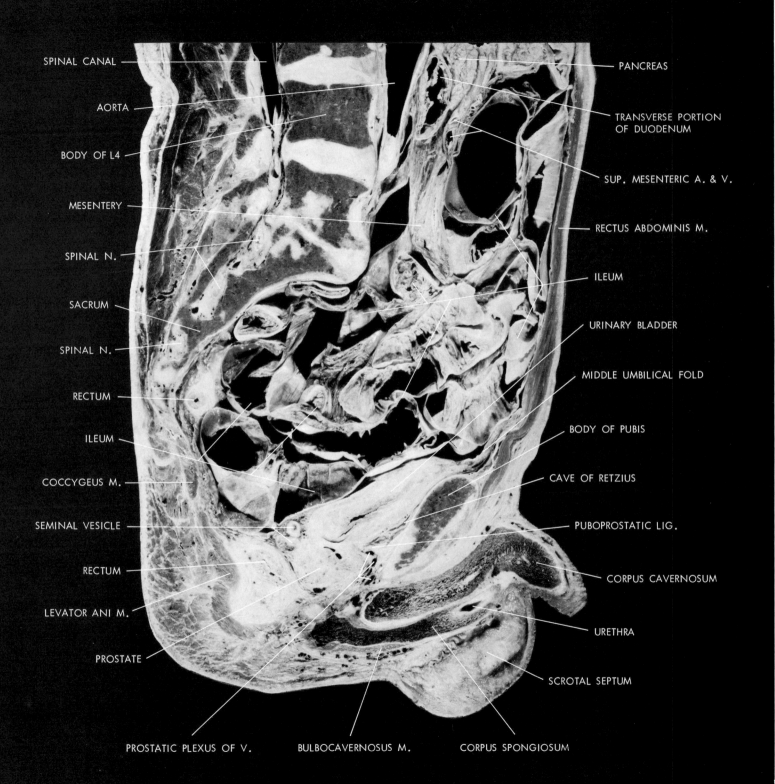

SPINAL CANAL

AORTA

BODY OF L4

MESENTERY

SPINAL N.

SACRUM

SPINAL N.

RECTUM

ILEUM

COCCYGEUS M.

SEMINAL VESICLE

RECTUM

LEVATOR ANI M.

PROSTATE

PROSTATIC PLEXUS OF V.　BULBOCAVERNOSUS M.　CORPUS SPONGIOSUM

PANCREAS

TRANSVERSE PORTION
OF DUODENUM

SUP. MESENTERIC A. & V.

RECTUS ABDOMINIS M.

ILEUM

URINARY BLADDER

MIDDLE UMBILICAL FOLD

BODY OF PUBIS

CAVE OF RETZIUS

PUBOPROSTATIC LIG.

CORPUS CAVERNOSUM

URETHRA

SCROTAL SEPTUM

SAGITTAL
SECTION
A-28

Male Pelvis

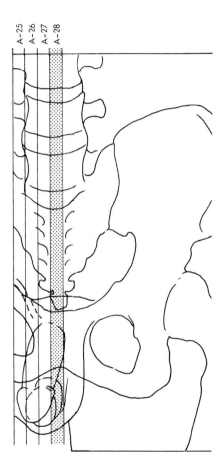

A-25　A-26　A-27　A-28

Index

Items in this index generally are listed under the nouns rather than the descriptive adjectives; for example, to find brachialis muscle, see "Muscle(s), brachialis." Page numbers in *italic* indicate illustrations. Structures of Chapter 4 (Male Pelvis and Perineum) and Chapter 5 (Female Pelvis and Perineum) are designated as male and female, respectively.